HATHA YOGA

A Comprehensive Guide

Ram Jain & Michèle Hauswirth

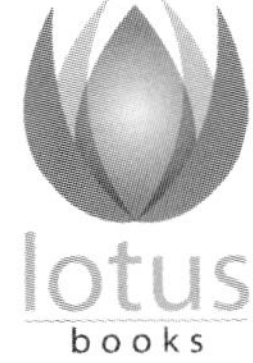

First published in 2017 by **White Road Publications**
info@whiteroadpublications.com

Reprinted in 2022 by **Lotus Publishing**

Reprinted in 2026 by **Lotus Books**
1607 N. Market Street, Champaign, Illinois 61820
Phone: 1-800-747-4457

Cover & Interior Design Tina Pedersen
Printed & Bound in the United States of America by Versa Press
Revisions Maarten Noteboom
Photographs Kees Penders
Make-up Edyta Zielinska

Medical Disclaimer

ISBN: 978-1-7182-3973-9 (print)

10 9 8 7 6 5 4 3 2 1 L1023

Table of Contents

Foreword

By Biff Mithoefer

In working with yoga practitioners and teachers over the years, I've consistently asked myself the questions: "What is it that people most need from their practice?" "What is missing in our lives that yoga can help us to rediscover?"

It's clear that the answer isn't looser hamstrings or firmer abs. Despite what we are often led to believe, these things have no real effect on our lasting joy. No goal or achievement can bring us true joy. True joy comes from, as Ram reminds us, "the union of self with the reality of self." This is self-realization, the place from which equanimity, joy, and peace can grow. When we can see ourselves as we truly are, letting go of the stories of how and who we are told we should be, we can accept ourselves. This self-acceptance is what we are all longing for.

Ram, with his many years of experience, speaks of the true essence of yoga. He reminds us that yoga isn't about reaching someplace outside ourselves, but about remembering who we are. We are often told in our modern practices that asanas need to be practiced with a goal in mind. We are told that we need to be deeper in a posture, or we need to perfect our balance poses, but Ram suggests that we must return to the most basic of all yoga instruction: "sthira sukham asanam," or "asana is a steady and comfortable pose." This seemingly simple phrase is not only about how we should practice our asanas, but it is also about how we can move through life. We need to be steady in our intention, both in our practice and in our lives, and we need to be comfortable with who we are.

This, for me, is the greatest gift that yoga has to offer the world right now, the possibility to be comfortably at peace with who we are and our place in the world. It is only from this place of acceptance that equanimity and compassion can grow.

I'm grateful to Ram and Michèle for bringing these principles back to us in a way that's accessible to all who are interested in connecting with the true source of yoga's potential to bring healing to the world.

INTRODUCTION

India's ancient blessing to the world is yoga. After all, yoga benefits everyone physically, mentally, and spiritually. And after having studied and taught yoga for many years, and trained thousands of yoga teachers, we feel truly blessed with yoga's increasing popularity, which brings so many positive benefits to more and more people all around the world. We believe, though, that we all can benefit even more from the practice of yoga—and yoga asanas (yoga postures) in particular—if we understand how the ancient principles of a yoga asana practice affect body and mind.

What are the ancient principles of yoga practice? Are you following them? These days most yoga styles are really yoga-inspired exercises. And because exercise is good, yoga-inspired exercise will benefit you. Such exercise, though, is not yoga asana practice in the traditional and most effective sense. In fact, today's physical practice of yoga has drifted far from the original teachings. Yet, even though we live in today's modern world, in fact *because* we live in today's modern world, the traditional teachings of yoga still apply and are relevant. Correctly understood and applied, they will yield even greater and more long-lasting results for your general well-being than will many of the more modern variations of asana practice.

What are the differences between traditional yoga asana practice and yoga-inspired exercise? What are their effects both on body and mind? With the support of scientific research, you will learn the answers in this book. Our purpose is to make you aware of the immense physiological benefits an asana practice can bring if you practice according to ancient, classical principles. To simplify the terms *classical asana practice* or *asana practice according to ancient principles*, we will be using the term *Hatha Yoga*. Even though Hatha Yoga is fairly recent in the long history of yoga practice, it provides the foundation for most yoga practices and styles that exist today. Its essence fully integrates the ancient principles of yoga. Hatha Yoga includes asanas, pranayama, mudras, bandhas, and shat kriyas. For the sake of simplicity and convenience, though, unless mentioned otherwise, in this book the term Hatha Yoga refers solely to the practice of yoga asanas.

The principles of Hatha Yoga are in harmony with what modern physics calls the Principle of Minimal Action. This principle explains that nature does not waste energy. Floating in water happens only when you do less and less. For this reason, you can swim only if you first learn how to relax and float.

A common mistake for yoga practitioners is the image- and goal-oriented attitude of perceiving the picture-perfect posture as the goal. We must not forget, however, the basic principle that the asana is achieved naturally, through simple harmony between body and mind.

This book will show you how the classical principles of a yoga asana practice are proven by modern scientific and scholarly research. Although science and yoga may seem far apart, during the last few decades, science has shown that many seemingly outrageous claims of yoga are true. One example is yogic control of the heartbeat and body temperature through breathing and concentration techniques. In fact, many of the effects of body–mind practices such as yoga and meditation have been scientifically researched during the last few decades and have been found to be highly effective in countless ways. We will explore these in greater depth.

The knowledge within this book is based not only on years of research, study, and practice but also on a deeply integrated background of having grown up in a traditional, spiritual environment in India. For in India, much traditional knowledge is passed down orally. The author has been exposed to yoga, Vedic philosophy, and spirituality since birth. He shares here what he has learned from various teachers as well as from classical yoga texts. He wishes to support the ancient principles of yoga and yoga asana practice with modern explanations and provide solid ground for the claim that if practiced correctly, yoga asanas can counter and prevent many of our modern-day ailments. If we integrate the universal principles of yoga into our daily practice, we will lead more healthy and balanced lives.

First you will learn the physical and mental benefits of a Hatha Yoga practice. Only then will you approach the most central topic of this book—something a majority of yoga teachers and practitioners struggle with—sequencing.

How can you sequence a yoga class or personal practice in a comprehensive, holistic way? This will become easy once you see how to classify asanas according to their effects on the physical and energy bodies. You will learn the ancient principles of sequencing of asanas according to their corresponding chakras (energy centers).

Because each body part or region of your body corresponds with one of the seven main chakras, this approach will provide you with a great tool for classifying, understanding, and sequencing asanas.

You will, however, learn more than how to classify asanas and how to build up a holistic and comprehensive Hatha Yoga practice. This book illustrates detailed descriptions of over 200 asanas, with their respective instructions, alignment cues, modifications, and variations. To complete the sequencing section, we provide you with a few sample sequences. We designed these according to the sequencing system you will learn.

Once you have this knowledge, you can then sensitively and intelligently provide the best sequences for various class lengths, goals, and experience levels.

For now you are invited to read, investigate, and, most importantly, try out these principles and techniques. Then, let your own experience be the judge. Please feel free to skip ahead to the practical part if you like. Consider trying out the sequencing system as you do your practice or prepare for your class. Also, feel free to read and digest the in-depth information in the first five chapters whenever you feel like it, and at your own comfortable pace.

After all, the practice of yoga is exactly meant to be that: a practice. As Swami Vishnu Devananda once advised, "An ounce of practice is better than tons of theory." Or, as B.K.S. Iyengar so profoundly stated, "It is through the alignment of body that I discovered the alignment of my mind, self, and intelligence."

After reading, experiencing, and experimenting with the information and principles in this book, you will

- understand the philosophical and historical background of Hatha Yoga and its relevance and applications in our modern times;
- understand the immense effects of a holistic Hatha Yoga practice on health and well-being;
- get an impression of the medical and scientific studies supporting the health benefits of Hatha Yoga practice;
- recognize the structure and elements for safe, fulfilling, and holistic Hatha Yoga practices; and

- learn the technique to instantly design customized Hatha Yoga sequences for different levels, themes, goals, and class durations.

How to Use This Book – Goals and Limitations

No two people are the same. No two bodies are the same. No two yoga practices are the same. To learn yoga, you need a teacher and personal feedback and guidance. A book, no matter how great it may be, can never replace a competent teacher. Even if you are an experienced practitioner of many years, a dedicated and experienced teacher will be able to guide you better and further than you can by yourself with the help of a book.

That being said, a book can still be a great tool for deepening your understanding, acquiring new concepts and techniques, developing skills, and evaluating different yoga practices. Only very few of us are fortunate enough to have a great teacher who provides constant and continual support and guidance. Most of us will have to acquire a great deal of knowledge through self-study and self-practice.

This book is intended to help and guide those of you who already possess a basic knowledge and practice of yoga asanas. As you progress, make the practice of yoga a part of your daily life and maybe even start to teach yourself; this book will be your companion for your self-practice at home and when designing classes and sessions. It will serve as a guide on your journey of understanding and applying sequencing.

We wish that this book will provide you with much knowledge. First we want you to learn an easy-to-understand and easy-to-apply system for creating holistic asana practices. Also we want you to learn how to keep yourself and your students safe. For this reason, we have also included many notes on alignment, how to modify and adjust asanas, and also in what circumstances to avoid certain postures.

What are the limitations of this book? As stated, we are all unique. There is no one solution that fits everyone. Whenever in doubt, especially concerning safety and injury prevention, consult with a senior teacher or physician. You can also ask your student to check with his or her physician before beginning yoga practice. We suggest to not rely solely on the information provided in this or any other book!

The instructions provided in this book are given with the assumption that the practitioner is in good physical and mental health and not pregnant. Yoga classes and programs for people suffering from serious diseases or chronic ailments and for pregnant women should be approached with specialized knowledge, and the information in this book does not focus on such cases.

Another challenge in this book is the choice of spelling and names of yoga asanas and yoga exercises. The names of yoga postures in Sanskrit have been translated into the English alphabet and are phonetic representations of original Sanskrit names. These phonetic translations have been affected by regional accents. We have tried to find a middle way between the traditional names and spelling and the modern and most common names and spelling of asanas and yoga exercises.

According to our understanding, for example, Headstand should be phonetically represented in English as Sheershasan, to give an indication of the right pronunciation. Most commonly, however, you will find this posture spelled as Sirsasana. This spelling would be correct if there were a dot below each s to indicate the pronunciation as sh. But translations from Sanksrit to English are faulty by design, because usually this dot (and other so-called diacritical marks) are not part of the English alphabet and therefore have been left out for reasons of simplification. So as a middle way, you will find Headstand spelled as Shirshasana. Doing so at least provides a clear indication that this asana should be pronounced with a sh. Also, sometimes certain postures have entirely different names, due to the many different traditions and lineages. Here again, we have followed the Hatha Yoga lineage to a certain degree, but also sometimes have given preference to names from the more contemporary Ashtanga and Vinyasa traditions. Our choices have been adopted with the purpose of making this a very practical and easy-to-use book: avoiding unnecessary confusion and making it easy to combine with information available in other books and other media.

A Short Note on the Role of a Teacher

This book is designed not only as a guide for your own practice, but also as a companion for those of you who are already yoga teachers or want eventually to become one. For this reason, we would like to start off with a short note about the role of a teacher.

Every teacher holds the power to influence his or her students' journeys. This influence can be small and forgotten over time. It can even be non-existent. In the worst case, it can be negative. But this influence can also be positive and life-changing. It can forge a connection of trust that lasts a lifetime. Keeping that in mind, we should strive for the latter. Do not, though, expect such an outcome, and simply perform your duty as a teacher to the best of your ability. If you stay humble, recognize your role and responsibility as a teacher, and remember that your students will always be your best teachers, then teaching will become an enriching part of your life that will keep you curious and motivated.

It is easy to become confused between the role of a teacher and the role of an instructor. An instructor is someone who simply provides or explains instructions about how to do an asana or exercise. Mostly an instructor will stand in front during much of the class and demonstrate the asanas for students to follow. An instructor is more concerned with what to do and how to do it, and will follow a set pattern, a sequence, or instructions. A yoga teacher, though, is more concerned with helping each student meet his or her goals in coming to the yoga class. A yoga teacher walks around the class watching, helping, correcting, and adjusting students. You should make a clear choice about which you wish to be.

Teaching—as opposed to instructing—means putting the students' interests first. A teacher is attentive and responsive to the students' possibilities and restrictions, needs and emotions. Even though we are teaching a yoga class to a group of people, we must recognize their individualities and refrain from having any expectations of what our students could or should be doing, or what they are thinking of us. Honor and respect all differences, and always remember that at this moment you are teaching your student yoga, but tomorrow he or she might be your teacher in another discipline.

When we ask our students in our yoga teacher-training courses which quality of a teacher they most highly admire and remember fondly one of the all-time favorites is that the teacher cares about them. Another quality often mentioned is integrity. Integrity means that you do what you say and you say what you do. We are all human, we all have weaknesses, and nobody expects that because you are a yoga teacher, you have mastered all yogic principles to perfection. So integrity simply means that you practice and try to integrate what you teach.

If you have come to yoga and developed a passion for it, do not lose your regular practice. Do not lose your humility and reverence for the practice as you get busy with teaching. At the same time, do not think you have to master every single asana. Do not think you have to be perfectly calm and serene before you can start to teach. Simply be as honest and kind with yourself as you are with your students. Follow your own path. Being an advanced yoga practitioner does not make you an advanced teacher. There is a big difference between knowing something and being able to explain and transfer that knowledge to students. Your constant efforts to help your students and to continue on your own path without pretension will show your integrity and earn their trust. Always remember: Your students do not care about how much you know until they know how much you care.

Part I

The Roots: Background of Hatha Yoga

Chapter 1

The Broad View – Yogic Philosophy

According to surveys conducted in 2015, over 35 million people worldwide practice yoga. Not satisfied with mere fitness, these people are seeking holistic well-being, vitality, vigor, flexibility, and strength. After all, all these are needed for living a peaceful and balanced life. To meet this increasing demand, over 50 different yoga styles have sprung up out of Hatha Yoga in the last few decades. Most of these styles focus on the physical aspects of yoga, namely postures and breathing exercises.

Yoga, however, is much more than the practice of yoga asanas (poses) and pranayama (breathing techniques). It is an ancient discipline that monks and ascetics on the Indian subcontinent are said to have developed more than five thousand years ago. Unlike many modern practitioners, these "fathers" of yoga were not concerned merely with physical results. The entire practice was holistic—embracing all aspects of human nature. These original yogis had complete perfection as their goal. This meant physical, mental, and spiritual perfection. They wished to have control over not just the body but also the vital energies, senses, and mind.

To understand and practice yoga holistically, it is beneficial to understand the philosophy behind it. Often yoga is defined by its literal translations: "to unite," "to join," or "to meet." Following the literal meaning, yoga is often mistaken to be "union of body and mind" or "union of body, breath, and mind." Yoga indeed does mean union: union of the self with the reality of self. Or in other words, self-realization. Thus, self-realization is the ultimate goal of the practice of yoga.

Self-realization is described as the state when you become free from the illusions of the material world and understand the true identity of your existence. In other words, when you find the answer to the question of "Who am I?" you have realized your Self. But you might think you already know who you are. You might say, "I am John." But you are not John—John is a name or a label you have been given. So then, who are you? You might say, "I am a doctor." But being a doctor is a profession that you pursue. So the question remains—who are you? This time you might say, "I am my personality," but your personality developed over time and it will keep evolving. You did not have a personality when you were born, but you were alive nonetheless, so you cannot be your personality. By now, you can understand that it is difficult to answer this question because we do not know who or what we really are. Instead, we identify ourselves with the labels or roles we have in our life.

Yoga is the path through which we can become aware of our true Self. This path requires mastery of the body, senses, and the mind. When we achieve mastery over body, mind, and senses we can become free from our ego. Ego is our attachment to the ideas that we create of ourselves and the world around us. This ego is created through our limited senses and our limited minds. For this reason, ego is also very limited. The ego filters all of our perceptions. It makes us see only what we want to see. If we were to wear a pair of purple sunglasses, we would see everything through the purple glass—even a white shirt would appear purple. If we want to see the real color of the shirt, we need to remove the glasses. Similarly, to see and understand the reality of Self, we need to let go of the ego and master our senses and the mind.

India's traditional writings on yoga also describe this ego-free state. The *Bhagavad Gita* explains that when you achieve the state of yoga, your mind or consciousness is focused only on the Self. In this state, your mind stops wandering around searching for pleasures, and identifies instead with the everlasting and blissful Self. This yogic state shines forth only under certain conditions. Your mind must become disciplined by understanding and discriminating between reality and illusion. It is only then that Self-awareness realizes its own eternally liberated and separate status.

"

> *A person is said to have achieved yoga, union with the Self, when the perfectly disciplined mind achieves freedom from all desires, and becomes focused only on the Self alone." (Bhagavad Gita, 6:4)*

The *Katha Upanishad* describes yoga as the highest state: where your five senses, mind, and intellect are still and under control. When these faculties become still, you realize the truth or reality of the Self and become free from the illusion of the world:

"

When the five senses are stilled, when the mind is stilled, when the intellect is stilled, that is called the highest state by the wise. They say yoga is this complete stillness in which one enters the unitized state, never to become separate again from reality. He who attains this is free from delusion (Maya)."
(Katha Upanishad, II: 3: 6–11)

According to Maharishi Patanjali, the author of the *Yoga Sutras*, yoga stops (nirodhah) the movements (vritti) of the mind (chitta). Here, Patanjali speaks of the mind's movements as mental disturbances arising from the mind's egoic attachments and desires. You experience these mental fluctuations as waves of happiness and sadness—and varying degrees of fulfillment. But once you realize the Self, your mind settles permanently into a stillness that is free from these disturbances.

"

Yoga ceases the movements of the mind." (Yoga Sutras, 1:2)

As the above scriptures reveal, yoga is the state where the mind and senses abandon their ego-oriented quests for pleasure and realize the reality of the Self. To fulfill this goal, the scriptures offer four yogic paths. Each is a non-sectarian practice suitable for humans with various personalities, possibilities, and capabilities. You may follow one or several of these paths to reach the goal of Self-realization.

Raja Yoga: The path of control. In this practice, you bring body, mind, and breath under control to let go of ego and realize the Self. Hatha Yoga, including the practice of asanas, is a part of Raja Yoga.

Jnana Yoga: The path of knowledge. In this practice, you surrender your ego through acquiring knowledge, which removes ignorance and illusion and leads to understanding the reality of the Self.

Bhakti Yoga: The path of devotion to the Divine. This is the path of surrendering your ego to whatever is your perception of Divinity. In this way you start to realize the reality of the Self.

Karma Yoga: The path of selfless duty. When you follow this path, you do your duty to the best of your abilities, without attachment to results or rewards. This helps you let go of your ego and leads to Self-realization.

Over the last few thousand years, yoga has enriched mankind with specific practices that—independent of any underlying philosophy—anyone can apply. If you apply all of these practices (or a majority of them) you can speak of a yogic lifestyle. However, it is each and every person's free choice to make it a lifestyle or to simply pick practices and values as they naturally see fit. After all, an essential quality of yogic teaching is its independence from religions and sects. Even though yoga philosophy teaches certain concepts such as karma and reincarnation, it does so in a non-sectarian way. In this way, yoga remains open to all different religions and beliefs. This strong anti-sectarianism can be found in most of the texts of Hatha Yoga. One example is in the Dattatreyayogasastra, the first text to teach a systematized Hatha Yoga:

"

> *Whether a Brahmin, an ascetic, a Buddhist, a Jain, a Skull-Bearer, or a materialist, the wise man who is endowed with faith and constantly devoted to the practice of yoga will attain complete success." (Dattatreyayogasastra, 3.1.2 - verse 41)*

The entire body of Hatha Yoga displays this non-sectarian view, making the methods and aims of yoga, its moral and ethical guidelines, as well as all its practices available to all.[1]

Chapter 2

Hatha Yoga and the Principle of Least Action

Hatha Yoga is a branch within Raja Yoga, the yoga of control, which is one of the four paths of yoga. Hatha Yoga developed from the principles of Raja Yoga. The goal of Hatha Yoga, as in Raja Yoga, is to achieve samadhi. Samadhi is a state of freedom from attachments, ego, and the illusions of the material world. At first it is a temporary state. Gradually it becomes permanent.

According to the Raja Yoga tradition, you must first purify your nature and habits. This involves returning to a pure and non-violent existence by observing and cultivating moral observances and habits. These are called the yamas and niyamas. Only after you master these can you proceed to the practice of asanas, pranayama, and meditation. According to the *Hatha Yoga Pradipika*, though, you should start with the physical practices first. This is because most people will find it easier to master the mind through the body than to purify their character, habits, and mind directly through the observance of yamas and niyamas.

For this reason, the main practices of Hatha Yoga are asana and pranayama. Their main goal is to purify body and mind and prepare you for further spiritual practices. In the previous chapter you have seen that you can practice the asanas independently of any philosophy. Further down the road, you will also learn how and why the practice of asanas can be done to achieve maximum physical, mental, and spiritual benefits. Being and staying healthy is a central concern in yoga. This is because when you have a healthy and strong body and mind, you possess the greatest vehicle for spiritual development. Other practices within the Hatha Yoga traditions—such as mudras, bandhas, shat kriyas, and mantras—were all developed as supplements to the practice of postures and breath control.

A common misconception of the word *hatha* is that it literally means "sun" (ha) and "moon" (tha). This has no resemblance with any word used in Sanskrit for sun and moon, and even though this definition of the term *Hatha* has been quite prevalent, it is simply a misconception. It came about because of a short passage within the *Hatha Yoga Pradipika*, where Swami Svatmarama speaks of how the physical practices can impact the flow of energy in the body, in particular the two primary (lunar and solar) energy channels of Ida and Pingala. These channels can be compared to the complementary forces that make up life: male and female, hot and cold, sun and moon. And the practice of Hatha Yoga purifies and brings balance between the Ida and Pingala channels. However, Svatmarama stresses that this balancing is just one effect of Hatha Yoga and that the goal, as in yoga in general, is the attainment of samadhi, or "oneness of mind."

The word *hatha* actually means "stubborn" or "forceful." So Hatha Yoga means the forceful or stubborn practice of yoga. It is a discipline you practice to purify and control your body. As a result, you gain control over the mind as well. When you stubbornly stick to the practice, you cultivate willpower and overcome fears and other mental interferences. For example, when you practice asanas, you do not remain only within the comforts of easy postures and well-known routines. Rather, you try to overcome fears and thoughts such as "I cannot do this." When you first learn to do Headstand, you may encounter fears and doubts whether you may ever accomplish the pose. However, as a practitioner of Hatha Yoga, you glue yourself to the goal, stubbornly devoted to learning the pose. Even as your body falls and your mind tells you that it is too difficult, you stubbornly continue to practice until you become steady and comfortable in the asana.

Simultaneously, as you practice asanas, you do so according to Patanjali's ancient definition of yoga asana practice, *sthira sukham asanam*, which literally means "asana is a steady and comfortable pose." This is because only in such an effortless and comfortable posture can you merge your attention (mind) with the infinite. Only through effortlessness are you in tune with your true nature and nature around you. This ancient definition is in sync with a law of nature that in modern times has become well known as the Principle of Minimal Action.

An example of the principle is when you try hard to stay on the surface of the water, you sink. When you relax and give up, you float. It is one of the most fundamental principles of nature, and all of nature acts according to this Principle of Least Action, as it is called in physics. Mathematicians formulated the principle during the first half of the 17th century. They observed that light travels at different speeds through different media and that light always chooses the path that takes the least time. How does the light know which path to take? They understood that nature will always follow the path that requires the least amount of energy and time. In fact, nature aims to conserve energy.

The Chinese also observed the same principle and called it Wu Wei (minimal action). Wu Wei lies at the basis of Tai Chi and Kung Fu. It refers to the cultivation of a state of being in which our actions are quite effortlessly in alignment with the ebb and flow of the elemental cycles of the natural world.

The same principle lies at the foundation of yoga asanas. You practice each asana most naturally when you ease into it with the least physical and mental effort. In this way you remain in sync with your own nature and the larger flow of nature all around you. When you practice Hatha Yoga and your body is in a restful and regenerative mode, you are acting according to the most basic and natural principle of the universe. You thus act in harmony with the totality of natural law.

But wasn't Hatha Yoga just defined as a stubborn and forceful practice? How, at the same time, can you also aim for least effort as well as mental and physical ease and comfort? That seems quite contradictory. You must distinguish, though, between cultivating a stubborn and forceful willpower for the practice and practicing forcefully. In Hatha Yoga you do the first. You stubbornly dedicate and devote yourself to the practice, overcoming mental limitations and distractions from your senses. You become stubborn about what you decide to do. And you practice easefully and steadily when you perform the asanas. In its essence, Hatha Yoga is about stubbornly finding the balance between ease and force, or between Yin and Yang.

CHAPTER 3

THE EVOLUTION OF YOGA ASANAS

"

By the practice of yoga one gains contentment, endurance of the dualities (of pleasure and pain), and tranquility. These teachings should not be given to all and sundry, but only to those who have the appropriate qualifications to learn with respect. Let no one declare this most secret doctrine to anyone who is not a son, who is not a pupil, who is not of a tranquil mind." (Maitri Upanishad, 6.29; 300 BC)

All sources suggest that knowledge of yoga practices was kept secret for millennia. Therefore it is extremely difficult to make a conclusive statement about the age and variety of yoga asanas. The practice of yoga asanas was until quite recently reserved for ascetics. It was passed down from teacher to student in the so-called guru–shishya (teacher–student) tradition.

In the guru–shishya tradition, the guru personally initiates the student. In turn, the student has proven himself to be competent and eager to learn the secrets of a particular lineage. This principle of learning under the direct supervision of a teacher was deeply rooted in the yoga tradition as well as in the general education system in India. The ancient yoga texts—the *Vedas*, the *Upanishads*, the *Yoga Sutras*, and all subsequent texts—were written knowing that only readers under the guidance of an experienced teacher in the lineage would be able to understand and practically benefit from the knowledge. This explains why the ancient classical texts mention asanas and meditation practices but do not explain them in detail.

Early References

Some of the first references to yoga can be found in the *Vedas*, a collection of mantras that seers cognized thousands of years ago. Orthodox Hindus consider the four *Vedas* to be the source of all later religious and philosophical teaching in India. The oldest of the four is the *Rig Veda*, with the other three being the *Sama Veda*, the *Yajur Veda*, and the *Atharva Veda*. All are believed to have been composed between 1500 and 500 BC. The *Vedas* contain knowledge about spiritual and practical life. They are not yoga texts as such, but lay the foundations for yogic ideas developed in later texts.

The word *yoga* appears in the *Rig Veda*, defined as "yoking" or "discipline." It describes, though, no systematic practice. The term *yoga* turns up again in the *Atharva Veda*, where it refers to the means of harnessing or yoking the prana (life force) by the practice of pranayama (yogic breathing exercises to control and expand prana). This is the first known textual reference to physical yoga as a practice.

The word *Upanishad* means "sitting down near" and refers to a student sitting close to their master to receive secret and sacred teachings. The *Upanishads* were composed after the *Vedas*. Although there were some 200 of them, only 12 are considered principal *Upanishads*, which are believed to have been composed in the period from 800 to 300 BC. Of the 12 principal *Upanishads*, the word *yoga* occurs in only four. In the *Taittiriya Upanishad* (ca. 700 BC) the word *yoga* appears in an analogy of a bird. Scholars think that this use of the word *yoga* refers to quietness of mind brought about through contemplation.

The first time in history we find a written explanation of yoga is in the *Katha Upanishad* (500–400 BC). This text describes yoga as the science of controlling the senses. It states that in yoga, the mind is stilled and Brahman (God) or the Supreme Self is realized. It says that this leads to spiritual liberation, liberation from the circle of life and death.

The *Svetasvatara Upanishad* (500–400 BC) offers some practical advice on how to practice yoga. The scripture describes the most conducive environment; how to breathe; and how to keep the body in a straight posture by holding the chest, neck, and head erect. It states that by silently chanting Om while focusing on its meaning, we will learn to control the senses, and by repressing and regulating breathing through the nostrils and observing subtle movements of the body, we will restrain the mind. Dedicated practice, it advises, will lead to freedom from disease, old age, and death. According to the *Svetasvatara Upanishad*, the first step toward the goal of liberation occurs when the body becomes light and healthy; when the mind becomes free from desire; when the yogi develops a shining complexion, sweet voice, and pleasant odor; and when his or her excretions become meager. These changes suggest that through the practice of yoga, a certain physical purification takes place because such a healthy body is not gained by sitting alone. We can reason that this is one of the first textual references to the practice of asanas.

> "
> *From the conquest of posture, so by mastering asanas, an invincible, unconstrained freedom from suffering due to the pairs of opposites (such as heat and cold, good and bad, pain and pleasure) is attained." (Yoga Sutras, 2.48)*

In the *Yoga Sutras*, Patanjali describes asana as "a posture" to be practiced prior to attempting pranayama or meditation. He provided the first reference to the term *asana* as we understand it today. He does not, though, describe any asana in detail, but states simply that an asana should be steady and comfortable (sthira sukham asanam). Only in such an effortlessly comfortable posture can the practitioner merge their attention (mind) with the infinite (the Self or God). This, after all, is the goal of yoga.

According to Patanjali, only once the postures are mastered may one continue to the practice of breath control. As Patanjali states, the practice of asanas in a comfortable and steady manner makes your body strong and immune to disease. Estimates of the date of the *Yoga Sutras* range from 500 BC to 200 AD. It is clear, however, that Patanjali did not originate the teachings in the *Yoga Sutras*. Rather, he inherited a huge mass of earlier teachings from the *Upanishads* and the *Bhagavad Gita*. Patanjali's contribution was to condense, refine, and systematize these teachings.

Light on Hatha Yoga

Today many people tend to associate all yoga with the term Hatha Yoga. This is rightly so in the case of the term *yoga asanas*, because the practice of yoga asanas has indeed become more systematized and accessible through the development of Hatha Yoga. There have been many, though, who have attained the state of yoga without practicing Hatha Yoga. Furthermore, the practice of yoga asanas existed long before the various practices that belong to Hatha Yoga were defined in writing.

Sanskrit texts ranging from the 11th to the 13th century AD mention mudras and bandhas[2] that would appear later in Hatha Yoga texts. The *Goraksha Shataka* (13th–14th c. AD) proclaims that there are 8.4 million postures, as many as there are species of living beings on this planet. According to Goraksha, the author, 84 of these postures have been selected by Lord Shiva as the main ones. Two of these, Siddha Asana and Padma Asana (which are later on included in the Hatha Yoga tradition), he considers to be of the highest importance for meditation. It is for this reason that he describes them.

The *Shiva Samhita* (1500 AD) mixes philosophy with specific practices. It also speaks at length about the chakras (centers of spiritual power in the subtle body) and nadis (subtle channels in your body that transmit energy) systems. The work mentions only four asanas, but many mudras and pranayama techniques. All these texts written between 1100 and 1500 AD[3] either mention Hatha Yoga by name—without explaining any techniques—or they describe mudras, bandhas, and a few asanas but do not call these techniques Hatha Yoga.

The turning point in the definition of physical yoga practices is the *Hatha Yoga Pradipika* (which translated means Illuminating Hatha Yoga or Light on Hatha Yoga). It was written in the 15th century AD by Swami Svatmarama, and is a compilation of around 20 texts, including the ones mentioned above. It is among the most influential of three surviving texts on Hatha Yoga.[4]

The *Hatha Yoga Pradipika* is the first text that introduces all the techniques taught in earlier works under one umbrella. It defines and discusses asanas, pranayama, mudras and bandhas, kumbhaka (breath retention), and nadanusandhana (concentration on inner sounds) as Hatha Yoga practices. The *Hatha Yoga Pradipika* also discusses the shat kriyas (six internal cleansing practices) that became characteristic of Hatha

Yoga. Furthermore, the *Hatha Yoga Pradipika* is the first available text on yoga to name and describe non-seated asanas. It also emphasizes, as does the *Yoga Sutras* of Patanjali, the importance of asanas for physical well-being:

> "
> *It is the first limb of Hatha Yoga and asanas are therefore described first. Asanas should be practiced for steadiness of posture, health and lightness of body."*
> *(Hatha Yoga Pradipika, 1.19)*

The *Hatha Yoga Pradipika* merely refers to the rich traditions of postures originating from the sages and then goes on to mention and describe only 15 asanas. Of the 15 asanas, 8 are varieties of sitting or lying postures, and 7 are non-seated positions. The verses describing asanas are derived from a variety of earlier texts: the *Dattatreyayogasastra*, the *Vivekamartananda*, the *Vasisthasamhita*, the *Yogayajnavalkya*, and the *Sivasamhita*. No source text has yet been identified, however, for 3 of the 7 non-seated asanas: Uttanakurmasana, Dhanurasana, and Matsyendrasana.[5]

Although the *Hatha Yoga Pradipika* is known as the ultimate textbook on Hatha Yoga, it is important to know that it is not an extensive guide to Hatha Yoga. It simply intends to provide basic information on the topic. In his book, Swami Svatmarama stresses the importance of an experienced teacher from whom the proper practice of Hatha Yoga should be learned. Without the guidance of the teacher, these exercises cannot be utilized to their full potential. Svatmarama emphasizes that the true meaning of yoga cannot be gained by merely reading textbooks. It must rather come from personal experience gained under the supervision of a guru. As the *Hatha Yoga Pradipika* states,

> "
> *A yogi desirous of success should keep the knowledge of Hatha Yoga secret; for it becomes potent by concealing and impotent by exposing."*
> *(Hatha Yoga Pradipika, 1.11)*

Pre-Modern References

Although by this time we can see that a refined and extensive system for yoga asana practice was emerging, the early texts were deliberately vague and lacking in detail. This was because yoga was considered sacred, and only after students had proved their worth and dedication would this esoteric knowledge be revealed to them by a teacher. This is because the writings were purposely kept vague to ensure secrecy. Recently, though, more texts on the practice of yoga, yoga asanas, and Hatha Yoga have started to appear. Though united in their yogic goal, these texts reveal many discrepancies due to the different schools and lineages that have developed over time. One example of these is the great variation in the number and selection of asanas mentioned in classic and pre-modern works.

For instance, the *Gherand Samhita*, assigned to the 17th or 18th centuries, was the first book to really lay out the details of the entire Hatha Yoga system. Like *Goraksha Shataka*, it states that there are 8.4 million asanas. Only 84 of these asanas does it deem to be superior, of which a mere 32 are said to be sacred in the world of mortals. Along with 32 primary asanas, it describes many forms of pranayama, 25 mudras, bandhas, and shatkarmas (internal cleansing) techniques.

Another example is the *Hatha Ratnavali*, the first book on yoga to actually list 84 asanas. It was written by Srinivasa, a yogi from South India. It dates from the 18th century. The text is strongly influenced by the *Hatha Yoga Pradipika*. The list of 84 asanas begins with Siddhasana (Accomplished Pose) and ends with Shavasana (Corpse Pose). It mentions 84 asanas, but describes, in all, only 36. Another text, the *Jogapradipika*, written by Jayatarama of Vrindavan in 1737, is the only other pre-modern text known so far that also names and describes 84 asanas. The names of the asanas, though, differ considerably from those listed in the *Hatha Ratnavali*.

As mentioned earlier, the discrepancies between the names and numbers of asanas indicate an extensive tradition of asanas as well as the existence of different lineages and sects. It is apparent that the number 84 was symbolically significant for authors of both ancient and classical yoga texts. The number 84 traditionally signifies completeness, and in some cases sacredness. Even though many classical and pre-modern works refer to 84 asanas as an auspicious number, it is apparent that such a unified tradition never existed. The discrepancies in texts, traditions, and lineages may seem confusing. However, they are merely a sign of the rich and diverse traditions of yoga.

Nonetheless, key concepts have remained somewhat stable and should be kept in mind as we move further:

- Yoga leads to control of your body, mind, and senses, and its final goal is self-realization.
- Yoga is non-sectarian and open to anyone and everyone. As practitioners it is our completely free choice to pick any path, any technique, and any method as long as it serves us and leads us toward a more conscious and healthy existence.
- To reap the full and intended results and move toward the final goal (if you wish to), yoga should be practiced humbly, with dedication, and under the supervision of a teacher.
- The practice of yoga asanas is highly beneficial for physical well-being, making the body strong and healthy in preparation for further spiritual practices.

Millions of modern yogis and yoginis have experienced the benefits claimed by the ancient texts. These benefits have ignited yoga's explosive rise and popularity. In the chapters that follow, we will explore why and how a yoga asana practice can be such a powerful tool for holistic well-being.

Part II

Medical Facts: Hatha Yoga for Holistic Health

According to yoga philosophy, health is the balance and proper functioning of all physical, mental, and energy systems. Asanas were conceived in ancient times to promote holistic health by stimulating and balancing the internal body systems and maintaining homeostasis.

As yoga became popular, the focus of the practice started to shift. As a result, some of its original principles began to become diluted. The original purpose of yoga asanas was to keep the internal physical body and the energy body healthy and in balance. Asanas were specifically developed for this reason. These days, though, yoga practices generally focus on toning and stretching the musculoskeletal system. It is important to remember that the changes in bodily appearance through regular practice of yoga asanas are side effects and should not be mistaken for the main goal. The main difference between a Hatha Yoga practice and a modern yoga asana practice is how the asanas are performed. Classically, asanas are defined as steady, comfortable poses. As soon as the asanas are performed in a dynamic way, without steady holds, we enter the realm of modern asana practice. Ancient scriptures define asanas with the words *sthira sukham asanam*, which defines the state where body and mind are steady and comfortable in a pose.

To sum it up, an asana practice according to Hatha Yoga principles:

1. aims to keep the internal body healthy and in balance rather than focusing on weight loss, toning, and shaping the exterior physical body; and

2. performs asanas with long, comfortable, and steady holds, rather than in a vigorous or dynamic manner.

Chapter 4

Hatha Yoga and Your Body's Systems

In this chapter we will see how—according to Hatha Yoga principles—a yoga asana practice affects the systems of your body. We will also discover if and how these effects differ from the effects seen from regular exercises or dynamic yoga asana practices.

Hatha Yoga and the Autonomic Nervous System

The autonomic nervous system is also known as the involuntary nervous system. It maintains homeostasis in your body. Homeostasis is the maintenance and balance of relatively stable conditions within your body's internal systems, despite changes happening inside and outside your body. The autonomic nervous system branches into the cardiac muscles, smooth muscles, and various endocrine and exocrine glands. It therefore influences most tissue and organ systems in your body.

Your autonomic nervous system consists of two subsystems: the sympathetic and the parasympathetic nervous systems. Your sympathetic nervous system prepares your body for action. It is famous for its fight-or-flight response. For example, if a dog attacks you, your heartbeat will quicken, your pupils will dilate, and the majority of blood will be sent to your muscles to prepare you either to fight or to flee. All your body's systems are put into emergency mode in order to manage and survive the immediate situation. Meanwhile, all your internal functions not related to the threat, such as regular functions for growth and healing of your body, are put on hold.

Your other subsystem is the parasympathetic nervous system. It brings your body into a rest-and-digest mode. It counterbalances your sympathetic nervous system, restoring your body to a state of calm and activating regular functions such as the secretion of saliva in your mouth or digestive enzymes in your stomach.

Only one of these two subsystems can be active at a time. They alternate according to the need and situation. The balance between these two systems is of utmost importance. In a healthy person, the transitions between the two systems are regular, smooth, and swift.

Apart from external and psychological factors, the sympathetic nervous system is also activated when you use your muscles or breathe more heavily. More vigorous and dynamic yoga asana styles will trigger your sympathetic nervous system.

Comfortable exercises, as well as slow and conscious breathing, on the other hand, will engage your parasympathetic nervous system. Likewise, a Hatha Yoga practice—with steady and comfortable postures and calm, conscious breathing—will bring you into resonance with your parasympathetic nervous system. In this state the proper functioning of all your internal organs and glands is ensured. They will receive an abundant blood supply.

We all know that stress is unhealthy. It triggers the sympathetic nervous system, which then creates more stress. This stress-induced cycle causes most common chronic diseases. After all, when your sympathetic nervous system is active, your body is in survival mode. Your heart rate increases, the blood supply to your internal organs is cut and redirected to your major muscles, and your respiration becomes quick and shallow. At the same time the stress hormone cortisol floods your bloodstream. Over time, this can lead to various vascular disorders such as hypertension and a depressed immune system.

With today's busy and stressful lifestyle, most of us receive little benefit from stimulating the sympathetic nervous system through vigorous exercise, at least not exclusively. If you are already too often and too long in a state of sympathetic arousal, you need to train your body and mind to easily relax into and stay within a parasympathetic mode more frequently.

Some elements within a Hatha Yoga practice promote rest and rejuvenate your system, and others raise your heartbeat, challenge you, and bring you into a sympathetic state. This is one reason Hatha Yoga is so important for your body. By consciously relaxing from the sympathetic nervous system into your parasympathetic nervous system during Hatha Yoga, you begin to effortlessly accomplish these transitions.

The Sun Salutation in the beginning of the practice serves as a good example. This cycle of asana-like steps is meant to warm up your body. Through the dynamic performance of the Sun Salutation, the sympathetic nervous system perks up. After 5 to 10 minutes of Sun Salutations, though, you lie down in Shavasana (Corpse Pose) and allow your breathing and heartbeat to calm down. This is the important shift when the parasympathetic nervous system takes over. Similarly, a dynamic Kapalbhati breathing (a form of pranayama breathing also known as Shining-Skull) excites the sympathetic nervous system, whereas the more calming Anulom Vilom (also known as Alternate Nostril Breathing) engages the more calming qualities of the parasympathetic nervous system.

For this reason, long holds during Hatha Yoga practice are essential. Holding an asana with comfort and ease for a certain duration brings you into rest-and-regenerate mode. Not all asanas are easy and effortless, though. Challenging asanas raise your heartbeat and respiration rates. When followed by a relaxation pose such as Corpse Pose, Child's Pose, or Crocodile Pose, however, your body learns how to shift from sympathetic to parasympathetic mode.

A good yoga practice involves poses and exercises that cycle through the accelerator and the brake so the autonomic nervous system gets a thorough workout. This is why a true Hatha Yoga practice does three things. First, it often challenges the body in order to warm up or in order to learn different postures and exercises and therefore activates the sympathetic nervous system. Second, it always includes elements that bring your body and mind back into a parasympathetic state. Third, it develops an awareness between the contrasting states of relaxation and excitement. Through understanding this, you increase your capability to shift from one state to the other in your daily life as well. Therefore Hatha Yoga helps to prevent imbalance between the sympathetic and parasympathetic systems. As you realize your energetic flexibility, you develop the ability to achieve states of inner balance and harmony, as well as improved health for your entire body.

How Hatha Yoga prevents and removes stress

Stress is a reaction to an internal or external stimulus. This stimulus disturbs your physical or mental equilibrium. It leads to an overly activated sympathetic nervous system and floods your body with adrenaline. Meanwhile, your respiration rate, heart rate, muscle tension, and blood pressure increase. This in turn increases stress and anxiety, making it a vicious circle.

Often stress can become such a habitual part of life that you do not even recognize it anymore. And as discussed above, long-term stress will eventually have damaging effects on your health. You may not always be able to control the sources of stress, but you can learn to modify your reactions to it. Through the calm and mindful practice of Hatha Yoga you can re-establish healthy breathing patterns and learn to relax. By learning to relax and consciously experiencing relaxation, you can recognize early signs of stress in your daily life and learn to respond more calmly and consciously. Through this natural growth, you will gain relief from stress and stressful situations.

This is important both for mental health and for physical well-being. When stressed, all bodily functions such as digestion, excretion, sleep, and so on are thrown out of balance. When stress becomes a chronic condition, we can suffer from a wide variety of bodily effects. Indigestion and hyperacidity are just two. In fact, many studies have proven a direct link between stress and most of the common ills, such as diabetes, depression, anxiety, heart disease, high blood pressure, immune system diseases, and more.

One study explains the effects of yoga[6] as being brought about by yoga reducing accumulated stress-related wear and tear on the body. This subsequently restores your body's optimal balance, or homeostasis. Mel Robin, author of the acclaimed *Physiological Handbook for Teachers of Yogasana,*[7] agrees. He believes that the practice of yoga can increase control of the vagus nerve—which increases integration in the shifts between the parasympathetic and sympathetic nervous systems. This integration lessens the effect of stress on your body and mind. Certain yoga asanas, especially inverted ones, or any when the forehead rests on the floor, may shift the autonomic nervous system toward parasympathetic dominance, through stimulation of the vagus nerve.

Other studies have shown that yoga practices correct under-activity of the parasympathetic nervous and GABA systems (in part through stimulation of the vagus nerve) in addition to reducing accumulated stress-related wear and tear. GABA is a major neurotransmitter in the mammalian central nervous system and plays the principal role in reducing neuronal excitability throughout the nervous system. Many reports have linked stress and depression to low GABA levels. Scientists have measured GABA levels of yoga practitioners both before and after an hour-long yoga session focused on Hatha Yoga and related breathing. There were no extensive periods of meditation or pranayama. The study guidelines demanded at least 55 minutes of common yoga postures and exercises, such as inversions and backbends, twists and Sun Salutations. The scientists compared 8 yoga practitioners to a control group of 11 individuals who did no yoga but instead read magazines.

The results, published in 2007, were stunning. They showed that the brains of yoga practitioners displayed an average GABA rise of 27 percent. By contrast, the comparison group experienced not the slightest change. A follow-up study looked at subjects with no prior knowledge of yoga. They learned the Iyengar style from scratch and practiced it for three months. The findings, published in 2010, showed that even beginning yogis experienced major rises in the neurotransmitter, along with improved mood and less anxiety. The average GABA rise was less than in the previous study—13 percent versus 27 percent—about half as much. Still, the new yogis did better than the walkers (the control group).

This suggests that the practice of asanas and related breathing is more efficient in reducing stress and its long-term effects than exercise (moderate or vigorous) or any other leisure activity. The main influencs of yoga asana practice on stress are, as shown above, the activation of the rest-and-relax mode (the parasympathetic nervous system) and the direct increase of GABA neurotransmitters in the brain.

Hatha Yoga and the Circulatory System

Improved blood circulation

The heart is the most important organ of the circulatory system. Its foremost role is to pump blood throughout your body. An effective blood flow to all the tissues in the body is essential for the proper functioning of internal organs and processes. Many people do not realize that blood flow to most parts of the body depends partially on gravity and posture. Therefore a sedentary lifestyle, poor posture, and imbalanced movement patterns obstruct blood circulation. Luckily, Hatha Yoga offers a proven, effective cure.

Continuous slouching, for instance, can chronically compress your internal organs between the heart and large intestine. This obstructs blood circulation because the channels of blood flow tend to collapse. When this happens, the blood cannot properly carry out its functions of supplying tissues with oxygen, hormones, nutrients, and enzymes. Hatha Yoga poses, though, help to increase blood circulation, especially in areas prone to sluggish blood flow.

With poor circulation, white blood cells, which help to fight infection, may become stuck to the walls of the blood vessels. This weakens your body's ability to fight off disease. When the blood circulation increases due to the practice of Hatha Yoga, the number of circulating immune corpuscles increases and the amount of harmful germs decreases.

In this way, Hatha Yoga, by improving and varying blood circulation, helps to keep all internal organs functioning optimally by:

- ensuring a proper supply of oxygen, nutrients, and enzymes to cells and tissues; and
- supporting the immune system and increasing the immune response.

What about blood circulation during conventional exercise? Conventional exercise and vigorous asana practice raise the heart rate, forcing the heart to pump more blood per minute. Although the blood flow increases, the overall circulation of the blood does not. During conventional exercise, about 88 percent of the cardiac output ends up feeding the major muscles. At the same time all the other organs and tissues must get by on less fresh blood. In dynamic asana practice too, as soon as the sympathetic nervous system kicks in and stays in charge, the majority of the blood floods toward the major muscles and blood circulation, leaving little fresh blood supply for the internal organs.

Improved blood circulation to the brain

Most traditional yoga books state that Headstand is the king of asanas because of its immense health benefits, especially for the brain.

This ancient wisdom still applies. Inversion therapy uses inverted poses to increase blood flow to the brain. Naturally, then, the brain receives a boost of oxygen and glucose. These immensely stimulate its productivity. In fact, recent studies state that inversions can improve the brain's performance by 14 percent.[8] Inversions performed regularly over a certain period of time will improve concentration, memory, observation, and clarity of thought. They will also counteract depression and anxiety. Furthermore, inversion therapy may even play a serious role in arresting the brain's "aging process,"[9] even preventing or delaying dementia.

This medical proof is encouraging. It again demonstrates the timeless truth of what had been perceived thousands of years ago by the sages in ancient India. Inversions, and especially Headstand, promote prolonged agility, health, and mental vigor. But why should we make the effort to do Headstand? Why not simply lie on an inversion table, hang upside down, or lean inverted against the wall? When practicing Headstand with tools and a wall, we tend to invert the body for longer than it might be comfortable handling the change in blood pressure and the weight on the neck and head. Furthermore, in propping up our Headstand, we will not develop the coordination and strength required to safely perform inversions. It is for these reasons that Headstand is recommended as part of a balanced Hatha Yoga routine. Even though inversion therapy may be beneficial for certain conditions and purposes, a balanced yoga asana practice including inversions will, in the long term, be more effective and beneficial for holistic health. As always, in order to reap the benefits of inversions, hold the posture steadily and comfortably so that your body becomes exposed to the effects on the internal systems.

Regulation of Blood Pressure

Normal blood pressure is important for good health. When it drops too low, the brain receives insufficient blood, and we become so dizzy and weak that we faint. In extreme cases organs can fail, producing breakdowns such as heart attacks. High blood pressure has its own hazards—mostly long term rather than immediate. It stresses the heart and artery walls. In doing so, it may lead to an increased risk of stroke, heart attack, and kidney failure. Fortunately, there are sensors in your body called "baroreceptors." These take pressure readings of the blood vessels and make suitable adjustments in blood pressure.

Your baroreceptors' sensitivity and responsiveness indicate your state of health. When the baroreceptors are more sensitive, they sense and respond earlier. Slow and controlled breathing[10] increases the sensitivity of these sensors. This results in a more fine-tuned control of heart rate and blood pressure.

Also, inverted asanas, typical in Hatha Yoga, increase the sensitivity and responsiveness of these baroreceptors, which in turn can lead to prolonged improvements in blood pressure. For example, Shoulderstand stimulates one particular kind of sensor. This sensor lies in the carotids, major arteries running through the front of your neck. Their job is to carry blood to the brain. The carotid sensors help this process along. They make sure the brain receives enough blood. During Shoulderstand, the chin presses deeply into your neck and upper chest, clamping down on the carotids and making the local pressure very high. When this happens, the sensors embedded in the arterial walls monitoring the changes in blood pressure set off alarm bells within your body. Your body thinks that the delicate tissues of the brain are under too much pressure from too much blood. They order the heart to pump less often and less hard. So the blood vessels expand and relax and blood flows at a more leisurely pace.

Something similar happens within the right atrium of your heart during any inversion pose. In this right upper chamber of the heart, blood enters from the veins. A sensor located here determines the atrium's fullness. When pressure is low, the sensor signals the heart to beat faster, increasing blood flow. When pressure is too high, the heart slows down. Inversions dramatically increase the blood flow to your right atrium from the feet, legs, and lower torso. This activates the sensor, and the heart slows down.

However, this happens only if the pose is held steadily for at least 30 seconds—easily and comfortably. Beginners learning inversions such as Headstand or Shoulderstand often feel nervous or unbalanced. So they use a lot of muscular tension to hold themselves up. Because this activates the sympathetic nervous system, blood pressure does not decrease, but instead increases. This is why those who already suffer from high blood pressure should not do inversions at all, or build them up very slowly under the supervision of their physician. Otherwise, their blood pressure may rise even more, which can be problematic. Teachers should be aware that beginning students will not experience the full benefits of the inverted poses until they can practice them with ease. As soon as your practice advances to that stage, you will harvest the full benefits of inverted poses.

Research has shown that conventional exercise, performed moderately, decreases blood pressure as well. Similarly, vigorous yoga asana practices can lower blood pressure because of the aerobic workout they provide. However, an aerobic workout has one main side-effect. It revs up the sympathetic nervous system. And this, as we now know, can lead to its own problems.

Hatha Yoga and the Lymphatic System – Detoxification

The lymphatic system plays important roles. It removes wastes and toxins while maintaining your body's immunity against pathogens. It does this by circulating lymph—a transparent fluid containing white blood cells and proteins. Lymph circulates around your body and drains fluid from the spaces in between cells. These are spaces where the cells dump their wastes and where other toxins and debris can accumulate. If these wastes build up, you begin to feel stiff, swollen, heavy, and lifeless.

The lymphatic system relies on the intrinsic muscle contractions of the lymph channel walls. It also depends on large-muscle activity in your body. In fact, contracting any muscle helps move lymph along. Yoga asanas, though, because they work every part of your body, are especially effective. Attention to your breath and to the compression and expansion of the solar plexus region during asanas further distinguishes asana practice from other forms of exercise. The breath is a lymphatic pump in itself. Conscious breathing helps direct lymph through the deep channels of the chest.

Yoga asanas work in three ways to increase the flow of lymph and relieve lymphatic congestion:

1. Inversions reverse the effect of gravity and drain lymph and used blood from your legs.
2. Twists (as well as forward, backward, and side bends) stimulate the flow of lymph up through the core of your body.
3. Contracting and releasing large muscles move lymph through your body.

To eliminate toxins is one of the key qualities and purposes of Hatha Yoga. Practicing asanas steadily and comfortably promotes this because it increases blood and lymph flow. Does this apply to a more dynamic and vigorous asana practice as well? To a certain extent, yes. This is because of the varied movements of your body.

However, as soon as a practice or exercise becomes strenuous, the production of lactic acid increases. As your body performs strenuous exercise, you begin to breathe more rapidly. This is because you are attempting to get more oxygen to your working muscles. Your body likes to get most of its energy from oxygen, but when the oxygen supply is too low to fuel what the muscles need, your body finds another way. It burns glucose, which produces lactic acid as a waste product. As the muscles continue to work, lactic acid accumulates. When your body cools down after practice or exercise, your lymphatic system has to work hard to carry away the lactic acid. After strenuous exercise your body might even feel stiff, swollen, and heavy because of the built-up load of lactic acid.

In Hatha Yoga, though, you avoid this build-up of lactic acid. After all, you perform asanas easily, so that your muscles get enough oxygen. For this reason, even when you work on challenging asanas, it is important to sequence the practice well. You need to make sure to include sufficient moments of relaxation. For example, when the heart rate becomes too high and you begin to breathe fast and perspire, it is time for a relaxing asana. This will normalize the heart rate, allow your breath to calm down, and minimize the formation of lactic acid.

Hatha Yoga and the Respiratory System – Oxygenation

Proper oxygenation of your cells is another important aspect of good health. Cells need oxygen to generate energy. To get enough oxygen to your cells, you must improve the blood's absorption of oxygen. Research has shown that deep breathing into the lower part of the lungs increases this oxygen absorption. This in turn is beneficial because, even with fewer inhalations per minute, the blood receives more oxygen. The blood then is able to better supply oxygen to all tissues of your body. A study on yoga practitioners showed that they adapted better to lower oxygen levels due to high altitude than did the control group, which did not practice yoga. The deep and conscious breathing that is typical in yoga seems to aid efficient ventilation: the amount of oxygen reaching the heart per minute.[11]

In daily life we often breathe too shallowly and therefore use only a small fraction of our lung capacity. After each normal exhalation, more than four times the amount of air we move with every inhalation and exhalation stays in the lungs. That stagnant air pooling at the bottom of the lungs dilutes and pollutes each fresh, oxygen-rich inhalation. You can easily imagine how this decreases the efficiency of each ventilation. Through deep, steady, and slow breathing during asana practice and breathing exercises, the old air pooling in the lungs is pushed out. This results in a more efficient blood oxygenation. This effect is more pronounced with breathing exercises where the emphasis is on exhalation, as with Anulom Vilom and Kapalbhati.

Another effect of slow and deep breathing is that the ratio between oxygen and carbon dioxide in the blood changes. By slowing down breathing, the relative level of carbon dioxide increases. Higher carbon dioxide levels in the blood dilate the blood vessels in the brain, leading to more generous blood flow. So the calm and comfortable practice of Hatha Yoga leads to an increased blood supply to the brain, which in turn allows the brain to absorb more oxygen.

Through increased respiration, the ratio of oxygen to carbon dioxide is changed in such a way that there is too little carbon dioxide in the blood. As a result, the small arteries and arterioles of the brain become constricted, which restricts its blood supply. At the same time, the red blood cells, responsible for transporting oxygen to all cells of your body, develop a greater affinity for oxygen. So heavy breathing not only causes blood vessels to constrict but also causes the red blood cells to become more reluctant to release oxygen to the cells. As a result, the brain receives less oxygen, even though the blood is oxygenated sufficiently.

So sometimes, vigorous exercise and breathing exercises without proper preparation can lead to a deprivation of oxygen in the brain, which can result in dizziness, light-headedness, panic attacks, and even fainting. We try to breathe even faster, increasing the carbon dioxide deficiency even more. This effect is commonly referred to as "hyperventilation." It can be helped by breathing into a plastic or paper bag, so that the carbon dioxide expelled with exhalation gets reabsorbed by the lungs and enters the blood to balance the levels of carbon dioxide and oxygen again.

If you incorrectly practice some yogic breathing exercises with active inhalation, rather than only active exhalation, you may trigger these same effects of hyperventilation. Kapalbhati (Skull-Shining Breath) is an example of this. If practiced incorrectly it becomes a different kind of pranayama, the so-called Bhastrika (Bellows Breath). Bhastrika is an advanced pranayama exercise, which is suitable only for experienced practitioners, and if practiced by beginners these same effects of hyperventilation may occur.

In Hatha Yoga, the lungs' capacity to absorb oxygen and the blood's capacity to distribute oxygen optimally improve. In conventional exercise or vigorous asana practice, even though the respiration rate increases, the oxygenation of the cells is less efficient, causing us to breathe even more rapidly in an attempt to provide enough oxygen.

The relation between inhalation and exhalation also has a direct effect on the autonomic nervous system. Whereas inhalation activates the sympathetic nervous system, exhalation activates the parasympathetic nervous system. Thus, breathing patterns and exercises that focus on exhalation and retention have the inherent quality of activating the parasympathetic nervous system. They therefore have a calming and rejuvenating effect on your body and mind.

When your body and mind are at ease, you breathe (one inhalation and exhalation) 13 to 15 times per minute. This means your body breathes around 22 thousand times per 24 hours. Whenever your respiration increases due to physical or mental stimulation, the flow of blood and other vital fluids increases as well. This in turn increases neuromotor activity, and neuromotor activity causes your body to utilize more energy. Subsequently, you need to absorb more glucose through food. These demands on your body do not affect your body as you grow up. After reaching maturity, however, they manifest as wear and tear. As this wear and tear continues, repair mechanisms and energy levels slow down. This results in stress and strain on your body.

According to the ancient Tantric scriptures *Shiva Swarodaya* and *Gyan Swarodaya*, the human lifespan is measured not in years, but in number of breaths. At the rate of 15 breaths per minute, a human life is made up of 946,080,000 breaths—a full 120 years.[12] By slowing down our breathing and maintaining a normal breathing rate of no more than 15 breaths per minute, we can conserve energy, increase our vitality, and maybe even live longer.

Hatha Yoga and the Metabolism

One of the many myths about yoga is that it stimulates the metabolism and causes weight loss. Nowadays health is often measured and defined by the level of fitness, and fitness is measured as the ability of the heart to pump an increased amount of blood per beat. According to ancient Indian sciences such as Ayurveda and Hatha Yoga, though, health is the balance of all bodily systems.

The purpose of asanas, then, is not to increase cardio fitness levels or metabolism. In fact, the intention and the effect of Hatha Yoga prove to be the exact opposite. In 2006, a study in Bangalore[13] showed that regular Hatha Yoga practice reduces the basal metabolic rate. This is the minimum number of calories your body burns, whether at rest, working out, or lying down. This metabolic rate differs from person to person, and these calories are the absolute minimum amount of energy that your body needs to stay alive and to execute all involuntary activities such as digestion, respiration, circulation, waste removal, and temperature regulation.

A team of scientists studied more than 100 men and women. They prescribed a diverse Hatha Yoga routine. The men and women—their average age 33 years—followed the prescribed routine for at least six months. The team reported that a regular yoga practice cut the basal metabolic rate by an average of 13 percent. The results were even more pronounced when broken down by sex. On average, the men decreased their resting energy by 8 percent. The women showed reductions of 18 percent—more than double the metabolic declines of the males.

At first sight, this metabolic slowdown might seem like a negative effect. After all, a lower metabolic rate means burning fewer calories. Does this mean that by practicing asanas one will gain weight? That will depend on eating habits, physical activity, and lifestyle. If you look closely, you will observe that, in general, yoga practitioners are lean. Many of them practice only yoga. The secret of weight loss or maintaining an ideal weight has nothing to do with a fast metabolism, but with mind and psyche. The regular practice of asanas affects the mind and desires. These in turn help to curb overeating and stress-related eating.

Furthermore, slowing your metabolism through calorie restriction may possibly protect against cancer, cardiovascular disease, and diabetes. It might even help you live longer. How does calorie restriction prolong life? Some evidence suggests that your lifespan cannot be increased simply by preventing obesity and its consequences. Although preventing obesity by increasing physical activity does prevent premature death, it does not significantly extend lifespan. The possible increase in lifespan is believed to be a result of restricting calories.[14]

These positive effects seem intimately tied to the metabolic slowdown that occurs over time when you restrict your calories. Many animal studies show that calorie restriction can extend lifespan. Systematic reviews and studies involving human subjects also suggest that calorie restriction, and moderate physical activity, may dramatically slow down the aging process. Eating less glucose makes your cells function in ways that support health and longer life.[15]

In summary, recent studies suggest that lowering your metabolic rate, if combined with calorie restriction, leads to longer life. Thus, combining Hatha Yoga, which has been shown to decrease the metabolism, and a calorie-restricted diet seems to be a formula for better health and longer life.

Do conventional physical exercise and vigorous asana practice support this process as well? Your body needs glucose for normal functioning, and when you exercise you need more glucose. You get glucose mainly from your diet. The more vigorous the exercise, the more food you need to intake. Thus, contrary to Hatha Yoga, strenuous physical exercise or vigorous asana practices increase dietary needs and the metabolism.

Hatha Yoga and the Spine and Joints

Yoga keeps your spine young. And you are only as young as your spine is flexible. These are common statements in the yoga world. They are supported by science. According to medical studies, yoga can slow down the deterioration of spinal discs. Physicians in Taiwan[16] reported on a study of 36 subjects. Half of the participants had taught Hatha Yoga for at least a decade. The other half were in good health. The two groups were of the same sex and similar in age. The physicians scanned all their spines and carefully inspected the discs for signs of damage. The results showed that the yoga teachers had significantly less degenerated discs than did the control group.

The intervertebral disc consists of an outer ring made up primarily of type 1 collagen and fibrocyte/fibroblast-like cells. This composition gives the disc the ability to resist tensile forces. The inner core, because of its composition, increases the disc's stiffness. This provides resistance to compression. As you age, though, the disc becomes more fibrous and disorganized and starts to wear out and become thinner. You can no longer see the difference between the disc's outer ring and its inner core.

Now, the intervertebral disc is poor in blood vessels. It gets indirect nutrients from two places: through diffusion from the bone marrow across the cartilaginous endplate, and through the outer ring, from the surrounding blood vessels. Scientists speculate that the various positions held by your spine during yoga practice delay disc degeneration by increasing the ability of nutrients to diffuse into the disc. It is also possible that the tension and compression of the disc during yoga exercises stimulate the growth and prevent the aging of discs. The difference in total disc scores between the yoga practitioners and the control group in the above-mentioned pilot study clearly shows that the long-term practice of yoga means fewer age-related changes in the intervertebral discs.

In addition to increasing the density and health of intervertebral discs, Hatha Yoga also greatly increases body awareness and improves posture. This has long-lasting effects on joint flexibility and health. Practicing asanas can prevent arthritis, which is the wear and tear of joints in the back, neck, hips, fingers, or knees. In a healthy joint, a well-lubricated lining of cartilage covers the ends of bones. This cartilage gets worn down most commonly by sports injuries, poor body posture, or dysfunctional movement patterns. Yoga asanas bring awareness to formerly unconscious postural habits. This new awareness provides the whole body with an entirely new range of movements. This in turn prevents joints from stiffening. By gentle and controlled movement, lubricating synovial fluid is distributed over the surface of the cartilage that covers the bones, keeping the cartilage well lubricated and healthy.

Hatha Yoga's varied movements keep your spine and joints well lubricated. As a result, you remain younger, stronger, and more flexible. In conventional exercise, the variety of movements is less, and more often than not these movements are neither gentle nor very controlled. Therefore the joints experience wear and tear, and the aging process of your spine is not slowed down. Dynamic and vigorous asana practices are in this case better for your joints and spine than conventional exercise. They provide a large and varied range of motions for your spine and joints. Further, these motions are generally done in a controlled manner.

Chapter 5

Hatha Yoga and Internal Organs & Glands

The effects of Hatha Yoga on the autonomic nervous system, blood circulation, blood pressure, oxygen levels, metabolism, and toxin elimination have been explained. One thing, though, is missing in most of the scientific studies about yoga: an explanation of how and why these positive results are achieved.

To keep the body in a state of holistic health, the ancient yogis believed that they needed to stimulate and balance the functions of the internal organs and specifically the endocrine glands. They did so with the practice of yoga asanas designed to directly influence the endocrine system. In the last few decades, this objective has not been given wide attention in the growing yoga community. But in recent years the claim that asanas can affect and stimulate the internal physical body has begun to be a subject for much research, which seeks a medical explanation for these effects.

In a study conducted at the Medical College of Trivandrum in Kerala, researchers concluded that the practice of yoga asanas, breathing exercises, and meditation leads to a decrease in total cholesterol levels in diabetes 2 patients. One way to explain these results is the activation of the parasympathetic nervous system. This, however, might not be the only explanation. The Kerala study states that "the dynamic stretching of the body during yoga asanas is postulated to rejuvenate pancreatic cells, increase insulin secretion and hence correct the impaired insulin secretion in chronic diabetes."[17]

A similar study conducted in Malaga, on the relation between Hatha Yoga, sleep quality, and hormonal modulation, states that, "the impact of a long-term yoga practice on specific endocrine and sleep quality parameters suggests a significant psychobiological modulation in long-term yoga practitioners, which may have interesting endocrine and clinical implications."[18]

These statements support the ancient belief that asanas have a direct and pronounced effect on the endocrine system and internal organs, therefore helping support your body's homeostasis. As mentioned above, there is no agreement yet on how the practice of steady asanas might in fact influence the endocrine system and internal organs. There are, however, three theories: the squeeze-and-release-effect theory, the sensory-triggers-to-the-brain theory, and the fascial-stimulation theory. All three theories demonstrate how a physical yoga asana practice based on classical principles can impact the health of your entire body, from the inside out.

The Squeeze-and-Release Effect

This first theory revolves around increased blood circulation. As your nervous system shifts into its parasympathetic mode while steadily and comfortably holding an asana, blood circulation to the internal organs and glands increases. The squeeze-and-release effect, however, intensifies the circulation to specific parts of your body. This effect can be explained by a simple example. Try squeezing your hand tightly for 20 seconds. As blood is pushed out, your hand becomes pale. As you release your grip, freshly oxygenated blood rushes into your hand through the arteries.

A similar effect takes place in all asanas. While holding a pose, certain regions are compressed. Blood drains out. When the pose is released, the body automatically sends an increased quantity of fresh blood (rich in oxygen and nutrients) to the formerly compressed regions. This effect works best with glands such as the thyroid, or organs such as the pancreas.

Other glands—such as the pineal, pituitary, and thymus glands—are not so exposed. Instead, they are protected in bony cavities. Even so, these glands can still experience the squeeze-and-release effect. This is because of increased pressure in your head (resulting from an increase in blood flow to the brain). By performing Headstand, the fluids within your skull become slightly compressed: intracranial pressure increases. This leads to a gentle squeeze and release once you come out of the pose. Headstand is considered beneficial for the functioning of your three master glands: the hypothalamus, the pituitary, and the pineal gland.

To summarize, this first theory explains the possible link between asanas and the endocrine system: asanas increase specific blood circulation in your body. Therefore, everything that organs or glands need from the blood (oxygen, glucose, hormones, and so on) will be more available and help to improve their overall function.

Like the monks in ancient India who spent hours seated in meditation every day, many of us lead sedentary lives. We spend much of the day seated in a car, at a desk, or involved in repetitious movement. Through increased vascular circulation triggered by the squeeze-and-release-effect, though, hormones reach their target organs or glands more quickly. This results in the activation of physiological processes that fine tune your body's homeostasis.

Sensory Triggers to the Brain

The second theory of how a yoga asana practice can impact the endocrine system and internal organs is based on triggers caused by the body's position. It is based on the observation that during asana practice, your body often assumes extreme positions that differ greatly from your daily postures of walking, sitting, and lying down. These positions trigger a nervous reaction in parts of the body that in daily life are mostly neglected. As a result, your body's own regulatory functions are stimulated.

To ensure homeostasis, your body constantly works to negotiate and balance external and internal disturbances. After all, these continuously threaten internal stability. In order to accomplish this self-regulation a communication control system is required. The basic type of such a control system is the feedback loop.

When your body receives a stimulus, such as pressure on the throat region during Shoulderstand, this feedback loop is activated. There are receptors everywhere in your body that monitor the environment and detect various changes, so-called stimuli. This is also the case in the throat region and in the thyroid gland, which is situated there. Information about the stimuli travels along the nervous pathway to the spinal cord or brain (depending on the location and nature of the stimuli). The responsible control center determines the appropriate response and course of action. In many cases this is the hypothalamus, which is situated in the brain.

So, the second theory is based on your body's finely tuned self-regulatory and healing system. By stimulating local nerves, this system becomes activated. The effect of these stimuli can be any endocrine or nervous reaction produced in order to maintain homeostasis in the location of the perceived trigger.

Fascial Stimulation

Fascia is the biological fabric that holds your body together, your body's own glue. It is the connective tissue that holds and at the same time separates bodily structures. It is found in individual muscle cells; in between bundles of muscle fibers; around our organs; and in our joints, ligaments, and tendons. Traditional Western medicine has ignored fascia until recently. Instead of understanding the intricate connection between all bodily tissues, it split the body into as many discernible single parts as possible. But fascia is one network in every sense. All these different names we give to elements within it—this tendon, that muscle, this organ, or that ligament—tend to hide the fact that your body is one unit. Every "part" is intricately linked by the connective tissue and fascia. Likewise, all your body's organs and all the viscera are suspended within this connected system.

The third explanation of Hatha Yoga's effect on our internal organs and glands finds a close relationship with an osteopathic technique called visceral manipulation. It was developed by French osteopath and physiotherapist Jean-Pierre Barral. Its basic principle is that everything in life moves, and that movement is life. The internal organs (viscera), muscles, ligaments, fascia, and blood vessels all move continuously. Every organ has its own intrinsic motion in three dimensions. And all the tissues need to be able to respond to movements around them. The tissues and organs need to be able to slide against and glide over each other. So your body needs to move in order to live. Any restrictions to your body's capacity to move will affect its health.

Habits of movement and posture, emotions and stress, trauma and injury, affect certain parts and structures of your body. Like the fly that lands on the spider's web and creates a vibration (a reaction) that the spider can feel at the other end of the web, every restriction and tension in one part of your body will have an effect within the web of fascia.

A full 90 percent of all musculoskeletal problems have a connection to the viscera. Over time, structural issues within your muscular system will start to influence the organs. Tightness and immobility start to develop within the fascia surrounding an organ and will impair its function, and vice versa. Compromised organs will cause reactions and changes in the musculoskeletal system. By applying gentle manipulations, the osteopath finds and releases tension and restriction to movement and allows the organs to move and work properly again.

A Hatha Yoga practice may have a similar effect on the viscera to that of the gentle palpations and manipulations during visceral manipulation. When you practice asanas, there is a lot of movement, compression, extension, and rotation in your trunk. By bringing movement to the fascia in the trunk you remove restriction and activate your body's self-correcting and self-regulatory system. By using movement to activate and release the fascia, you stimulate the internal organs and glands and improve their function.

Chapter 6

Hatha Yoga and the Seven Chakras

According to yogic philosophy, human beings have three bodies. All of them are interconnected via the vital life energy: prana. The three bodies are the physical body, the energetic or so-called astral body, and the spiritual body (or soul). The physical body in its entirety is connected to the energetic body, and furthermore every body part individually is associated and connected with an astral counterpart.

As we know, asanas work on the physical body in various ways. They ensure and enhance homeostasis. They do so by bringing your body into a parasympathetic state. Further, the practice of asanas exerts an immediate effect on internal glands and organs, increasing and balancing their functions. Also, asanas influence and stimulate the astral body.

An important aspect of the astral body is the chakra system of energy centers. In yoga, we focus on the seven major chakras. These exist along the line of your spine. Each one connects to its specific glands or organs of the physical body, as well as areas of the mind that influence personality. According to yogic scriptures, health and well-being blossom when energy flows in a balanced way through each of the seven major chakras. The astral body also includes about 72 thousand astral energy nerves: nadis. The three main nadis—the Sushumna Nadi, the Ida Nadi, and the Pingala Nadi—coincide with the spinal column.

The astral body is intricately connected and intertwined with the physical body. Every physical action has an influence on the astral body and therefore on the chakras. Some influences are more direct and pronounced. Others are subtle and materialize over time. The astral and physical bodies are in a constant state of connection and exchange. The energies of the astral body and the physical body influence each other and their processes. So a malfunctioning gland or organ has an effect on the rest of the physical body as well as on the corresponding chakra.

In the physical body, blood flows through veins, capillaries, and arteries. In the energy body, prana flows through the nadis, which are energy pathways. There are many ways we absorb this prana: breathing is one of them. So when we breathe in, we inhale prana. When we expand the breath and improve the quality of it, we are expanding and improving the quality of this vital life force within and around us. Yoga asanas and breathing exercises improve and expand the flow of prana through the chakras. When all chakras are in balance, then the astral and physical bodies are in a state of holistic health and equilibrium.

When prana is prevented from flowing naturally, either becoming blocked or overactive at a certain point, it can create disharmony on both physical and emotional levels. Yoga postures, when performed according to Hatha Yoga principles, stimulate specific chakras. For example, Bridge Pose and Shoulderstand stimulate the energy at the throat chakra. This in turn activates and stimulates physical and subtle responses. Subtle energetic qualities of the Vishuddha Chakra (the throat chakra) govern your ability to speak, listen, and express yourself as a higher form of communication. They govern creativity, faith, and a feeling of freedom and liberation.

Some of the physical responses of Hatha Yoga we discussed in a previous chapter can be explained from a scientific viewpoint. Other effects, however, are more subtle. For example, by practicing Kakasana, Crow Pose, we stimulate the Svadhishthana Chakra. There is no immediate physical pressure on the organs and glands (kidneys and gonads) related to this chakra. Yet, through the stimulation of the chakra, the physical counterparts are stimulated and balanced as well.

Your body is a single system, interconnected so complexly that it is difficult, even impossible, to fully appreciate. So whatever you do, whichever asana you practice, your whole body is involved. Therefore the entire body also reacts. Yet each of the main internal organs in the trunk as well as glands in the physical body can be linked to one of the seven main chakras. And each asana balances the function of its corresponding chakra, organ, and gland, and of the whole body.

The Seven Chakras and Their Physical and Mental Properties

Sahasrara means "thousand." The Sahasrara Chakra resembles a lotus with a thousand petals located at the crown of your head. This chakra is referred to as the Crown Chakra and is considered to be the center of spirituality, awareness, and enlightenment. It allows for the inward flow of wisdom and brings the gift of cosmic consciousness. This is also the center of connection with supreme consciousness.

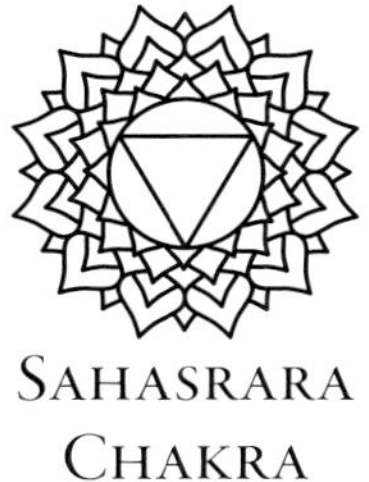

Sahasrara Chakra

Ajna means "foremost," and the sixth chakra, the Ajna Chakra (pronounced "Agya") is located about 4 inches behind the eyes, at the center of your head. It is also known as the Third-Eye Chakra. This is the center of perception. Your capability to perceive and understand are dependent on the condition of this chakra.

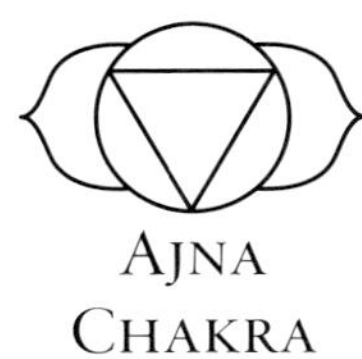

Ajna Chakra

In the physical body, the Sahasrara and Ajna Chakras correspond with the hypothalamus, the pituitary gland, and the pineal gland, located in the brain, as well as the eyes, ears, and the nose.

Vishuddha means "especially pure," and the fifth chakra, the Vishuddha Chakra, is located at the base of the throat. It is the center of communication, sound, and the expression of creativity via thought, speech, and writing. The possibility for change, transformation, and healing are located here. It is associated with the element akasha, or ether, and the sense of hearing, as well as the action of speaking. Because of its physical location, it is also called the Throat Chakra.

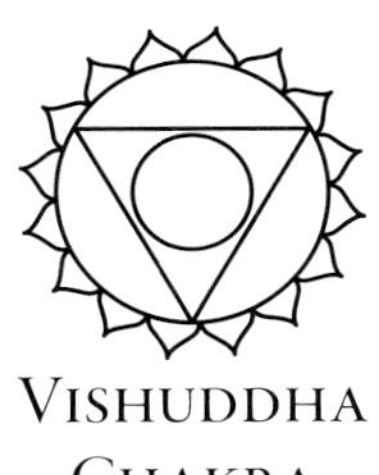

Vishuddha Chakra

The Vishuddha Chakra is connected to the thyroid and parathyroid glands, as well as the larynx and tongue in the physical body.

Anahata means "unstruck" or "unhurt" and refers to non-attachment. The Anahata Chakra is located in the center of the chest, near the heart. It is associated with the element air. The Anahata Chakra is also associated with love and compassion and is therefore often referred to as the Heart Chakra.

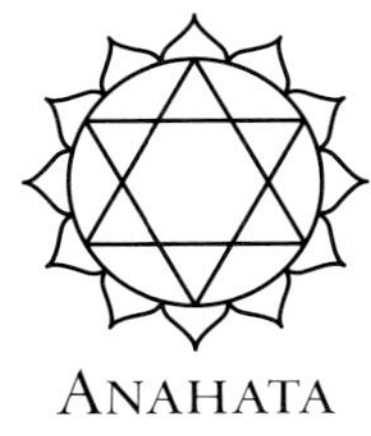

Anahata Chakra

The Anahata Chakra is connected to the heart, the lungs, and the thymus gland in the physical body.

Manipura literally translates as "place of shining gem" and is the name of the third chakra, the Manipura Chakra, located at the solar plexus (between the belly button and bottom of the rib cage). The Manipura Chakra is related to the fire element in your body. Ego, energy, will power, aggression, and intellect are the qualities of this chakra, which often is referred to as the Solar Plexus Chakra.

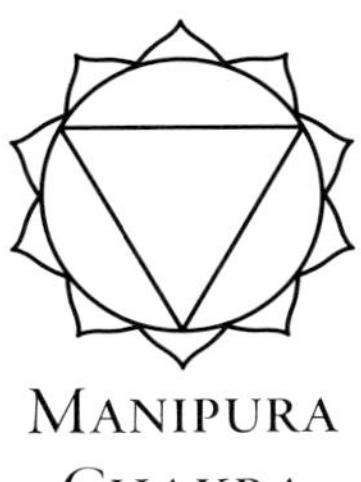

Manipura Chakra

The Manipura Chakra is connected to the stomach, gallbladder, liver, spleen, and pancreas in the physical body.

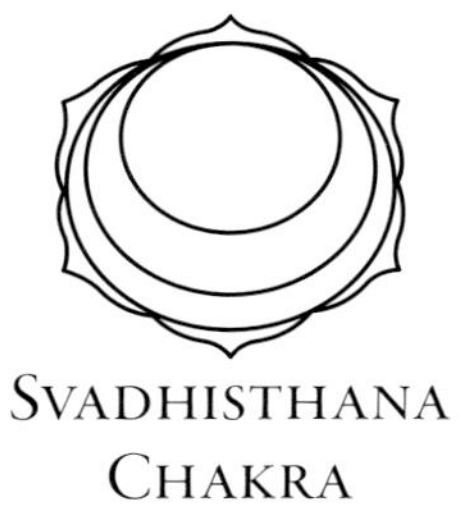

Svadhisthana Chakra

Svadhishthana means "dwelling place of the Self" and is the name of the second chakra, the Svadhishthana Chakra, located at the lower abdomen, four finger breadths below the belly button. This chakra is also known as the Sacral Chakra and governs sexuality, desires, and pleasures. It is associated with the element of water and the act of procreation.

The Svadhishthana Chakra is connected to the urinary tract, kidneys, and gonads (ovaries, testes) in the physical body.

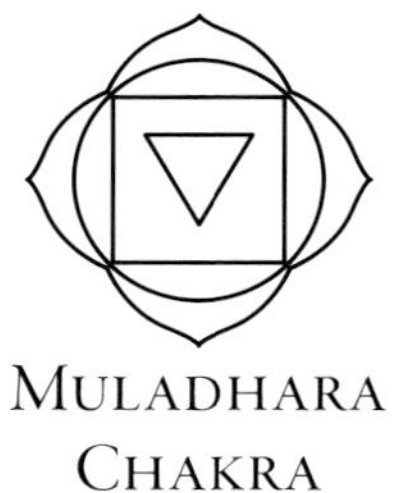

Muladhara Chakra

Muladhara means "root support," and the first chakra, the Muladhara Chakra, is located at the base of your spine, between the perineum and the coccyx. Muladhara is considered the foundation of the energy body and is also referred to as the Root Chakra. Kundalini awakening begins here, because it is the base from where the three main nadis—Ida, Pingala, and Sushumna—emerge. It is the most instinctual of all chakras. It governs instinct, safety, survival, and grounding. It is associated with the element of earth and the action of excretion.

The Muladhara Chakra is connected to the large intestines and adrenals in the physical body.

Mostly, the physical location of an organ or gland corresponds with the location of its corresponding chakra in the astral body. There are some exceptions, however. The adrenals, for example, correspond with the Muladhara Chakra, even though their physical location would suggest the Svadhishthana Chakra. This has to do with the functions of the adrenals. The adrenal glands are in charge of survival. The Muladhara Chakra is the primary chakra: the chakra of instinct, survival, and stability. The sexual glands (gonads and ovaries), however, are associated with creation and creativity, which link to the Svadhishthana Chakra. The truth is that we can survive without our sexual glands, but we cannot live without our adrenal glands.

So, the location of an internal organ or gland is not sufficient to determine its corresponding chakra. Another factor we have to look at is its element. So even though the stomach and the kidneys are more or less at the same level in your body, the stomach is related to the Manipura Chakra, while the kidneys, because of their functions involving the water element, are related to the Svadhishthana Chakra.

The Seven Chakras and Their Corresponding Asanas

Chakra	**Sahasrara**	**Ajna**	**Vishuddha**	**Anahata**	**Manipura**	**Svadhishthana**	**Muladhara**
Location	Crown	Third eye	Base of throat	Center of chest	Solar plexus	Lower abdomen	Perineum
Element		Gross energy & matter	Space	Air	Fire	Water	Earth
Associated activities & emotions	Intelligence Intuition Perception Devotion Awareness		Communication Expression Inspiration	Attachment Emotions Compassion	Energy Ego Aggression	Creativity Sexuality Desires	Survival Primal instincts Stability
Associated organs	Brain Eyes Nose Ears		Tongue Larynx Lymph nodes	Lungs Heart	Stomach Gallbladder Spleen Liver Small intestines	Urinary tract Kidneys	Large intestines Prostate
Associated glands	Hypothalamus Pituitary gland Pineal gland		Thyroid Parathyroid	Thymus	Pancreas	Gonads (ovaries/testes)	Adrenals
Asanas of the Basic Sequence	Shirshasana		Sarvangasana Halasana	Ardha Setu Bandhasana (Pawanmuktasana) Matsyasana Sukha Gomukhasana	Paschimottanasana Purvottanasana Bhujangasana Shalabhasana Dhanurasana Ardha Matsyendrasana	Sukha Kakasana Trikonasana	Vrkshasana Tadasana

Part III

Practicing Effectively: Guidelines for a Holistic Hatha Yoga Practice

Chapter 7

The Importance of Preparation

If you want to build a house that lasts for a lifetime, you first need to pour a strong foundation. The most beautiful and artfully crafted castle cannot last on a foundation of sand. Likewise, a yoga asana practice needs a strong foundation. This foundation ensures benefits that exceed mere physical toning and bring you into realms of true holistic well-being. The benefits of a practice built on a foundation of principles and discipline are many. This is true on the physical, mental, and spiritual levels. A holistic asana practice is a balanced practice because it creates harmony between the physical, mental, and energy bodies. A balanced practice should always comprise several key elements, and benefits greatly from a conducive setting.

Establishing a Conducive Environment

Setting the environment

A favorable environment plays an important role. A calm, undisturbed environment deepens the effect of asanas, pranayama, and meditation.

- **Time:** Traditionally asanas were practiced either at dawn (brahmamuhurta) or at dusk (sandhya), when the rhythms of life are calm and gentle and temperatures are mild. Though dawn and dusk are ideal, one can practice whenever when one is not tired or sleepy, as long as it is not within 2 hours after a main meal.

- **Space:** The space used for asana practice is also of great importance. You should practice in an open, distraction-free, uncluttered space. There should be enough space around the mat and above your head. The space should be well lit and well ventilated.

- **Temperature:** Temperature affects your body as well as the mind. If it is too cold, the muscles do not become warmed up properly. They may contract and refuse to relax, and the mind might become dull and lazy. Pushing your body in this condition greatly increases the chances of injury or overload. Conversely, too much heat loosens up the muscles, and your body easily tends to push beyond its limits and to overstretch. The nervous system shifts into sympathetic mode as the heart beat increases. Ideally the temperature of the room should be mild—neither too hot nor too cold. You should feel comfortable wearing a t-shirt, without requiring a fan or a sweater. This ensures a proper temperature for the nervous system to relax into the rest-and-regenerate mode.
- **Clothing:** Traditionally asanas have been practiced wearing only a kaupinam, a rectangular strip of linen or cotton tied around the hips and genitals. Ideally one should wear clothes made of natural fabrics, to let the skin breathe and perspire freely. Most important is that you feel comfortable and relaxed in whichever attire you choose and that you do not pick clothes to impress or to try to fit in. The practice of asanas should be a practice with mindful attention and love toward yourself. Being too focused on how you look will keep your practice in the realms of the mundane and superficial, rather than leading you toward inner peace and self-acceptance.

Physical state

Asanas should not be practiced while you are sick or suffering acutely from severe disease or while you are fatigued. Practicing asanas with fatigue can lead to misuse of muscles and to injury. An adapted, gentle form of asanas can be, however, truly beneficial if you are recovering or suffering from chronic diseases or fatigue. Asanas should be practiced only after emptying the bowels and on an empty stomach. If the bowels are carrying feces, then asana practice may toxify your body due to "over-cooking" the feces. Traditionally, bowel-cleansing techniques such as basti or enema are performed before asana practice.

Mental state

According to Maharishi Patanjali, asanas should be performed with the mind free from desire, anxiety, anger, or fear. Practicing asanas when the mind is unstable, worried, anxious, or upset may cause injury or increase agitation. For a fruitful practice, you should train your mind to let go of any emotions and thoughts as you step onto your mat. Bring the awareness to your body and breath and postpone any thoughts to after your practice. By the end of the practice some of the negative emotions might have lifted already. You might have a new perspective on the same situation, without having spent your mental energy worrying or bickering. Keeping your mind set tightly on the goal of the practice will help to keep your mind stable. It is important, however, that the goal should be free from competition, seeking approval, or display.

Bend But Do Not Break — Avoiding Injuries

Contrary to the common belief that yoga is safe, many injuries can occur during asana classes or practices. Sometimes injuries happen due to improper guidance. At other times they may be due to the mistakes of the practitioner. It is exciting for teachers and students to see results and development. It is of paramount importance, though, to remember that our practice will enrich us holistically only if we refrain from putting our ego into the equation. As soon as the ego is there, measuring our yoga and our students' yoga by certain predefined parameters, our chance of actually doing more harm than benefit increases tremendously. This does not mean that we should always remain within our comfort zone, that we should not try to grow within our practice. It means that it should be done understanding the following six principles. These six principles, kept in mind at all times, provide a foundation for safe, healthy, and rewarding asana practice.

No two people are alike – The principle of individual differences

Everyone evolves according to his or her own nature. Because each body and mind is unique, each person's natural physical and mental response to yoga practice is different. It is natural that your motivation, coordination, endurance level, physical state, mental state, and body type will influence your yoga practice. No two people will display exactly the same alignment in an asana. Each will assume the unique alignment that is natural for him or her. The natural duration of the hold will also vary from person to person. Thus, there is no single ideal alignment or duration of an asana that will be natural and most beneficial to everyone.

Expand your comfort zone – The principle of overload and the principle of progression

The physical condition of your body improves with optimal overload. Therefore you need to apply a greater than normal stress to the body in order to improve. This overload can be applied through increasing the duration of the pose or increasing the complexity of the asana. For example, if you have been holding Shoulderstand for 30 seconds for 2 months without increasing the duration or complexity, your body will become accustomed to the posture and the effect on the body will start to decrease.

On the other hand, if the overload is increased too much or too quickly, there is a greater chance for injury and a reduced chance of improvement. There is an optimal and unique level of overload for each person. You must therefore apply overload carefully and progressively. If you do not follow this principle, the possibility of overtraining and subsequent injury is high. You must decide on the progression of overload according to your physical condition, endurance, frequency, and motivation. Overload is effective only when your body experiences a challenge but still retains the ability to perform the movements with control and without any errors.

It does not get easier, you just get better – The principle of adaptation and the principle of use/disuse

Your body adapts to the increased time or complexity of an asana in a predictable physiological manner. By repeating the asana over and over again, your body adapts to the overload. As you become comfortable with your yoga practice, you will need to vary the program to stay aligned with the principle of overload. This way, you will continue to improve in strength, flexibility, balance, and stability. This principle also explains how by repetition even complex asanas will become easier as your body gradually adapts. This explains why, while learning Crow Pose, you may fall many times each day, and then suddenly be able to hold the pose effortlessly.

"Use it or lose it" is a common expression. It suggests that your body does not stay in one condition: it either improves or worsens. Whenever you abandon asana practice, any gains you have made in strength, flexibility, balance, and endurance will diminish. So you must adjust the overload according to your use and disuse of your body. So after having taken a break from regular practice, when you commence again, you will need to dial down the level a little, and then build up again.

The magic ingredient – The principle of rest

The effect of your practice takes place after your practice. Therefore rest is vital. Do not underestimate its importance. With rest you give your body a break and the chance to integrate, adapt, repair, and grow. Like your regular practice of any skill, your regular yoga asana practice trains your body to improve your performance and to increase the loading capacity of your body. With your regular Hatha Yoga practice your entire body grows stronger and more coordinated. When tissue rests after training, it repairs itself to be stronger than before. If you fail to rest enough, your tissues will weaken and injuries are likely to develop. How often your body needs to rest depends on your body type, health, and form of practice. So also the ideal amount of rest varies from person to person.

Chapter 8

The Five Fundamental Building Blocks

There are five important ingredients for a safe, fulfilling, and holistic asana practice according to the principles of Hatha Yoga. These five ingredients, or steps, are:

1. relaxation,
2. conscious breathing,
3. warming up properly,
4. true asana—finding steadiness and ease within the pose, and
5. proper sequencing of asanas.

Each practice or class starts with a short, initial relaxation. Lying down in Corpse Pose, focus on your breath and consciously relax each part of your body. Then, before starting any asanas, you first warm up your respiratory system and tune your mind and intention into the present moment. You can start the class or practice with two breathing exercises, Kapalbhati (for activating the sympathetic nervous system) and Anulom Vilom (for activating the parasympathetic nervous system). After warming up your respiratory system, proceed to warming up your spine, joints, and entire body. Only then begin your practice of asanas. An ideal warming-up exercise is the Sun Salutation.

Your practice of asanas that follows your warm-up aims for balance on two levels: a muscular level (by alternating forward and backward bends) and an internal level (by sequencing your asanas from the Crown Chakra on down). Your final period of relaxation after the practice gives your body and mind time to bathe in the effects of your practice and rejuvenate.

Step 1: Relaxation

No yoga practice is complete without sufficient relaxation. You should practice relaxation before beginning your session, while performing each asana, between asanas, and at the end of your session.

Relax before your practice: Your practice starts with initial relaxation. Lying down in Corpse Pose for 5 minutes prior to starting helps bring your focus to your body and breathing. It also regulates body temperature, blood pressure, and respiration rate. Further, it assists your body and mind to attune and prepare for the upcoming practice.

Relax throughout your practice: As stated in Patanjali's *Yoga Sutras*, a yoga posture should be steady and comfortable (*sthira sukham asanam*). Not only should your body be relaxed but your mind as well. Maintaining a relaxed state of mind allows your body to become more flexible, supple, and light. This helps you find and gradually expand your comfort zone and perform any asana with much more ease and control.

Relax in between each posture: Relaxation poses are practiced for 30 to 60 seconds in between sets of asanas. The main purpose of regular relaxation between poses is to prevent your body from jump-starting the sympathetic nervous system. Usually it is sufficient to fit in a relaxation pose after every two to four asanas. However, after a particularly challenging asana or exercises, extra relaxation moments are recommended.

Relax after your practice: A final relaxation at the end of your practice enables your body and mind to fully integrate the changes that have taken place during the practice. When tissues rest after training, they repair and heal and become stronger.

Relaxation Pose

Shavasana

Corpse Pose

Basic instructions

Lie on your back, with your legs straight and relaxed, feet mat-width apart, toes relaxed and dropped outwards.

Arms are apart at a 40-degree angle from your body, with palms facing upward.

Hands and fingers are relaxed.

Eyes are closed.

Your entire body is completely relaxed and heavy on the floor.

The mind is focused on breathing.

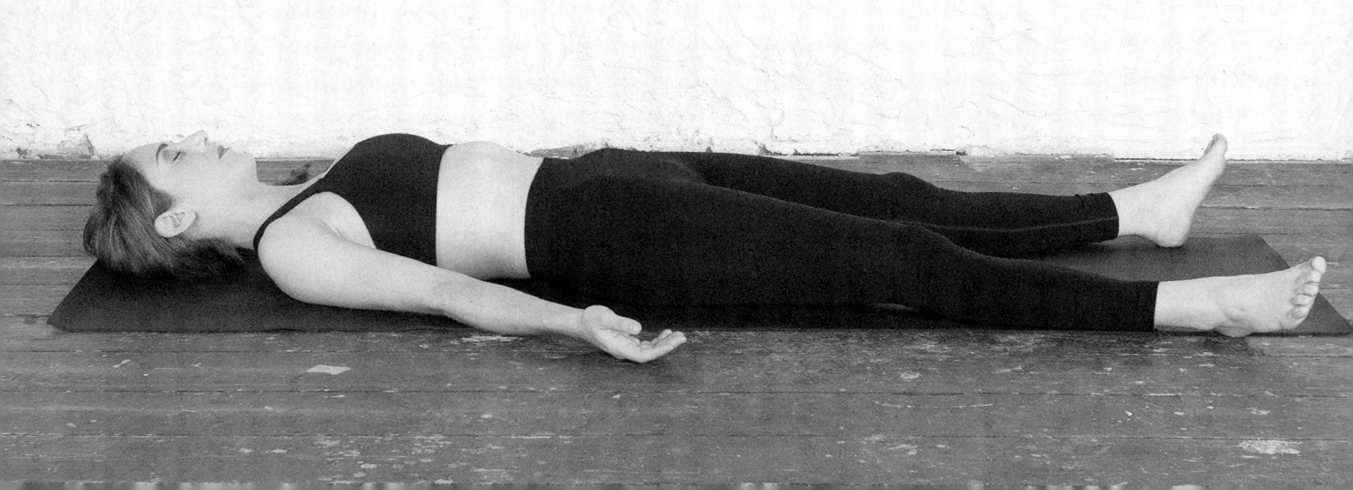

When to do

- for initial and final relaxation
- after breathing exercises
- after Sun Salutation
- in between or after supine asanas

Variation

Supta Baddha Konasana

Sleeping Bound Angle Pose

Lie on your back and bring the soles of your feet together, knees dropping toward the floor. Arms are apart at a 40-degree angle from your body, with palms facing upward. Hands and fingers are relaxed and eyes are closed. Take easy abdominal breaths, letting your body sink into the floor. (If you feel strain in your groin area or knees, you can place bolsters or cushions below your knees.)

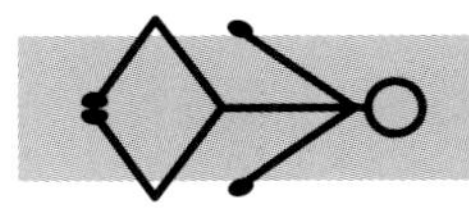

Relaxation Pose

Shashankasana (aka Balasana)

Child's Pose

Basic instructions

Sit on your knees, with your hips resting on your heels.

Bend forward and place your forehead on the floor, while keeping your hips on your heels. (If your hips are lifting off from the heels, separate your knees. If your hips are still not resting on your heels, make two fists and place them one atop the other, then rest your forehead on your topmost fist. You can also support your hips with a cushion.)

Your arms are resting on the floor, alongside your body.

Let your shoulders relax toward the floor.

Focus on easy, abdominal breathing.

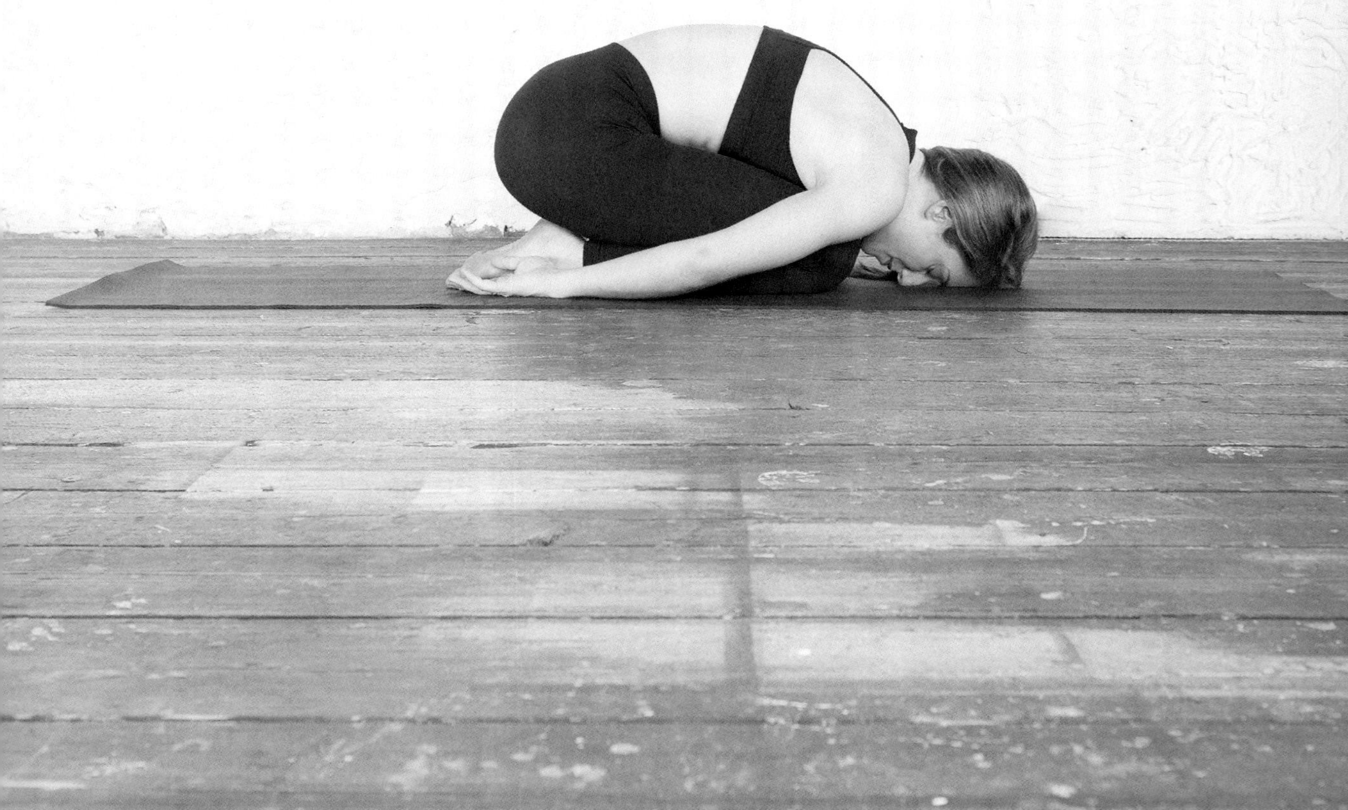

When to do

- before and after inversions
- in between seated asanas
- after extensive backbends
- in between hand balances

Contraindications & cautions

If you suffer from hypertension you are advised to avoid Child's Pose. In between seated asanas and after backbending you can do a seated variation of Child's Pose, where you sit on your buttocks and hug your knees to the chest, feet resting on the floor. Allow your spine to round and rest your forehead on the top of your knees.

If you have very low blood pressure you can do Child's Pose, but make sure to come up slowly to avoid becoming dizzy.

Variation

Khagasana

Hare Pose

Start seated on your knees, with your hips on your heels. Open your knees mat-width apart, keeping the big toes together. Walk your hands forward as you bend your torso forward. Keep your hips toward your heels and bring your forehead to the floor. For an extra stretch in your middle and upper back, you can also place your chin on the floor. Keep a gentle activation between your hands reaching forward and your hips sinking toward your heels, and breathe evenly.

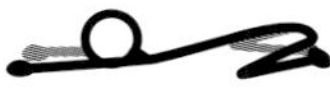

Relaxation Pose

Makarasana
Crocodile Pose

Basic instructions

Lie down on your stomach.

Make a cushion with your hands and place one cheek on top. (If your shoulder feels tight in this position, you can also keep your arms along your body, palms facing up and one cheek resting on the floor.)

Big toes of both feet are touching, heels are dropped outwards. Hips are relaxed.

Focus on breathing into your stomach and lower back.

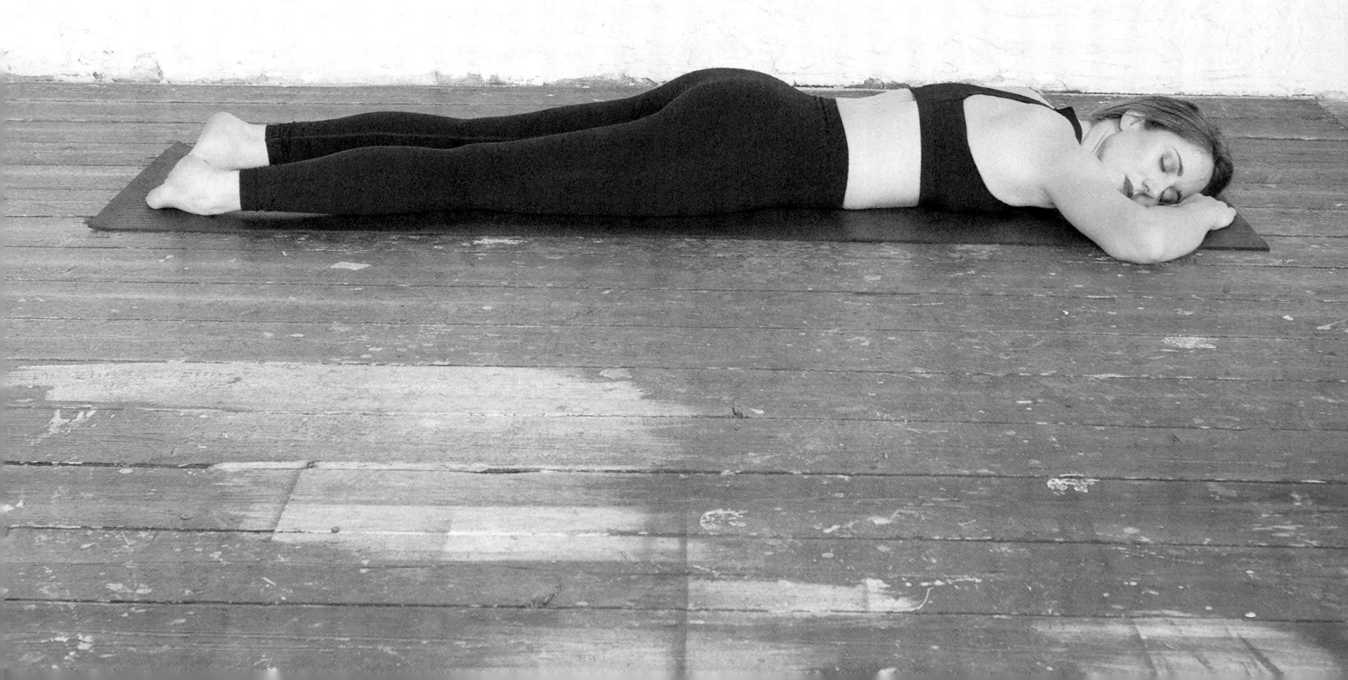

When to do

- in between prone backbending asanas
- during initial or final relaxation as an alternative to Corpse Pose

Variation

Sashtang Pranam Asana

Prone Prayer Pose

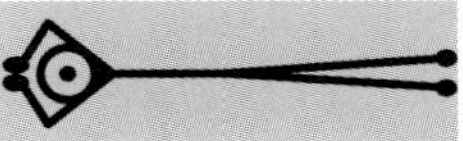

Lie down on your stomach, with your feet hip- or shoulder-width apart. Place your forehead on the floor and bring your hands in Prayer position above you on the floor. Close your eyes and breathe evenly.

Step 2: Conscious Breathing

Regular and conscious breathing is an important factor in the holistic practice of asanas. Breathing should be calm and effortless, which helps your body to stay in the parasympathetic zone. During the practice of asanas, the focus should be on diaphragmatic breathing, such as abdominal breath or full yogic breath. Starting the practice with some conscious breathing and breathing exercises helps to establish the mode of abdominal breathing and helps maintain that breathing pattern for the duration of the practice.

During most of the asanas and exercises in Hatha Yoga we maintain abdominal breathing. This is the most natural and effortless way of breathing. During some asanas in which the chest is expanded, such as Extended Cobra Pose, Cow Face Pose, or Camel Pose, to name a few, you can also practice full yogic breath, which is deep diaphragm breathing aiming to use the full lung capacity. Practicing full yogic breath in chest openers provides a gentle workout for the lungs while at the same time deepening the pose.

While you strive to hold the poses, you should avoid holding your breath. It is helpful to inhale with all the extensions and exhale with all the flexions. Breathing in with extensions helps stretch your intercostals and abdominal muscles while lengthening your body. Breathing out with flexions helps relax your intercostal muscles while engaging your core and abdomen and bending your body forward.

Before you start your asana practice, warm up your musculoskeletal system with Sun Salutations and some alternative exercises. But before that, warm up your respiratory system with two breathing exercises: Kapalbhati and Anulom Vilom.

Breathing Exercise

Kapalbhati

Skull-Shining Breath

In Sanskrit *kapal* means "skull" and *bhati* means "shining." Together they mean "shining skull." Kapalbhati is considered to be so cleansing to the entire system that, when practiced on a regular basis, the face shines with good health and radiance. In fact, traditionally Kapalbhati is one of the six internal cleansing exercises (shat kriyas) rather than a form of pranayama.

Even though it is traditionally classified as a cleansing exercise, Kapalbhati is an excellent breathing exercise to warm up the respiratory system and internally warm up your body in preparation for the following physical practice. It is an easier version of the pranayama Bhastrika and suitable for most levels of experience and fitness.

Basic instructions

Sit in a cross-legged position, with your spine straight and erect. Take an abdominal breath in to prepare for pumping.

Contract your abdominal muscles to forcefully exhale from the nose.

Relax your abdominal muscles naturally, for inhalation. Be cautious not to inhale actively, but instead release your abdomen and allow the air to be sucked in passively.

Repeat this for 3 sets, increasing pumping from 30 to 40 to 50 pumps per set.

In between sets, take a deep breath, and release, and then a gentle abdominal breath and retain the breath with increasing duration from round to round. So first 20, then 30, and in the last round 40 seconds. As you become more used to and skilled doing Kapalbhati, the pumping and the retentions can be gradually increased.

Benefits

Regular practice:

- cleanses the nasal passage, drains the sinuses, and eliminates accumulated mucus;
- greatly strengthens and increases the capacity of the lungs and intercostal muscles;
- removes bronchial congestion and spasm, while also helping to relieve asthma;
- removes stale gases and old oxygen in the lungs, due to the forced exhalation;
- massages the intestines, stomach, liver, spleen, heart, and pancreas through movement of the diaphragm and abdominal contractions;
- strengthens your abdominal muscles and improves digestion; and
- refreshes and invigorates your mind and increases alertness as a result of the increase of oxygen to your brain.

Contraindications & cautions

Kapalbhati should be avoided by those suffering from hypertension, anxiety, or panic attacks.

Breathing Exercise

Anulom Vilom

Alternate Nostril Breathing

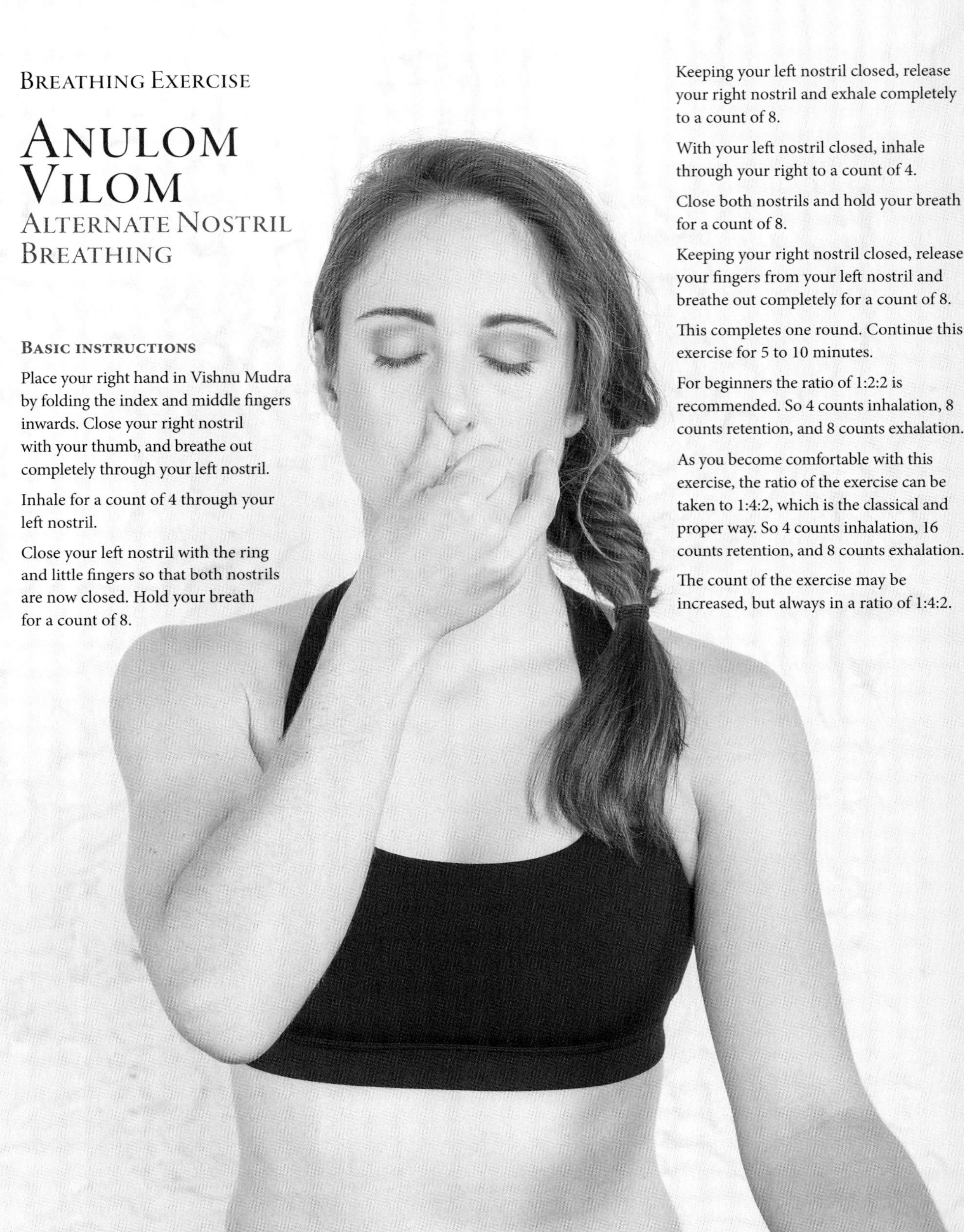

Basic instructions

Place your right hand in Vishnu Mudra by folding the index and middle fingers inwards. Close your right nostril with your thumb, and breathe out completely through your left nostril.

Inhale for a count of 4 through your left nostril.

Close your left nostril with the ring and little fingers so that both nostrils are now closed. Hold your breath for a count of 8.

Keeping your left nostril closed, release your right nostril and exhale completely to a count of 8.

With your left nostril closed, inhale through your right to a count of 4.

Close both nostrils and hold your breath for a count of 8.

Keeping your right nostril closed, release your fingers from your left nostril and breathe out completely for a count of 8.

This completes one round. Continue this exercise for 5 to 10 minutes.

For beginners the ratio of 1:2:2 is recommended. So 4 counts inhalation, 8 counts retention, and 8 counts exhalation.

As you become comfortable with this exercise, the ratio of the exercise can be taken to 1:4:2, which is the classical and proper way. So 4 counts inhalation, 16 counts retention, and 8 counts exhalation.

The count of the exercise may be increased, but always in a ratio of 1:4:2.

Benefits

Regular practice:

- cleanses and strengthens the entire respiratory system;
- expels more stale air and waste products from your lungs, because exhalation is twice the time of inhalation;
- decreases respiratory rate, prolongs exhalation, and thus leads to increased carbon dioxide levels in the blood, which in turn leads to improved oxygen absorption in the cells;
- helps to bring equilibrium between the solar and lunar energies in the body (The breath naturally alternates between the two nostrils, changing approximately every 2 hours. The breath in your right nostril is hot, symbolically referred to as the Sun or Pingala. It is catabolic and acceleratory to the organs of your body. The flow from your left, which is cool and referred to as the Moon or Ida, is anabolic and inhibitory to your body.);
- helps to balance the hemispheres of the brain;
- helps to calm the mind, making it lucid and steady, preparing it for meditation; and
- helps to purify the nadis, the energy paths in the astral body.

Contraindications & cautions

Anulom Vilom can be practiced by anyone and everyone, it is a truly beneficial breathing exercise. However, some should skip the retentions, and only alternate the breathing in and out. Skip the retentions if you are suffering from hypertension, anxiety, or panic attacks.

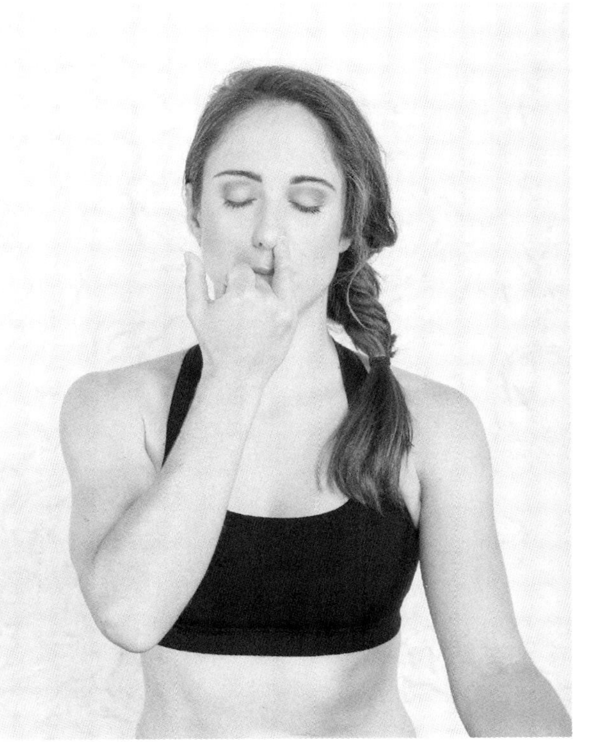

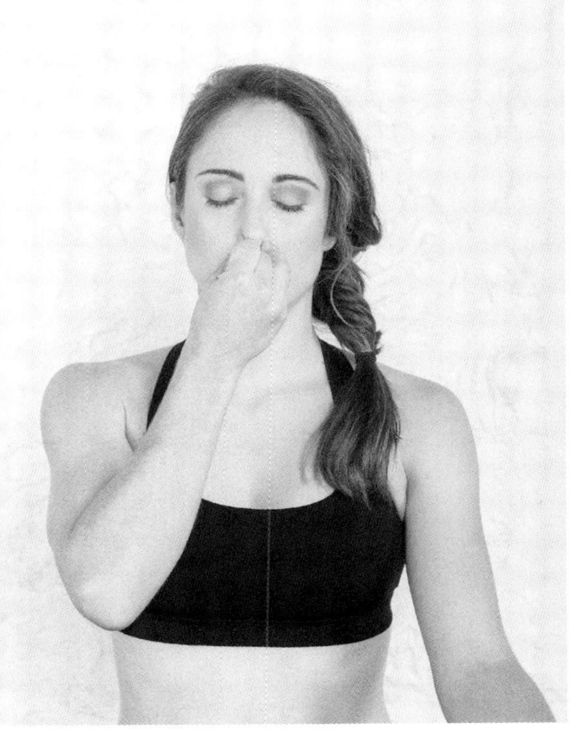

Step 3: Warming Up Properly

A proper warm-up is essential to prepare for asana practice and also to prevent injuries. Sun Salutations are a commonly practiced warm-up that primarily warms up the central nervous system and subsequently the major muscles and joints. The fluid and dynamic movements of the Sun Salutation, though, should not be confused with asana practice. Because the Sun Salutation is performed dynamically, it does not give the same benefits as steady asanas.

Traditionally, the Sun Salutation is performed with your back toward the rising sun, your spine and spinal cord warmed by the sun's heat. Each movement of the Sun Salutation proceeds in coordination with breathing: each motion connecting to an inhalation, an exhalation, or a retention. With a calm and contemplative mind, you should continue the Sun Salutation only until you begin to perspire. Engaging a vast variety of muscles and joints, warming up your spine and spinal cord, regulating the breath, and focusing the mind, doing the Sun Salutation is effective and should be repeated a minimum of six rounds.

A proper warm-up takes between 10 and 20 minutes. How long you need to warm up depends on various factors: the temperature of the room, your general physical condition, your previous activities (in the morning you need to warm up longer than in the evening after a day of activity), your age, and your injuries or health conditions. Generally speaking, the older you grow the longer you might need to warm up. So after Sun Salutations, other warming-up exercises such as leg raises (to activate the iliopsoas muscle) and dolphin (to strengthen the upper arms and back and practice the weight shift in preparation for inversions) can be added for variety.

It is important to remember that warming up always has to start with small, gentle movements. Initially, you should not even come close to the normal range of motion that you have when you are warmed up. Also remember that stretching with the goal of increasing your flexibility can be done safely only after you are completely warmed up. Only after several minutes, as you start to feel your body temperature rise, should you increase the speed and range of motion. In the course of the warm-up the intensity of the exercises has to go up. This can be achieved by increasing their speed, their range of motion, or their force.

SURYA NAMASKARA
CLASSICAL SUN SALUTATION

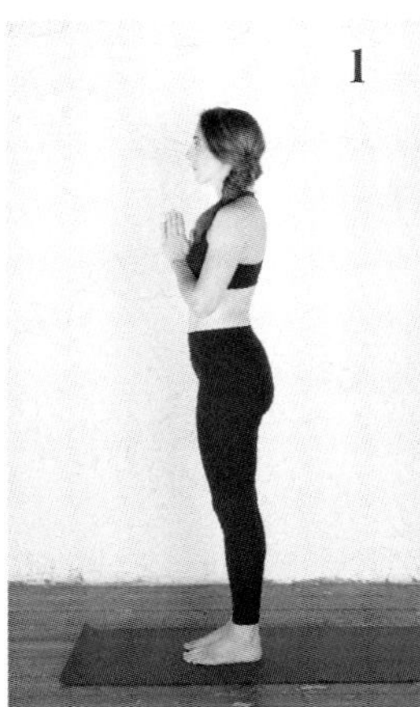

BASIC INSTRUCTIONS

Starting position: Stand straight, with spine erect and shoulders relaxed. Your feet are hip-width apart. Your knees are straight but not hyperextended; your arms are relaxed next to your body.

1. Breathe in and out, bringing your palms together in front of your chest.

Shoulders and elbows are relaxed.

Knees are straight but relaxed.

Back of your neck is long.

Reach up with the crown of your head toward the ceiling.

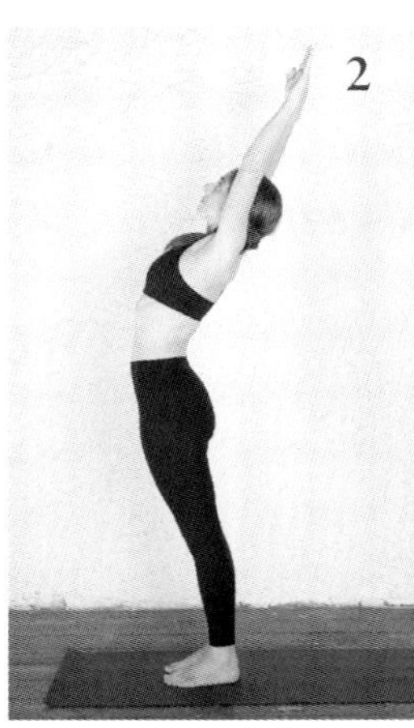

2. Breathe in and reach with your arms—up and backward.

Your arms are alongside your ears.

Look diagonally upward, do not drop your head back.

Knees are straight, hips pushing slightly forward.

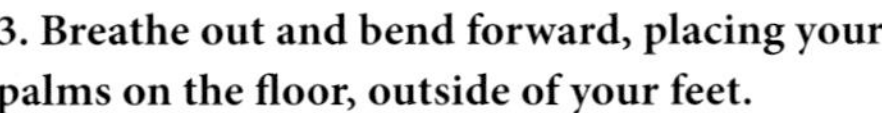

3. Breathe out and bend forward, placing your palms on the floor, outside of your feet.

If you cannot place your palms on the floor with your knees straight, you can bend your knees slightly.

Reach with your nose toward your knees.

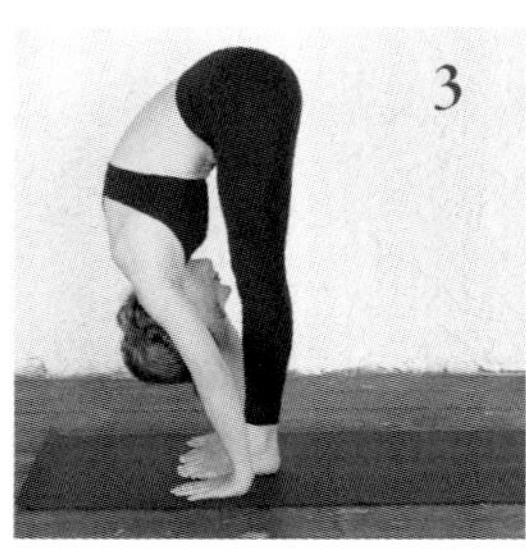

4. Keeping your hands there, inhale and bring your right leg back as far as possible.

Place your right knee on the floor, pointing your right foot.

Push your pelvis forward without losing the 90-degree angle of your left knee.

Open your chest, look diagonally upward while palms remain on the floor.

5. Hold the breath and bring your left leg back.

Your body is in a straight line from your head to your heels (push-up position).

6. Breathe out and drop your knees, chest, and forehead to the floor.

Without moving your body backward, bring your chest down to the floor between your hands. Then bring your forehead to the floor.

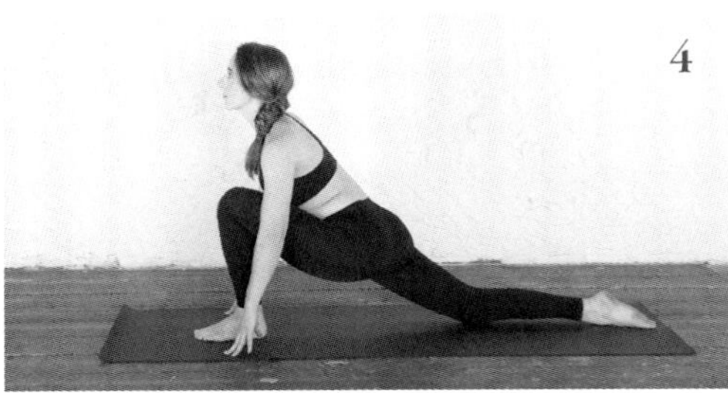

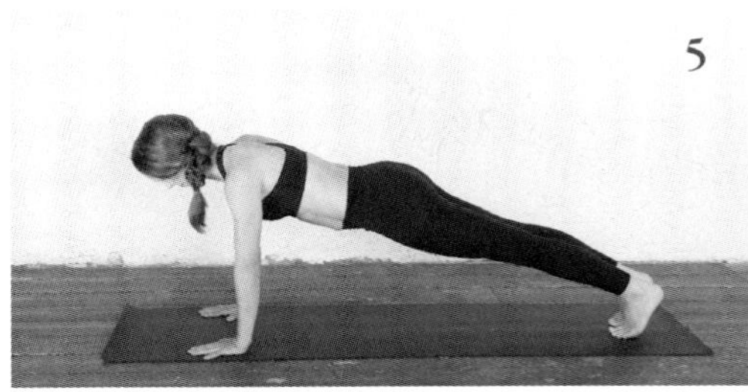

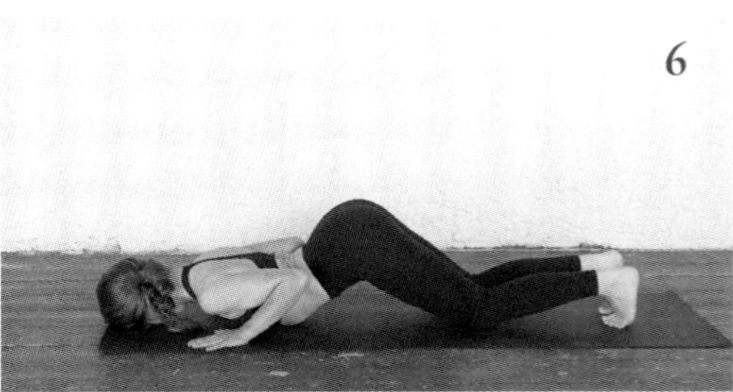

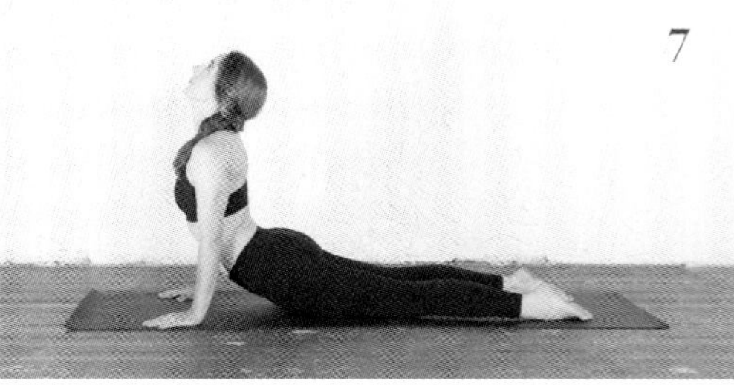

Knees, chest, and forehead are touching the floor; hips are off the floor.

7. Breathe in and scoop forward and up, looking up and backward.

Open your chest and look up and back without dropping the head.

Legs remain on the floor, feet are pointed.

Do not move your hands as you come into this position.

Elbows are slightly bent, tucked in toward your body, and your shoulders are pushing down.

8. Breathe out, curl your toes, and push your hips up to the ceiling.

Without moving your hands or feet, push your hips toward the ceiling.

Your hands are flat on the floor, heels can be slightly lifted off the floor. Head is between your arms. Look at your feet, trying to bring your chest to your knees.

9. Breathe in and bring your right foot forward in between your hands.

Keep your fingers and toes in one line.

Drop your left knee to the floor, point your left foot, and push your pelvis forward and toward your right heel.

Look diagonally upward—the same as in Position 4.

10. Breathe out, and keeping your hands where they are, curl the toes of your left foot and step your left foot forward, next to your right foot.

Nose in between your knees, hands holding your ankles.

Keep your knees straight.

11. Breathe in and reach with your hands out and upward.

Arch backward—the same as in Position 2.

12. Breathe out, and bring your hands in front of your chest.

This completes half a round. Repeat to the left (left leg stepping first back and forward) to complete one full round of Sun Salutation. Perform 6–8 rounds, then rest in Corpse Pose.

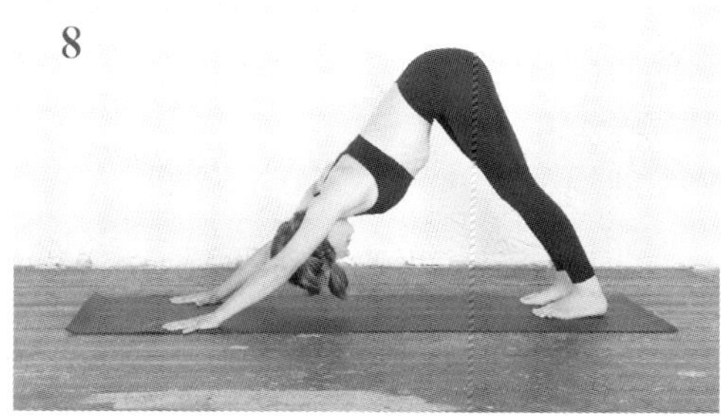

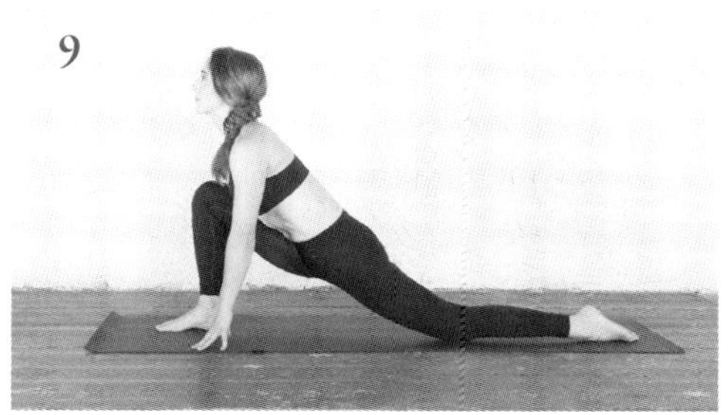

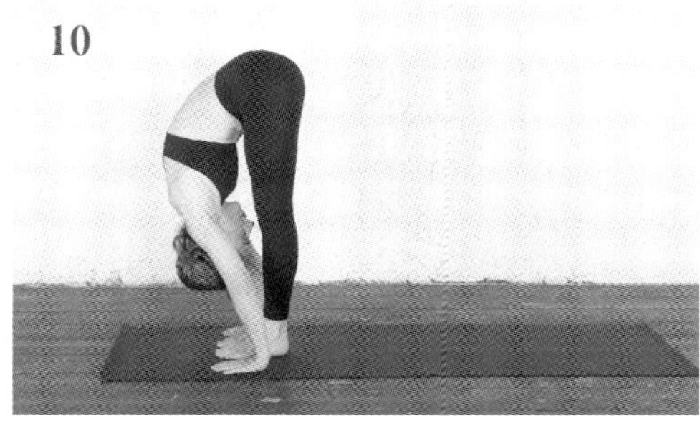

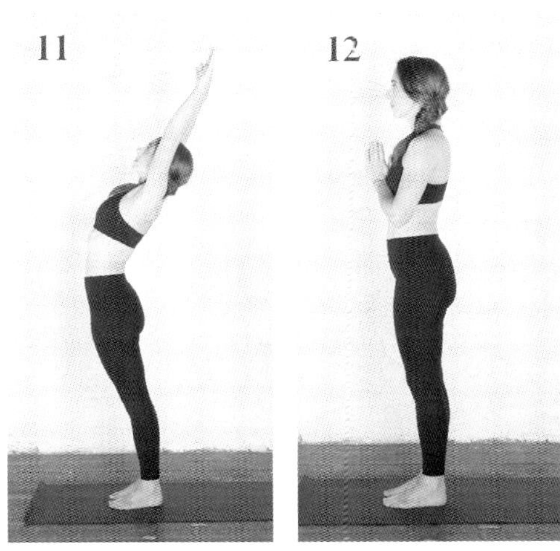

Warming Up
Double Leg Raises

Basic instructions

Lie on your back, with your feet together and flexed.

Keep your arms by your sides, with your palms facing downward.

Your hands are either tucked in toward your hips or under your hips for extra support.

Keep your back flat on the mat, with the back of your neck elongated and your chin tucked slightly in.

Lift both your legs up until almost perpendicular to the floor, and gently lower them down again (only as far as you can still keep the control in your abdomen and your lower back relatively flat against the floor).

Repeat 6 times, then rest in Corpse Pose.

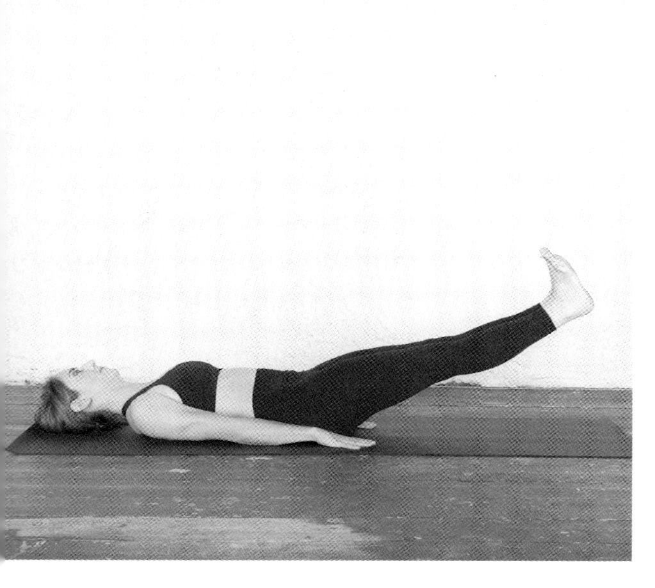

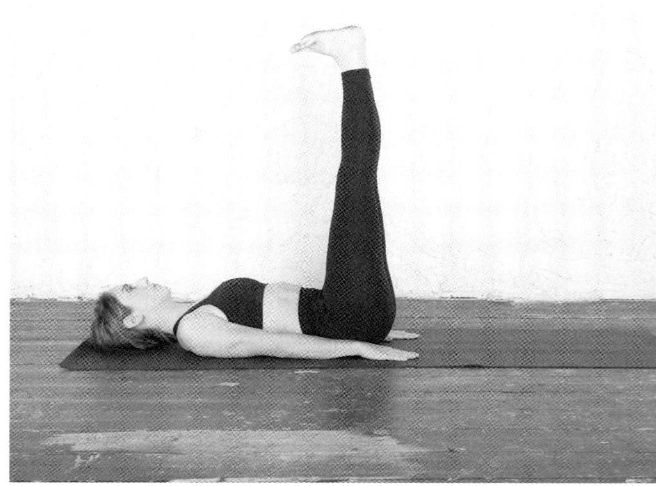

Warming Up
Dolphin

Basic instructions

Sit on your knees, with your hips resting on your heels.

Place your elbows on the floor, and keeping them in the same position, bring your hands forward and clasp them tightly.

Keeping your knees on the floor, lift your hips up (keeping your knees hip-width apart).

Make sure that your shoulders are right above your elbows, then walk your knees back, until they are positioned slightly behind your hips.

Curl your toes, straighten your knees, and push your hips up and backward.

Now move your torso forward, reaching with the chin to the floor, just in front of your hands.

From there, move your torso backward again, until your forehead hovers just above the floor behind your hands, with your hips reaching up and backward.

This completes one repetition. Repeat 10–15 times, then rest in Child's Pose.

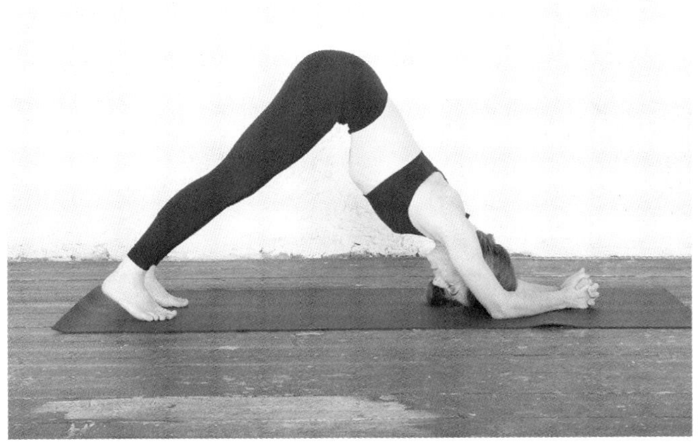

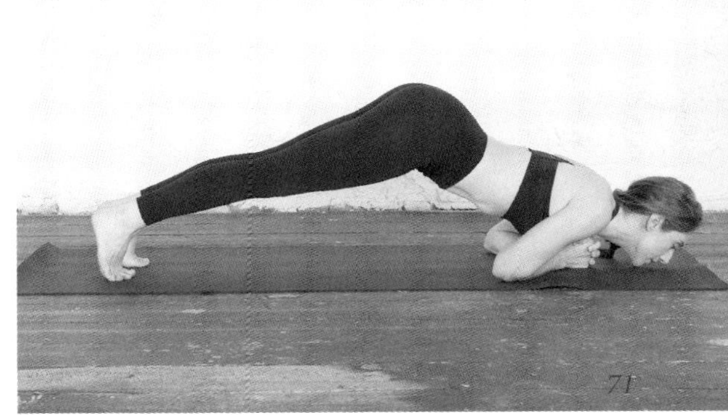

Step 4: True Asana – Finding Steadiness and Ease Within the Pose

Once your body is warmed up, the practice of asanas can begin. As explained earlier, holding the asanas in a steady and comfortable manner is essential in Hatha Yoga. The duration can be increased in relation to your progress. With regular practice, your ability to stay in a pose with ease will continue to develop. This being said, it is of course part of your journey to challenge yourself to stay longer, go further, or increase the complexity of the pose. These efforts should always be accompanied with conscious breathing and should never render you breathless, in pain, or feeling unwell.

Remember that a steady pose does not mean static or rigid. Even though the outer form of the asana may look still, your inner experience should not become an experience of confinement or rigor. As we have learnt earlier when talking about the effect of Hatha Yoga on our body's fascia: movement and life go hand in hand. So even though you are holding an asana steadily, you remain aware of the different directions of energy necessary to maintain the pose. You remain alert to the effects of the pose on your body and breath. As the asana is held, within your body there is a conscious and active process that brings you deeper into the pose or in other cases closer to the full expression of the pose. So even though you may look still, internally you are engaging and expanding in all directions, using your breath and consciousness to stay in the realms of ease and effortlessness.

Step 5: Proper Sequencing of Asanas

In a balanced yoga asana practice, it is important to include forward bends, backbends, inversions, side bends, twists, and balancing postures. It is also important to sequence the practice in such a way that all of these elements are included and especially that the forward bends and backbends are well balanced, taking into account their intensity and duration. This helps to create and maintain flexibility of your spine.

Often, students with chronic lower-back pain do not like to do backbends such as Cobra Pose and Bow Pose. They prefer doing forward bends because they experience immediate relief. However, chronic lower-back pain is often caused by a weak core and weak lower-back muscles. By strengthening and stretching these muscles as well as working on core awareness and strength, while maintaining a balanced ratio of forward and backward bends, during your asana practice, many cases of chronic back pain can be relieved.

When considering the effects on the internal organs and endocrine system, the principle of counter-poses is equally important. Some poses provide extra benefits when done in a specific order. Some poses exert a strong pressure on a specific body part, and the squeeze-and-release effect on that part is amplified by the proper order of poses and their counter-poses. For example, Upward Plank Pose becomes more effective if performed directly after a forward bend such as Seated Forward Bend.

Part IV

The Basic Structure: The Foundation for Hatha Sequencing

Chapter 9

Following the Natural Order

As we have seen in the chapter about the history of yoga, it is impossible to draw upon a unified and classical tradition of yoga asana practice. It is therefore also not possible to give a watertight explanation of why asanas should or even can be sequenced in any particular way.

When speaking about the art of sequencing yoga practices, what we can discuss, though, is that sequencing should be done in a comprehensive and consistent way, without becoming rigid and choreographed. And that we should practice asanas in a manner that reflects the core principles of Hatha Yoga: following the laws of nature, following the Principle of Minimal Action. We should aim to design sequences that create the most natural and effortless flow of prana through the body.

The sequence of yoga postures described in this book works from the Crown Chakra downward. This replicates the downward-descending, purifying element that purifies and stimulates your body. In doing so it creates space and the possibility for astral energies, such as the Kundalini Shakti, to rise upward.

Following these principles of natural order, on a merely physical plane we stimulate the nervous system in an organic and holistic way, starting with the brain and the spinal cord. They together form the central nervous system, which manages the entire body. By activating and stimulating the central nervous system, we subsequently activate the peripheral nervous system as well. So starting with the Crown Chakra and moving along the spinal cord in a downward direction, we activate the complete nervous system in a systematic manner and in a way requiring the least effort.

Another natural downward movement is excretion. One of the main purposes of asanas within the Hatha Yoga tradition is to purify the physical body. One of the most effective ways to do so is to ensure proper elimination of toxins on the physical and subtle levels. Improper elimination is usually caused by sluggishness and stagnation.

These lead to accumulated toxins and wastes, which in turn create imbalance and disharmony in the physical and astral bodies.

A yoga asana practice according to Hatha Yoga principles follows the downward movement of Apana Prana. Apana is considered to be the second-most important of the five vayus, or types of prana, in Hatha Yoga and Ayurveda. *Vayu* is a Sanskrit word that means “wind” and refers to the different movements of prana (life force) through the body. Apana Vayu is responsible for regulating the outward flow of prana from the body and governs elimination of physical wastes and toxins from the body. Yogis in ancient India who developed yoga asanas were convinced that maintaining equilibrium in the body results in good health. The first step toward this is making sure that your elimination processes work smoothly.

So the practice of yoga asanas according to Hatha Yoga principles is structured in such a manner that the chakras and their corresponding organs and glands in the physical body are stimulated in a top-to-bottom sequence. This ensures a holistic activation of the entire body and proper elimination of wastes and toxins.

Chapter 10

Chakra-Wise: The 17 Primary Asanas

The following sequence of 17 primary asanas is based on the teachings of Swami Sivananda (1887–1963). This sequence will provide the framework for your yoga practice or yoga class. Swami Sivananda was one of the pioneering teachers who made Hatha Yoga accessible to the broader public. Yet he did so by maintaining yoga's connection to classical teachings.

In the following pages we will provide a detailed overview of a well-balanced sequence. It is accessible both to beginners and to more advanced practitioners alike. The basic sequence comprises 17 asanas. Within this set of asanas, three of the relaxation poses (Corpse Pose, Child's Pose, and Crocodile Pose) are not included. This is because they have already been described in the previous chapter.

Each of the 17 asanas is assigned to its respective chakra. Accompanying each of the asanas you will find detailed benefits, instructions, cues on alignment, contraindications and cautions, and modifications.

By the time you have reached the chapter with the variations and have understood the principle of how to add and replace asanas, you will possess a detailed understanding of how to create hundreds of balanced yoga sequences based on these ancient principles.

Asana for the Sahasrara & Ajna Chakras (Crown & Third-Eye Chakras)

1. Shirshasana
Headstand

Benefits

Regular practice in a steady, comfortable manner within a balanced yoga asana program:

- stimulates the Crown and Third-Eye Chakras and therefore stimulates your pineal, pituitary, and hypothalamus glands, improving their overall function;
- activates your parasympathetic nervous system, ensuring the proper function of all internal processes such as digestion and elimination as well as hormonal balance;
- lowers your heart rate and blood pressure, and therefore gives your heart a rest;
- improves venous return of blood from your legs and therefore is highly beneficial for varicose veins and hemorrhoids;
- increases blood flow to and blood pressure within your head and therefore supplies your brain with an abundance of oxygen- and nutrient-rich blood;
- improves and corrects eye, nose, and throat ailments;
- corrects general fatigue and lack of vitality, and improves and prevents depression and anxiety;
- helps to prevent headaches and migraines;
- improves memory and concentration;
- improves digestion and cures constipation as it releases gravitational compression on the colon;
- improves blood flow to scalp and face and naturally revitalizes both;
- strengthens deep core muscles and back muscles; and
- increases upper-body and arm strength.

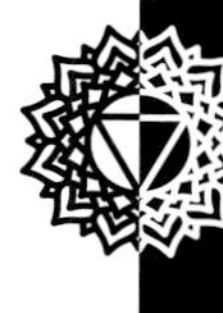

How to come into the pose

Sit on your knees and hold your elbows to measure the ideal distance. Then bring your arms to the floor under your shoulders.

Keeping your elbows there, bring your hands closer and interlock your fingers to form a cup.

Place the top of your head on the floor, with the back of your head held by your cupped hands.

Keeping your head and your elbows there, straighten your knees and lift your hips upward. Keeping your weight on your elbows, walk with your feet toward your head, keeping your knees straight. Keep walking until your hips are directly over your shoulders.

Slowly lift one foot at a time off the floor, bringing your knees in toward your chest. Hold this position for one breath, pushing your elbows into the floor.

Keeping your knees bent and together, slowly straighten both legs to the ceiling.

Focus on a point, keep pushing your elbows into the floor, and breathe slowly and deeply.

Coming out of the pose

To come down, keep one foot toward the ceiling, and, with control, lower the other foot to the floor.

Relax in the Child's Pose for 30 seconds.

Alignment cues

Ultimately the aim is to have your ears, shoulders, hips, and ankles in one straight line. This is ideal for long holds. As you start to learn the pose, though, refer to the alignment described a little further down in Modifications.

Maintain the majority of your weight on the top of your head, while your arms share the weight and provide a supportive base.

Draw away your shoulder blades from your ears, toward your waist, keeping your neck elongated and stable.

Duration of hold

Beginners: 10 seconds–1 minute

Intermediate: 1–5 minutes

Advanced: 5–15 minutes

Contraindications & cautions

- Hypertension
- Cardiovascular issues
- Neck issues
- Shoulder issues
- Recent surgery or inflammation in your head region (e.g. ears, eyes, nose, etc.)
- Arthritis or osteoporosis
- Brain injuries
- Lower-back and spinal issues (e.g. chronic pain, herniated disc, sciatica, SI-joint instability)
- Acute migraine or headache
- For asthma or other breathing disorders: hold only for short durations and skip altogether if it causes too much discomfort, nausea, or shortness of breath
- Practitioner younger than seven, because the skull is still a bit soft and it is safer not to place weight on it yet

Modifications

In the beginning phase, when learning Headstand, make sure to keep your feet slightly in front of your body. Do not aim for shoulders-hips-ankles alignment, because that increases the risk of toppling over. Until you can enter and exit the pose with control by yourself and hold for at least 1 minute, keep your feet slightly in front of you.

An easier and less intense pose, which still gives you the benefits of the inversion, is Half Headstand.

Asanas for the Vishuddha Chakra (Throat Chakra)

2. Sarvangasana
Shoulderstand

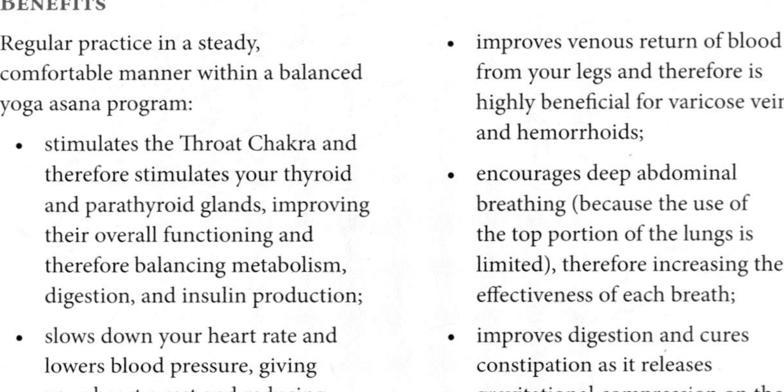

Benefits

Regular practice in a steady, comfortable manner within a balanced yoga asana program:

- stimulates the Throat Chakra and therefore stimulates your thyroid and parathyroid glands, improving their overall functioning and therefore balancing metabolism, digestion, and insulin production;
- slows down your heart rate and lowers blood pressure, giving your heart a rest and reducing strain on it;
- activates your parasympathetic nervous system, ensuring the proper function of all internal processes such as digestion and elimination as well as hormonal balance;
- improves venous return of blood from your legs and therefore is highly beneficial for varicose veins and hemorrhoids;
- encourages deep abdominal breathing (because the use of the top portion of the lungs is limited), therefore increasing the effectiveness of each breath;
- improves digestion and cures constipation as it releases gravitational compression on the colon;
- provides a gentle massage to the heart and lung region;
- strengthens the deep core muscles, legs, buttocks, and lower back; and
- increases upper-body and arm strength.

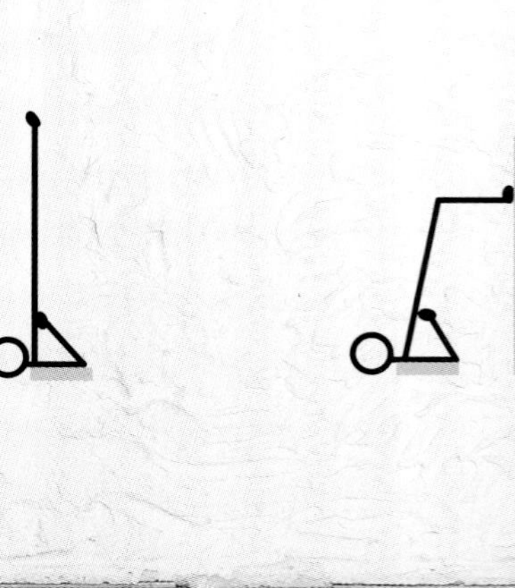

How to come into the pose

Lie down on the back, with your feet together and arms next to your body.

Keeping your head and neck on the floor, breathe in as you lift both legs to 90 degrees.

As you lift your hips up toward the ceiling, place your hands onto your hips and walk your hands up toward your shoulder blades.

Lift your hips up as high as you can, bringing your chest toward your chin.

Keep your back supported with your hands and make sure that your feet end up straight above your head.

Breathe slowly in this position and focus on the throat region.

Coming out of the pose

To come out of the pose, drop your legs slightly toward your head and place your hands on the floor. While keeping your head on the floor, use your hands as breaks and slowly roll down.

Alignment cues

Try to straighten the back as much as possible. If required, bring your hands closer to your shoulders and your elbows a little closer to each other.

Make sure that your feet are right above your head, with most of your weight on your shoulders.

Your neck should not be bearing your body weight, and should not be pressing into the floor but keeping its natural curve off the floor. To accomplish this, draw your shoulder blades toward each other, creating an arch in your neck.

Keep your legs and feet relaxed and hold the pose with the least effort possible.

Duration of hold

Beginners: 30 seconds–1 minute

Intermediate: 1–3 minutes

Advanced: 3–6 minutes

Contraindications & cautions

- Hypertension
- Cardiovascular issues
- Neck issues
- Shoulder issues
- Recent surgery or inflammation in your head region (e.g. ears, eyes, nose)
- Arthritis or osteoporosis
- Brain injuries
- Lower-back and spinal issues (e.g. chronic pain, herniated disc, sciatica, SI-joint instability)
- Acute migraine or headache
- Asthma or other breathing disorders: hold only for short durations and skip altogether if it causes too much discomfort, nausea, or shortness of breath

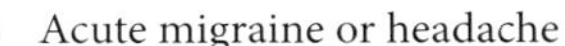

Modifications

It is recommended to place a folded blanket 3–5 cm thick underneath your shoulders to release pressure on your neck. By placing the blanket underneath the shoulder girdle, but keeping your neck off the blanket, you create a level difference that allows your body to straighten up more, avoiding over-flexion and therefore strain of your neck.

If you struggle to hold the pose, you can use the wall as support.

3. Halasana
Plough Pose

Benefits

Regular practice in a steady and comfortable manner within a balanced yoga asana program:

- stimulates the Throat Chakra and therefore stimulates the thyroid and parathyroid glands, improving their overall functioning;
- slows down heart rate and lowers blood pressure, therefore giving the heart a rest;
- activates the parasympathetic nervous system, ensuring the proper function of all internal processes such as digestion, elimination, and so on;
- improves exchange of oxygen and carbon dioxide in the lungs by making active use of the lower part of the lungs;
- improves digestion and cures constipation as it releases gravitational compression on the colon;
- strengthens deep core muscles;
- increases upper-body and arm strength;
- releases tension in the entire spine, especially the lower back and cervical region;
- stretches the hamstrings and glutes;
- creates flexibility in the shoulder joints; and
- massages all visceral organs by compression, and upon release of the pose floods organs with fresh, nutrient-rich blood.

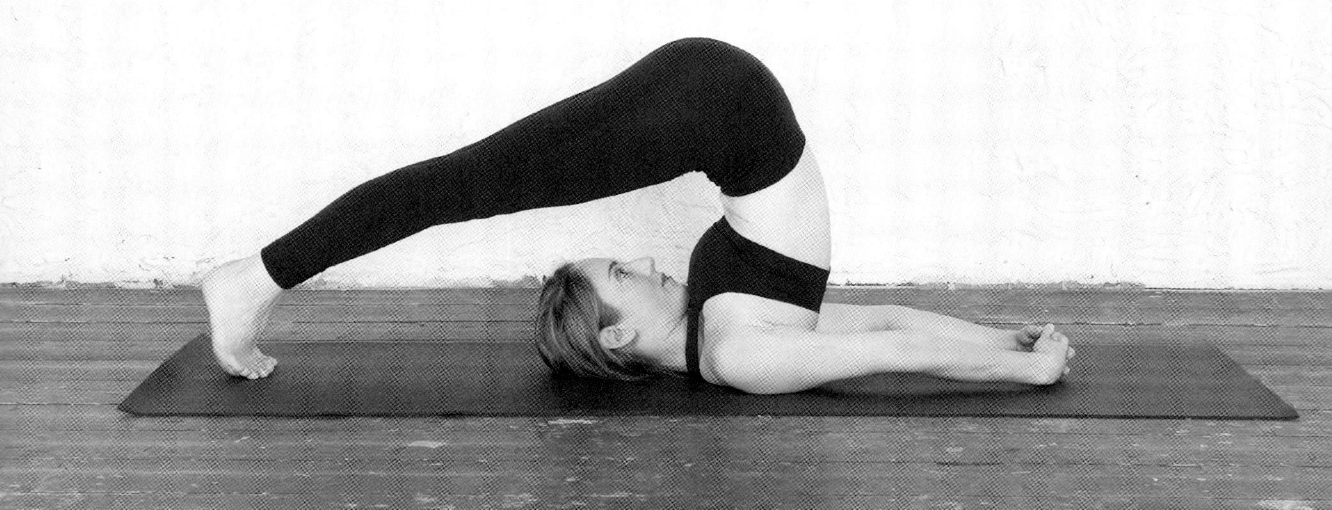

How to come into the pose

Lie down on your back, with your feet together and arms next to your body.

Keeping your head and neck on the floor, breathe in as you lift both legs to 90 degrees.

As you lift your hips up toward the ceiling, place your hands on your hips and walk your hands up toward your shoulder blades.

As your legs start to lift up, guide them toward your head. Slowly place your feet on the floor behind your head. Keep your knees straight, feet together, and feet flexed.

If your toes can reach the floor comfortably, you can interlock your hands on the floor behind your back.

Keeping your knees straight, gently push your heels away, and breathe evenly.

Coming out of the pose

Placing your hands on the floor and using them as levers, bend your knees slightly and slowly roll the back on the floor.

Alignment cues

Knees should be kept straight if possible.

Look straight upward toward the ceiling; do not turn your head.

Hips ideally are right above your shoulders.

Shoulder blades are drawn toward each other to release pressure on your neck.

Duration of hold

Beginners: 15–60 seconds

Intermediate: 30–90 seconds

Advanced: 90 seconds–3 minutes

A thumb rule for the duration of Plough Pose is half the duration of Shoulderstand. So if you hold Shoulderstand for 2 minutes, stay in Plough Pose for 1 minute.

Contraindications & cautions

- Hypertension
- Cardiovascular issues
- Neck issues
- Shoulder issues
- Recent surgery or inflammation in your head region (e.g. ears, eyes, nose, etc.)
- Arthritis and osteoporosis
- Brain injuries
- Lower-back and spinal issues (e.g. chronic pain, herniated disc, sciatica, SI-joint instability)
- Acute migraine or headache
- Asthma or other breathing disorders: hold only for short durations and skip altogether if it causes too much discomfort, nausea, or shortness of breath

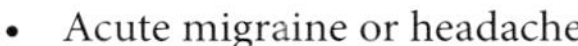

Modifications

Place a folded blanket 3–5 cm thick underneath your shoulders to release pressure on your neck (as in Shoulderstand).

If you cannot reach the floor with your feet, try opening your feet wider apart and gently placing down one foot at a time. Otherwise, support your feet on a block or against the wall. In this case, keep the support of your hands on your lower back.

Asanas for the Anahata Chakra (Heart Chakra)

4. Ardha Setu Bandhasana

Half Bridge Pose

Benefits

Regular practice in a steady and comfortable manner within a balanced yoga asana program:

- stimulates the Heart Chakra and therefore stimulates your heart, lungs, thymus, and lymph glands;
- stimulates your thyroid and parathyroid glands;
- slows heart beat and reduces blood pressure (if chest is raised high enough to press into the chin);
- stretches your spine in the opposite direction than in Shoulderstand and Plough Pose and therefore reverses the compression of the lumbar and thoracic regions;
- strengthens abdominal and lumbar muscles;
- rejuvenates and tones the legs and buttocks;
- stretches intercostals and can be therapeutic for asthma; and
- releases lower-back tension and pain and rejuvenates tired back muscles.

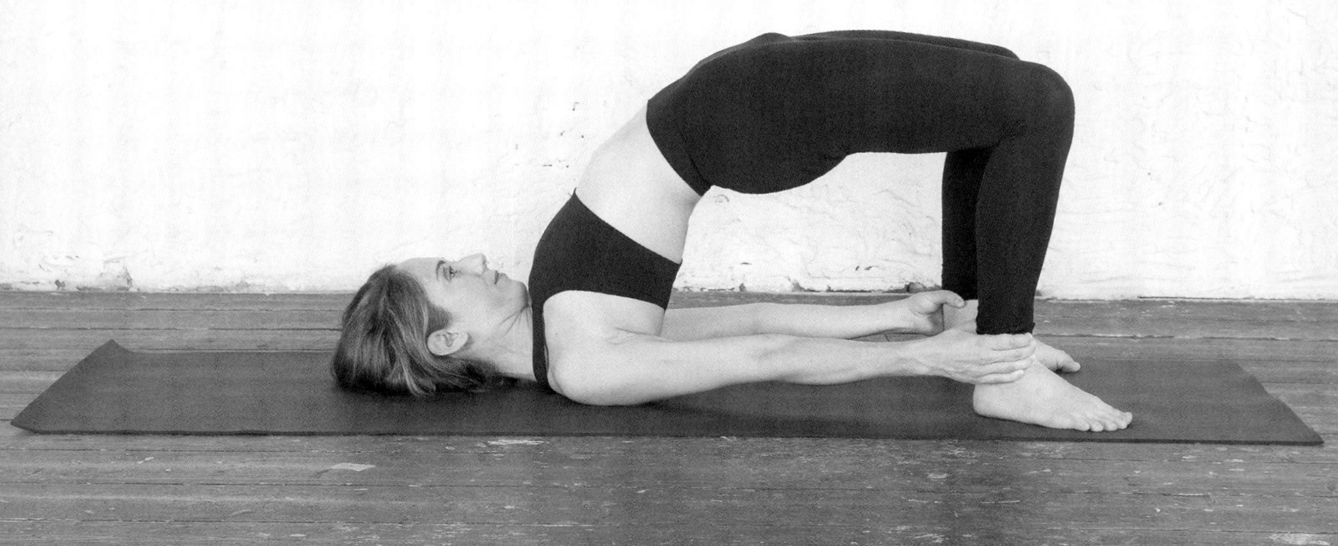

How to come into the pose

Lie down on your back, bend your knees, and bring your feet close to your hips. Keep your feet hip-width apart and heels on the floor.

Place your hands by your sides, palms facing downward.

Breathe in, push your hands into the floor, and slowly lift your hips up to the ceiling.

Reach with your hands toward your ankles and bring your chest toward your chin.

Keep lifting your pelvis upward and back toward your head, and breathe evenly.

Coming out of the pose

Place your palms flat on the floor and vertebra by vertebra roll the back down toward the floor.

Alignment cues

Keeping shoulders and head on the floor, draw your shoulder blades toward each other.

Knees should stay parallel, toes may point slightly outwards.

Knees and ankles should be at a 90-degree angle to the floor.

Duration

Beginners: 30 seconds–1 minute

Intermediate: 1–2 minutes

Advanced: 2–4 minutes

Contraindications & cautions

There are no general contraindications and cautions to this pose. However, respect your limit of movement and do not push further than that, as that can cause strain in your neck or knees.

Modifications

If you cannot hold your ankles while maintaining the correct alignment, you can also:

- keep your palms flat on the floor, next to your thighs, and then push your pelvis up as high as you can; or
- support your back by bringing your hands in the same position as in Shoulderstand (fingers pointing in toward your spine and thumbs up alongside your body).

5. Pawanmuktasana
Air-Releasing Pose (Supplementary Pose)

Air-Releasing Pose is practiced at this point in the sequence to provide a gentle counter-pose for Half Bridge Pose. It stretches the back, hips, and back of your legs, and when done properly helps to relieve excess gases from your stomach and intestines.

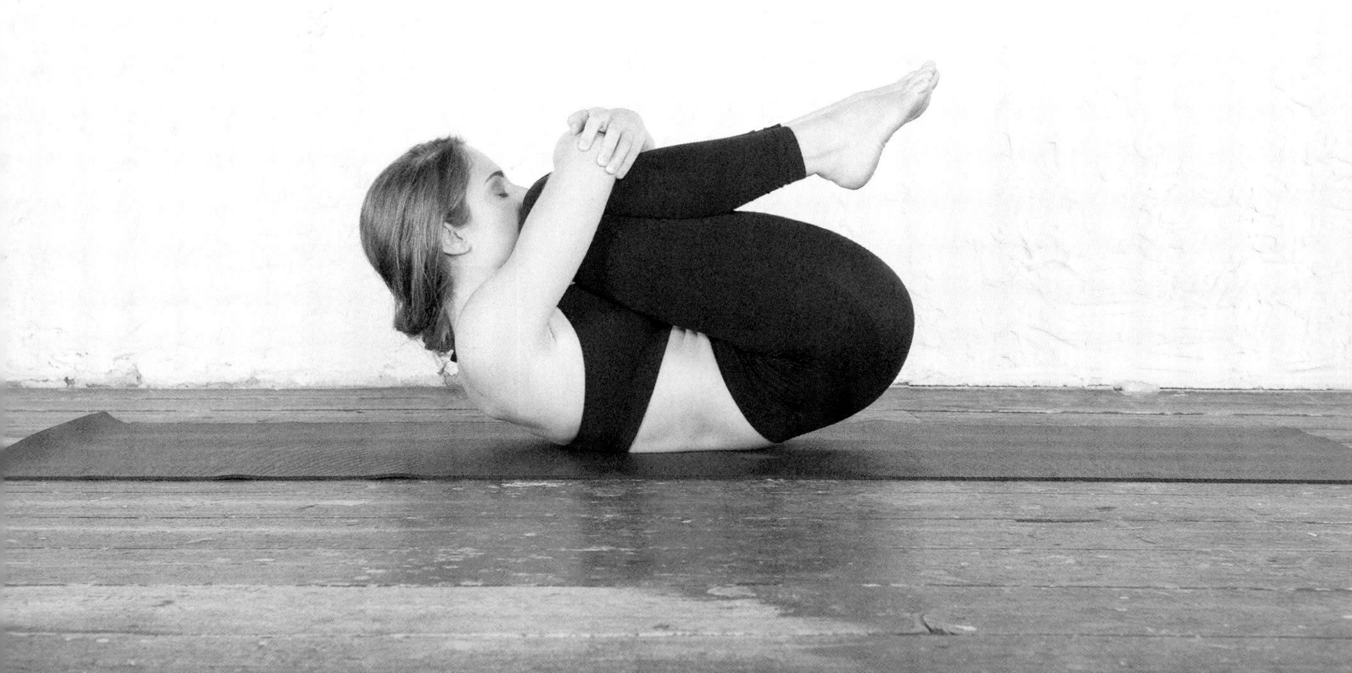

How to come into the pose

Lie down on your back and hug your knees to your chest.

Bring your nose to your knees, rounding your entire spine. Take deep breaths into your lower abdomen.

Alignment cues

Lower and middle back are resting on the floor. Tailbone and upper back are lifted off the floor in the effort to bring the nose and knees close together.

Feet and knees are parallel, and your arms are crossing over your kneecaps or shins.

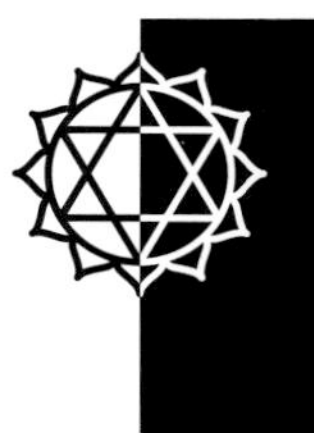

Duration

Hold for 30 seconds to 1 minute.

Contraindications & cautions

Abdominal issues (e.g. diarrhea, ulcer, menstrual pains, recent surgery)

Modifications

Keep your head on the floor if you have neck or shoulder pain.

Keep your knees apart if due to tight hips or hamstrings you find it difficult to draw your knees close to your chest.

6. Matsyasana
Fish Pose

Benefits

Regular practice in a steady and comfortable manner within a balanced yoga asana program:

- stimulates the Heart Chakra and therefore stimulates the heart, lungs, thymus, and lymph glands, making it esteemed as highly beneficial for boosting the immune system;
- stimulates the thyroid and parathyroid glands;
- encourages deep abdominal and diaphragmatic breathing and stretches the intercostals, therefore strengthening the lungs and increasing their capacity, resulting in higher athletic performance and better coping with respiratory conditions such as asthma and spasms in the bronchial tubes;
- relaxes the upper-back and neck muscles;
- strengthens and tones the arm and upper-back muscles; and
- reverses the compression caused by Shoulderstand, stretching the thoracic and lumbar regions of your spine in the opposite direction.

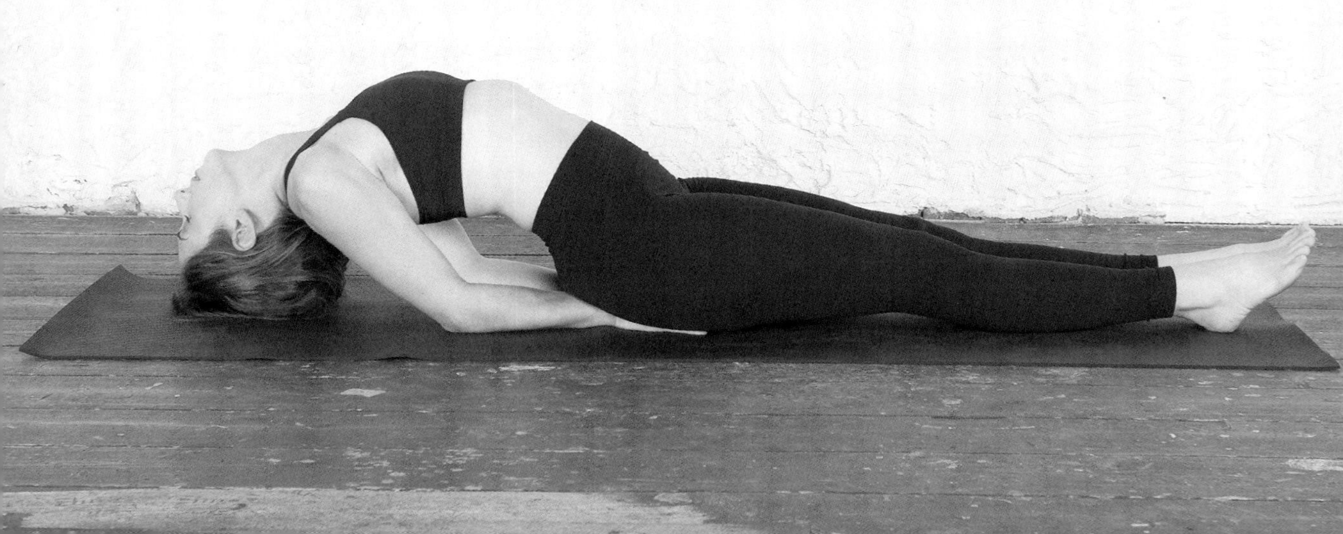

How to come into the pose

Lie down on your back—legs and feet together.

Place your hands under your hips, palms facing downward and elbows slightly outward.

Breathing in, look toward your feet and bring your weight onto your elbows.

Bring your elbows as close together as possible.

Breathing in, open your chest and drop your head back so that the crown of your head rests on the floor.

Taking deep breaths, expand your lungs and chest.

Coming out of the pose

Breathe in and lift your head to look at the feet. Breathe out and relax in Corpse Pose.

Alignment cues

Make sure your hands are below your hips. If your hands are too high or too low, the alignment of the whole pose will be off.

Make sure that your head is resting on the floor.

Do not lean on your head. Your head should be slightly touching the floor, but the weight should be on your elbows only.

Keep your feet and legs relaxed.

Open your chest as much as possible. Breathe as deeply as possible, taking advantage of the fact that the chest is thrown wide open.

Duration of hold

Beginners: 30 seconds–1 minute

Intermediate: 1–2 minutes

Advanced: 2–4 minutes

Contraindications & cautions

- Neck issues
- Acute headache
- Hypertension

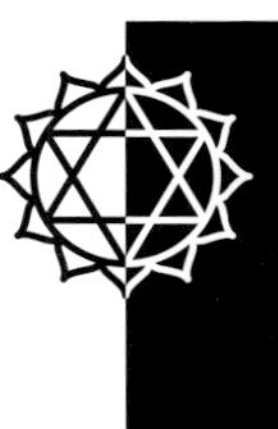

Modifications

If you feel dizzy or feel pain in your neck, you can rest your upper back or head on a cushion.

7. Sukha Gomukhasana

Easy Cow Face Pose

Benefits

Regular practice in a steady and comfortable manner within a balanced yoga asana program:

- stimulates the Heart Chakra and therefore stimulates the heart, lungs, thymus, and lymph glands—therefore boosting the immune system;
- encourages abdominal and diaphragmatic breathing;
- stretches intercostal muscles and therefore increases lung capacity, which results in higher athletic performance and better coping with respiratory conditions such as asthma;
- helps to straighten your spine and improve overall body posture;
- improves the condition of kyphosis (chronically hunched upper back or rounded shoulders); and
- removes tension in your shoulders as well as in your upper and middle back.

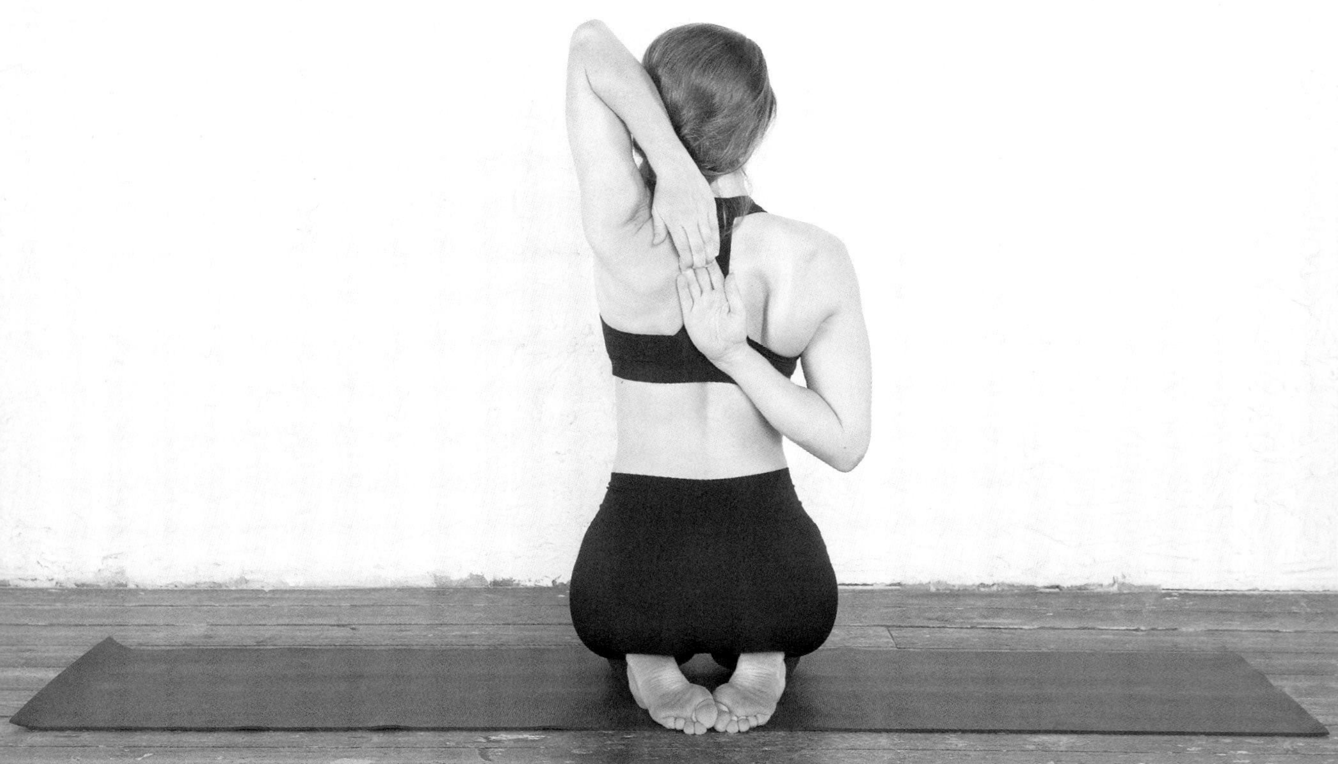

How to come into the pose

Sit on your knees, with your hips resting on your heels.

Extend your right arm to the side, bend your elbow, and place your hand in between your shoulder blades, palm facing away.

Lift your left arm over your head and bend your elbow to place your left palm in between your shoulder blades (palm touching the back).

Clasp your hands behind your back, in between your shoulder blades.

Coming out of the pose

Gently release the grip of your hands, roll your shoulders, and proceed to the other side.

Alignment cues

The back of your neck should be kept as straight as possible.

Your lower back should arch only slightly (retaining its natural curve).

Try to keep the elbow of your upper arm behind your head.

Duration

Beginners: 30 seconds–1 minute per side

Intermediate: 1–2 minutes per side

Advanced: 3–5 minutes per side

Contraindications & cautions

- Shoulder issues
- Knee issues: to decrease strain on knees, support your hips on a cushion or keep your legs stretched out in front of you

Modifications

If both hands are on your spine, but do not touch, hold on to a strap or towel to provide resistance.

If your lower hand does not reach to the center of your spine, do not attempt to clasp the hand. Instead gently clasp your elbow with the opposite hand and work on the rotation in the shoulder.

If sitting on your heels is not comfortable, use a block or cushion underneath your hips.

Asanas for the Manipura Chakra (Solar Plexus Chakra)

8. Paschimottanasana

Seated Forward Bend

Benefits

Regular practice in a steady and comfortable manner within a balanced yoga asana program:

- stimulates the Solar Plexus Chakra and therefore stimulates and balances the functions of the stomach, gallbladder, liver, spleen, and pancreas;
- improves digestion and elimination of toxins;
- increases peristalsis and combats constipation through the squeeze-and-release effect;
- regulates blood sugar levels, through regulating pancreas function;
- helps to balance the menstrual cycle and to improve blood circulation to the pelvic region, therefore helping to relieve symptoms caused by menopause and menstruation;
- slightly increases blood pressure toward your head and has a calming effect on the brain and mind and helps to relieve stress and anxiety;
- stretches the entire spine, especially the lumbar and thoracic spine, and therefore improves blood circulation in the back region and tones the spinal nerves; and
- improves flexibility of the lower back, hips, and hamstrings.

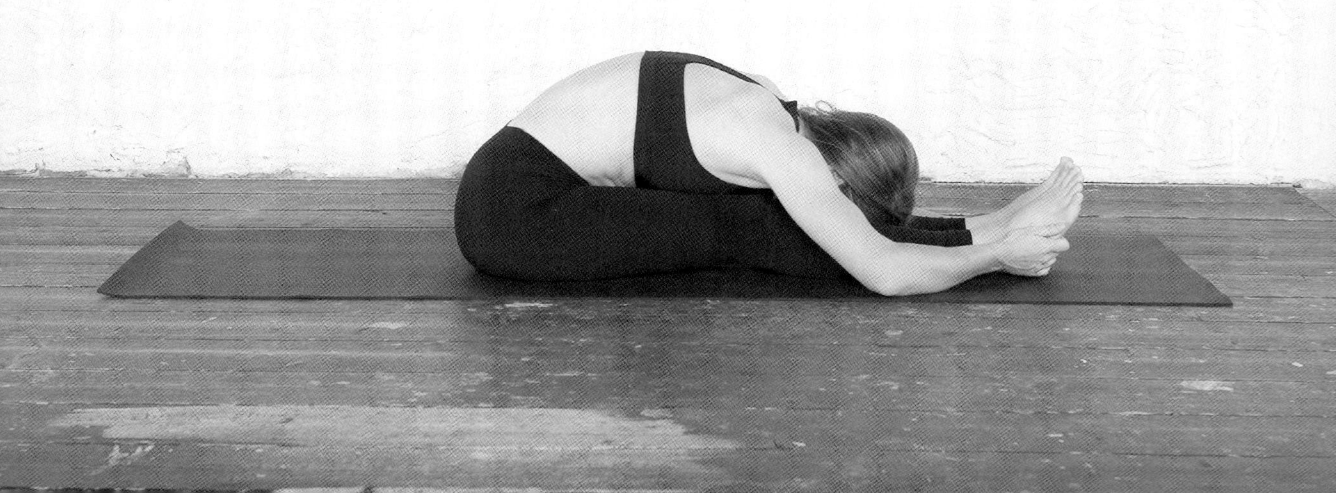

How to come into the pose

Sit with your legs together or hip-width apart, and straight in front of you.

Make sure you are sitting high up on your sitting bones.

Inhale and reach with both arms toward the ceiling, arms parallel to your ears.

As you exhale, keep on reaching forward, and bend forward, reaching with your hands toward your toes.

Bring your nose to your knees. If you are unable to reach your toes, hold your ankles, shins, or even your knees. Rest your elbows on the floor.

Coming out of the pose

Breathe in and slowly roll up, vertebra by vertebra, shoulders and head coming up last.

Alignment cues

Make sure you are sitting high up on your sitting bones; avoid rolling back toward your tailbone.

Hands are holding calves, ankles, or heels—wherever they reach comfortably. Keep your arms and shoulders relaxed and use your breath to move deeper in the pose. Do not use your arms to pull yourself downward.

Your elbows are resting on the floor or relaxing toward the floor.

Your back is rounded.

Your head and neck are relaxed. Reach with your forehead toward your knees or shins, and if possible rest it against your legs. (If necessary, you can use a prop to rest your head on for longer holds.)

Duration

Beginners: 1–2 minutes

Intermediate: 2–4 minutes

Advanced: 4–10 minutes

Contraindications & cautions

- Abdominal issues (e.g. diarrhea, ulcer, menstrual pains, recent surgery)
- Lower-back and spinal issues (e.g. chronic pain, herniated disc, sciatica, SI-joint instability)
- Hypertension: keep your head elevated above heart level

Modifications

If you are suffering from a herniated or compressed disc in the lower or middle back, or any other spinal issues (e.g. sciatica, SI-joint instability), be careful with this pose. If you are allowed to do forward bends by your physician, work on creating the movement from your pelvis and keep your spine as straight as possible (so do not round your nose to your knee).

If the lower back is tight, you can open your legs hip-width apart.

For tight hamstrings, you can bend your knees and support them with a block or folded blanket.

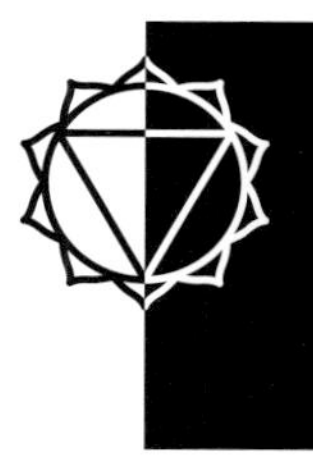

9. Purvottanasana
Upward Plank Pose

Benefits

Regular practice in a steady and comfortable manner within a balanced yoga asana program:

- works as a counter-pose to seated forward bends and increases the effect of these poses by increasing the blood flow to the stomach, gallbladder, liver, spleen, and pancreas;
- gives a gentle backbend to your entire spine, especially in the thoracic spine (chest opener);
- tones arms, shoulders, and wrists; and
- increases core strength.

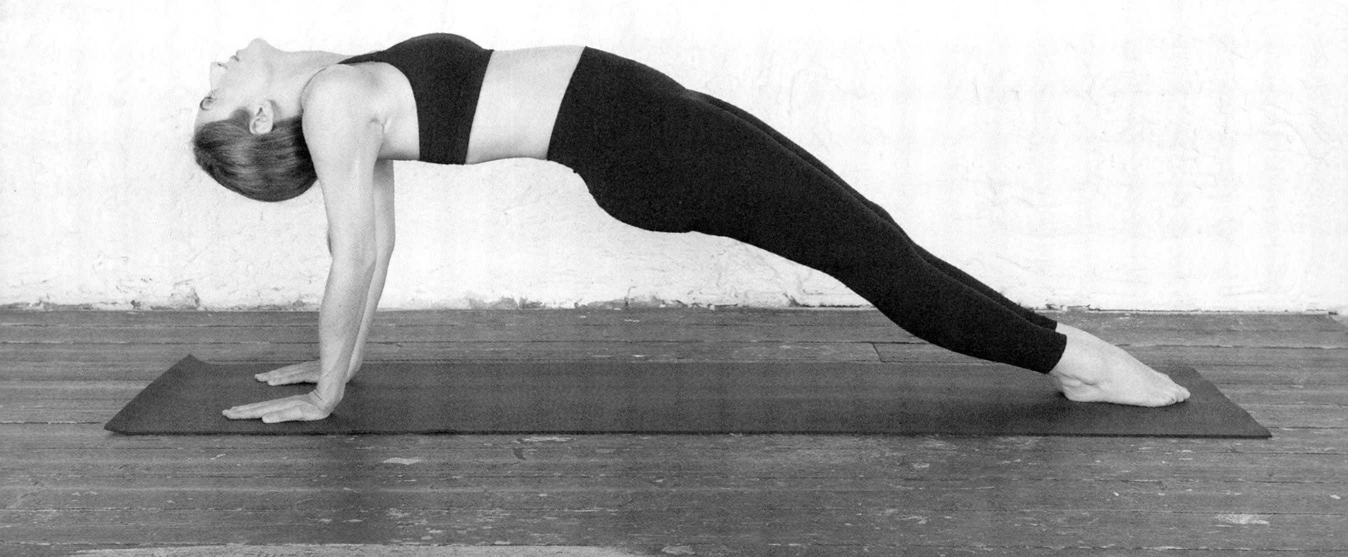

How to come into the pose

Sit with your legs straight in front of you.

Keep your hands next to your hips, fingers facing backward.

Pulling your shoulders to your ears, open your chest, lean back, and place your hands flat on the floor.

As you breathe in, point your feet, push your hips upward, open your chest, and gently drop your head backward.

Keep pushing your pelvis up toward the ceiling, feet into the floor, and allow your shoulders to roll back and your chest to expand.

Coming out of the pose

Breathing in, look at your feet as you bring your hips down. Then lie down on your stomach in Crocodile Pose.

Alignment cues

Activate your inner thighs to keep your legs parallel and close together.

Open your chest to the maximum and take deep breaths.

Your wrists and shoulders should be in one vertical line when you are in the pose. Make sure that when you are in the pose, your shoulders are not further back than your wrists, because this can strain your wrists. Also make sure that your shoulders are not in front of your wrists, as this will limit the movement.

Duration

Beginners: 10–20 seconds

Intermediate: 20–40 seconds

Advanced: 40–90 seconds

Contraindications & cautions

- Wrist issues
- Shoulder issues
- Neck issues
- Hypertension and hypotension

Modifications

If you have hyperextended elbows, turn your fingertips toward your feet.

If releasing your head backward is too heavy on your neck, causes dizziness, or is just not comfortable, you can look toward the ceiling.

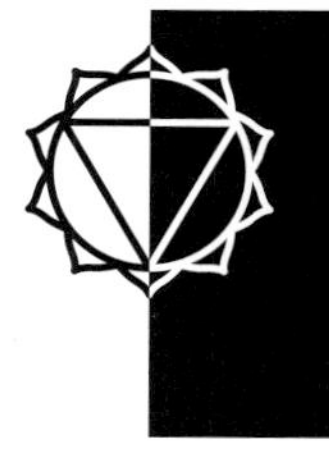

10. Bhujangasana

Cobra Pose

Benefits

Regular practice in a steady and comfortable manner within a balanced yoga asana program:

- stimulates the Manipura Chakra and therefore stimulates and balances the functions of your stomach, gallbladder, liver, spleen, and pancreas;
- tones all digestive organs and improves digestion, through abdominal pressure;
- increases bodily heat and therefore digestive fire;
- stimulates the contraction of your intestines and therefore helps to relieve constipation;
- regulates blood sugar levels, through regulating the function of the pancreas;
- tones and strengthens your lower-back muscles, therefore having a positive effect on chronic lower-back pain;
- tones your buttocks and inner thighs;
- stretches the thoracic region of your spine by expanding the rib cage;
- relieves hunchback and improves posture;
- tones your ovaries and uterus and can reduce menstruation problems;
- helps to reestablish a proper lumbar curve and can therefore be beneficial for sciatica; and
- reduces fatigue and lethargy.

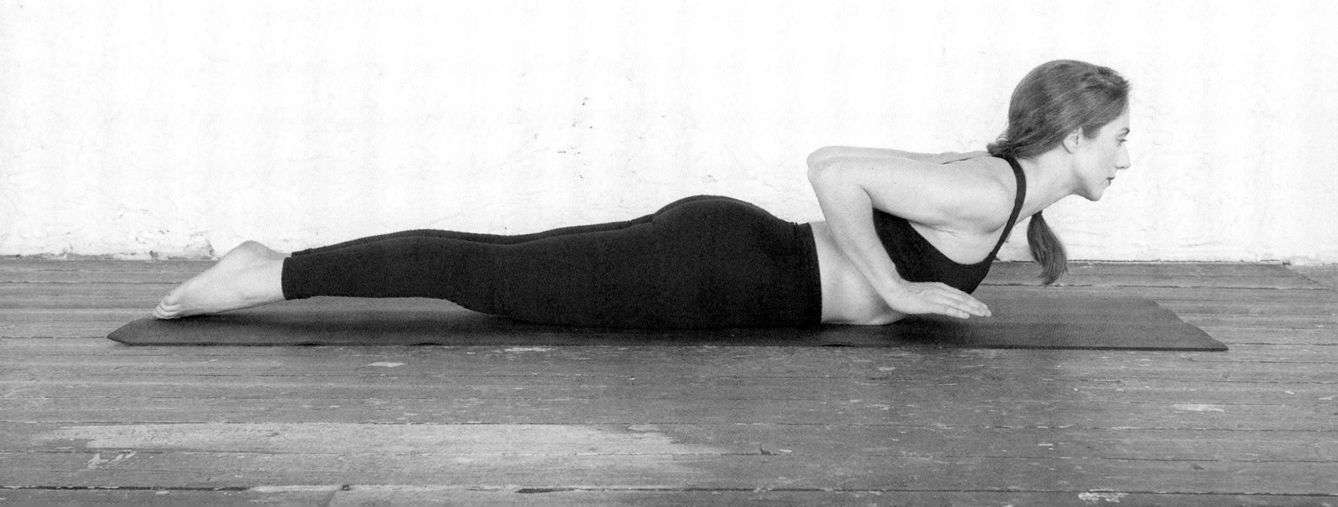

How to come into the pose

Lie down on your abdomen, with your legs and feet together, forehead on the floor.

Position your palms on the floor, next to your chest. Elbows are tucked in toward your body and pointing upward.

Breathe in, pushing your navel into the floor, and raise your head and chest off the floor.

Take easy, relaxed breaths as you hold the pose.

Coming out of the pose

Exhale and gently lower your upper body and head to the floor. Relax in Crocodile Pose.

Alignment cues

Keep your lower stomach, pelvis, and legs on the floor.

Squeeze your legs together, heels together.

Shoulders are down and away from your ears.

Keep your hands slightly off the floor.

Duration

Beginners: 30 seconds–1 minute

Intermediate: 1–2 minutes

Advanced: 2–3 minutes

Contraindications & cautions

- Abdominal issues (e.g. diarrhea, ulcer, menstrual pains, recent surgery)
- Cardiovascular issues
- Lower-back and spinal issues (e.g. chronic pain, herniated disc, sciatica, SI-joint instability)

Modifications

If you have chronic lower-back issues or even a herniated disc, a modified version of this pose might work well for you: Keep your hands on the floor and use them as support. You can even bring your elbows on to the floor just below your shoulders. It is important that you stabilize your back by engaging your core. Suck your belly button toward your spine as you hold the pose. Keep your shoulder blades drawn away from your ears toward your waist and look straight ahead.

11. Shalabhasana
Locust Pose

Benefits

Regular practice in a steady and comfortable manner within a balanced yoga asana program:

- stimulates the Solar Plexus Chakra and therefore stimulates and balances the functions of your stomach, gallbladder, liver, spleen, and pancreas;
- tones all digestive organs and improves digestion, through abdominal pressure;
- produces bodily heat and increases digestive fire;
- helps to control blood sugar levels through stimulating your pancreas;
- strengthens the biceps and deltoid muscles of your upper arms;
- strengthens your abdominal and lumbar muscles;
- strengthens and tones your buttocks and legs;
- stimulates your reproductive system;
- improves concentration and helps to relieve stress; and
- relieves hunchback and corrects posture.

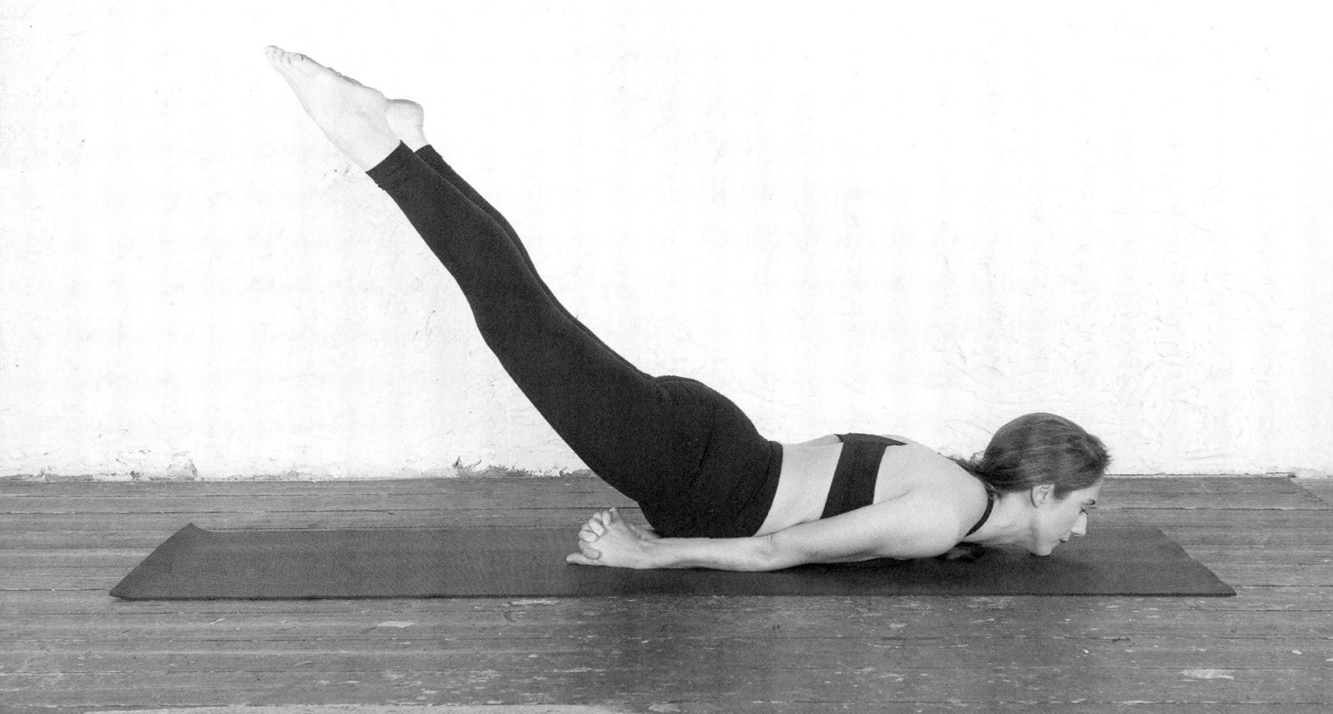

How to come into the pose

Lie on your side, interlock your hands tightly in front of you, and push them downward, below your pelvis (keeping your elbows as close as possible).

Roll over to lie on your chest and look forward, chin on the floor.

Keep your feet hip-width or even wider apart.

Inhale and lift both legs off the floor as high as possible, pushing your shoulders and arms into the floor.

Coming out of the pose

Breathe out and gently lower your legs to the floor. Release your hands and relax into Crocodile Pose.

Alignment cues

Elbows and wrists are as close as possible.

Shoulders are rolled inwards.

If you feel pain in your arms or elbows you can place a rolled blanket under your elbows.

If you feel tension in your neck or cannot place your chin flat on the floor, you can place a blanket underneath your chest.

You can modify your hand position as follows: making two fists next to each other or hands flat next to each other with palms facing downward.

Duration

Beginners: 10 seconds

Intermediate: 10–20 seconds

Advanced: 20–40 seconds

Contraindications & cautions

- Abdominal issues (e.g. diarrhea, ulcer, menstrual pains, recent surgery)
- Shoulder issues
- Cardiovascular issues
- Neck issues

Modifications

This is quite an intense and difficult pose. To build up toward it, you can first practice Half Locust Pose, as explained in the variations section further on in the book.

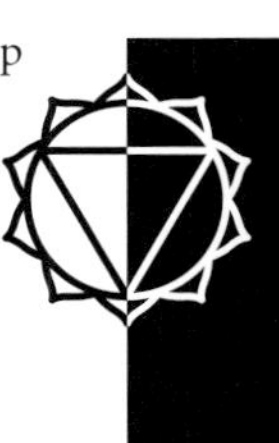

12. Dhanurasana
Bow Pose

Benefits

Regular practice in a steady and comfortable manner within a balanced yoga asana program:

- stimulates the Solar Plexus Chakra and therefore stimulates and balances the functions of your stomach, gallbladder, liver, spleen, and pancreas;
- tones all digestive organs and improves digestion, through abdominal pressure;
- produces bodily heat and increases digestive fire;
- tones, strengthens, and massages your lower-back muscles and therefore acts as a remedy to chronic lower-back pain;
- stretches and lengthens your abdominal muscles, psoas, and quadriceps;
- relieves hunchback and improves overall posture;
- opens your chest, stretches your intercostals, and therefore increases lung capacity and efficiency;
- increases mobility in your shoulder joints;
- improves rheumatism of your hips, knee joints, and hands;
- compresses your entire spine and rejuvenates your intervertebral discs and your central nervous system;
- stimulates reproductive organs, providing relief for women who regularly suffer from menstrual cramps;
- releases tension in shoulders and neck and therefore is beneficial for those suffering from tension headaches;
- helps to combat stress, anxiety, and fatigue; and
- increases vitality, concentration, and willpower.

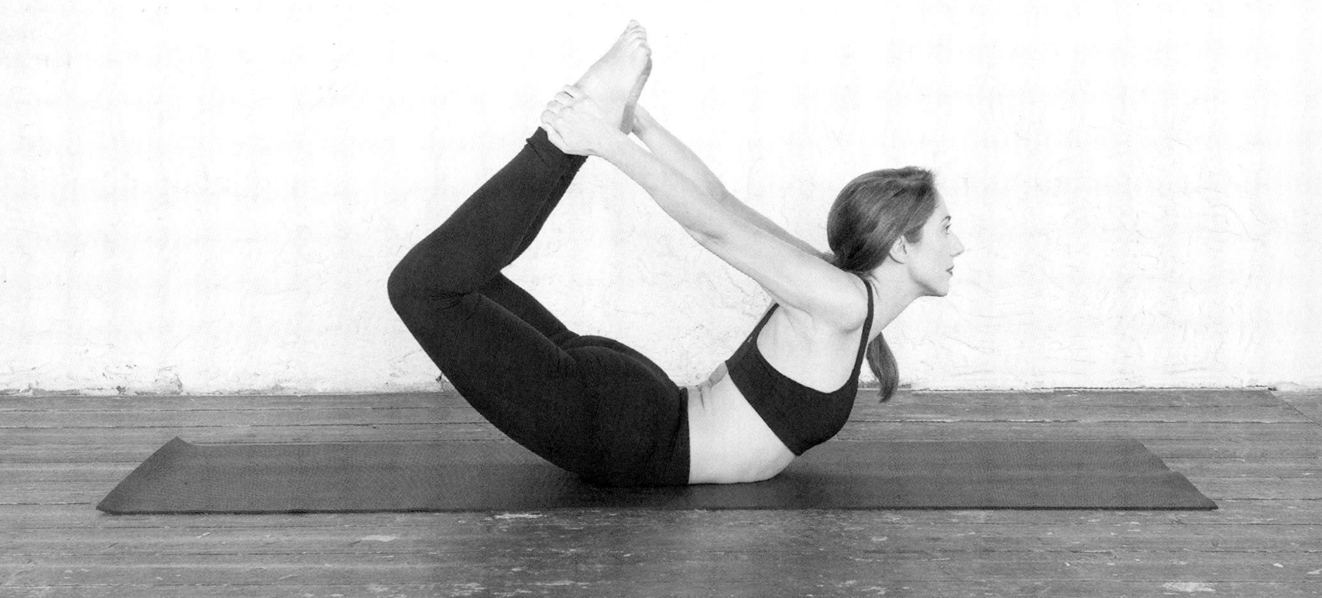

How to come into the pose

Lie down on your abdomen, with your forehead on the floor, knees shoulder-width apart.

Bend your knees and hold the ankles from the outside, with elbows straight.

Breathe in, push your feet into your hands, lift your chest and knees, and look diagonally upward.

Coming out of the pose

Breathe out and gently lower your chest and knees to the floor. Then release the grip on your ankles and lie down in Crocodile Pose.

Alignment cues

Elbows are straight. Use the opposing force of your feet kicking against your hands to lift yourself higher up.

Aim to keep your weight on your abdomen and bring your chest and knees into one line parallel to the floor.

Keep your neck extended from your spine. If flexibility allows, look diagonally upward, otherwise gaze forward.

Duration

Beginners: 10–20 seconds

Intermediate: 20–40 seconds

Advanced: 40 seconds–1 minute

Contraindications & cautions

- Abdominal issues (e.g. diarrhea, ulcer, menstrual pains, recent surgery)
- Shoulder issues
- Knee issues
- Cardiovascular issues

Modifications

If you have difficulties holding on to both ankles, you can practice Half Bow Pose, as explained in the variations section further on in the book.

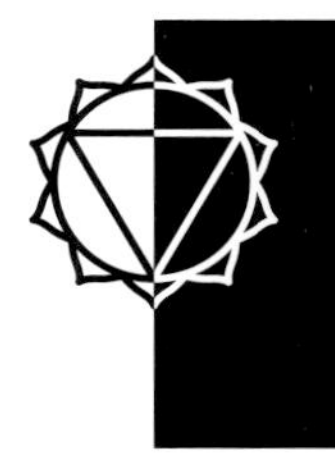

13. Ardha Matsyendrasana
Half Lord-of-the-Fishes Pose (aka Half Spinal Twist)

Benefits

Regular practice in a steady and comfortable manner within a balanced yoga asana program:

- stimulates the Solar Plexus Chakra and therefore stimulates and balances the functions of your stomach, gallbladder, liver, spleen, and pancreas;
- stimulates the functioning of your liver, having a detoxifying effect;
- aligns your spine as the ligaments attached to your spine stretch;
- rejuvenates and energizes your spine by massaging your intervertebral discs and causing more nutrients to diffuse into the discs, as well as stimulating the production of growth factors limited by aging;
- relieves back pain and stiffness from between your vertebrae;
- stimulates your pelvic region, providing a fresh blood supply to the reproductive organs and urinary system;
- massages your abdominal organs and increases your digestive juices;
- stimulates the functioning of your pancreas, and therefore balances blood sugar levels;
- relieves tension that may have built up in your back from forward-bending and backbending asanas;
- opens your chest and increases the oxygen supply to the lungs and therefore can have a therapeutic effect for asthma;
- relieves stiffness in your hip joints; and
- releases tension in your arms, shoulders, upper back, and neck.

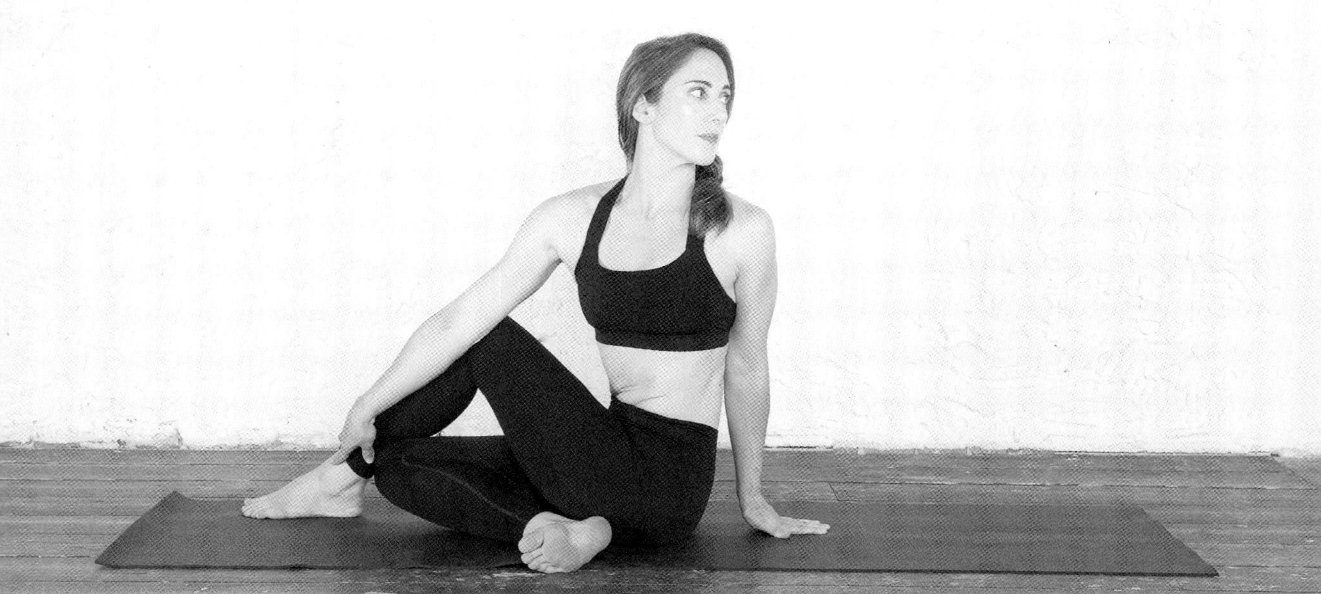

How to come into the pose

Sit with your legs stretched out in front of you.

Bend your right leg, bring the heel to your left hip, and make sure both hips are on the floor.

Cross your left foot over your right knee and place it on the floor.

Place your left hand behind your spine, palm flat on the floor (if possible).

Reach up with your right hand, bringing your right elbow to the outside of your left knee. If flexibility allows, you can hold on to your left ankle.

Twist gently toward your left, looking over your shoulder.

Coming out of the pose

Gently turn back, release your arms and unwind your legs. Then repeat on the other side.

Alignment cues

Keep both sitting bones on the floor, if necessary moving your lower heel out a bit.

Keep shoulders above hips, but do not lean on the hand behind your back.

Keep reaching out with the crown of your head, keeping your spine as erect as possible and the back of your neck elongated.

Duration

Beginners: 1 minute per side

Intermediate: 1–2 minutes per side

Advanced: 2–3 minutes per side

Contraindications & cautions

- Lower-back and spinal issues (e.g. chronic pain, herniated disc, sciatica, SI-joint instability)
- Abdominal issues (e.g. diarrhea, ulcer, menstrual pains, recent surgery)

Modifications

In case of any chronic back issue such as herniated disc, sciatica, or SI-joint issues, twisting should be approached with caution. The focus should be more on keeping the lower spine relatively straight and creating a gentle twist more in the thoracic part of the spine.

If, due to tightness in your lower back or hips, it is not possible to keep both sitting bones on the floor, straighten your lower leg.

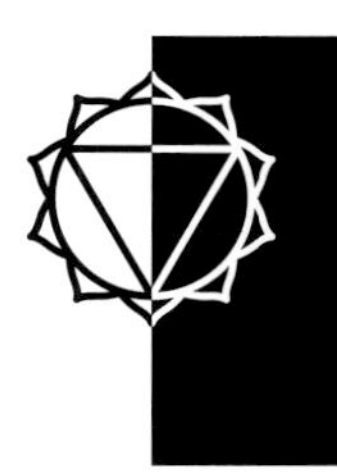

Asanas for the Svadhishthana Chakra (Sacral Chakra)

14. Sukha Kakasana

Easy Crow Pose

Benefits

Regular practice in a steady and comfortable manner within a balanced yoga asana program:

- stimulates the Sacral Chakra and therefore stimulates and balances the functions of your urinary tract, kidneys, and gonads;
- develops strength in the shoulders, arms, and wrists;
- benefits the circulatory system in the upper limbs and torso;
- opens the chest and stretches the intercostal muscles, therefore increasing lung capacity;
- increases core awareness, balance, and coordination;
- stretches and at the same time strengthens the groin and inner thighs;
- increases focus and concentration;
- removes fatigue; and
- increases vitality and willpower.

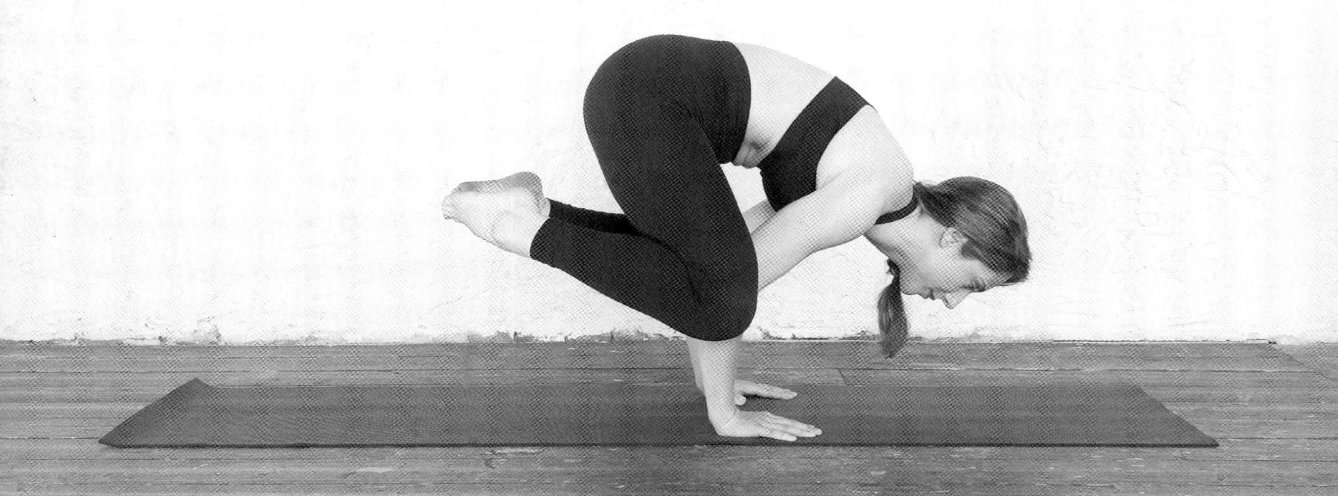

How to come into the pose

Sit on your toes, with heels (almost) together and knees apart.

Place your elbows in the crease of your knees (the fleshy part between lower and upper legs).

Keep your hands slightly higher than your knees, fingers spread widely and fingertips slightly pointed inwards.

Maintain this alignment as you shift your weight forward, placing your palms (shoulder-width apart) on the floor.

Focusing your eyes on a point half a meter in front of your fingertips on the floor, slowly lift your feet off the floor, one foot at a time.

Pulling both feet toward your hips, keep looking at a point on the floor approximately 1 foot in front of your fingertips.

Coming out of the pose

Shifting your weight backward, with control, place your feet on the floor and release your hands.

Alignment cues

Keep your core active by continuously lifting your heels up toward your buttocks.

Keep your back slightly rounded.

The angle between your hand and forearm should be 90 degrees. If it is not, lift your wrist slightly higher by placing a blanket underneath the lower part of your palm (so the upper part of palm and fingers are lower than the lower part of your palm and root of your thumb).

Duration

Beginners: 10–20 seconds

Intermediate: 20–40 seconds

Advanced: 40 seconds–1 minute

Contraindications & cautions

- Wrist issues
- Shoulder issues
- Knee issues
- Groin and hamstring issues
- Cardiovascular issues
- Hypertension

Modifications

If balancing is challenging initially, you can press the forehead against a cushion on the floor to practice the weight shift.

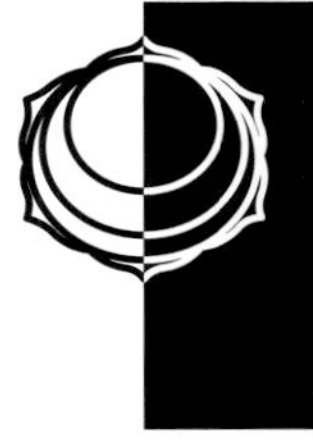

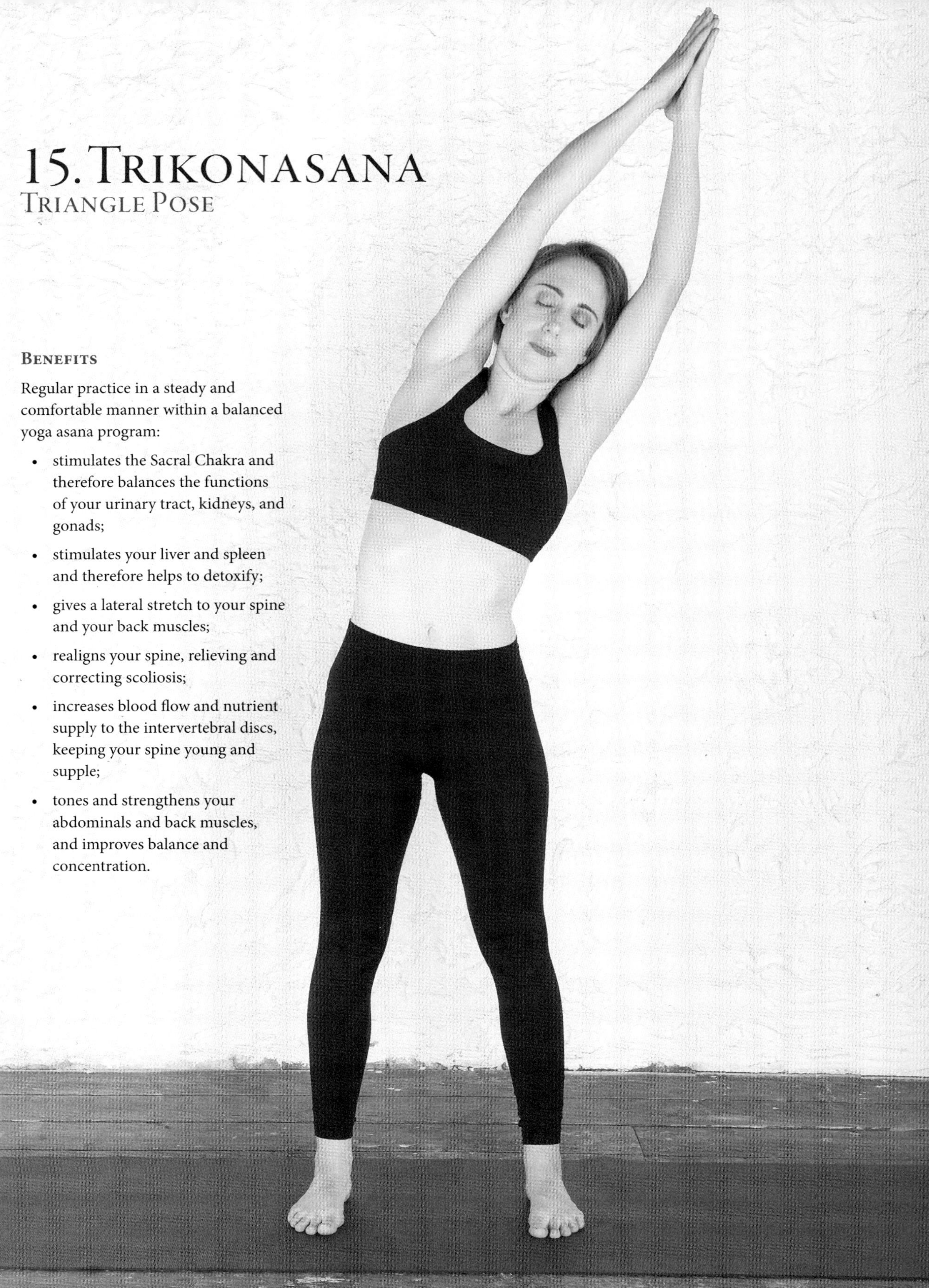

15. Trikonasana
Triangle Pose

Benefits

Regular practice in a steady and comfortable manner within a balanced yoga asana program:

- stimulates the Sacral Chakra and therefore balances the functions of your urinary tract, kidneys, and gonads;
- stimulates your liver and spleen and therefore helps to detoxify;
- gives a lateral stretch to your spine and your back muscles;
- realigns your spine, relieving and correcting scoliosis;
- increases blood flow and nutrient supply to the intervertebral discs, keeping your spine young and supple;
- tones and strengthens your abdominals and back muscles, and improves balance and concentration.

How to come into the pose

Stand straight, with your feet shoulder-width apart.

As you inhale, bring your arms up next to your ears and reach upward, extending and lengthening your spine.

Place your palms together, making sure that your hands stay in a straight line above your forehead.

As you exhale, press your right heel into the floor and reach up and out to your left side.

Extend your entire torso to your left, initiating the movement at the base of your spine and keeping both sides of your torso elongated.

Coming out of the pose

Inhale and return to the standing position. Relax your arms for a moment, then repeat on the other side.

Alignment cues

Keep your feet parallel and your hips square. Do not allow the hip to "pop" out to one side.

Make sure not to collapse at the rib cage, but keep reaching up and out.

Your hands are neither right above your head nor in front of your head. They are placed so that the roots of your thumbs are directly in line with your forehead, reaching up at the same time.

Shoulders will lift up, but make sure to keep the back of your neck elongated.

Duration

Beginners: 20–30 seconds each side

Intermediate: 30–45 seconds each side

Advanced: 45–90 seconds each side

Contraindications & cautions

There are no general contraindications for this pose, if practiced correctly. But this pose, even though it looks simple, is quite heavy. If you feel dizzy or start to sweat heavily, release the pose.

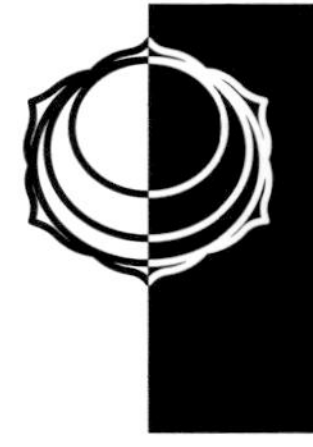

Asanas for the Muladhara Chakra (Root Chakra)

16. Vrkshasana
Tree Pose

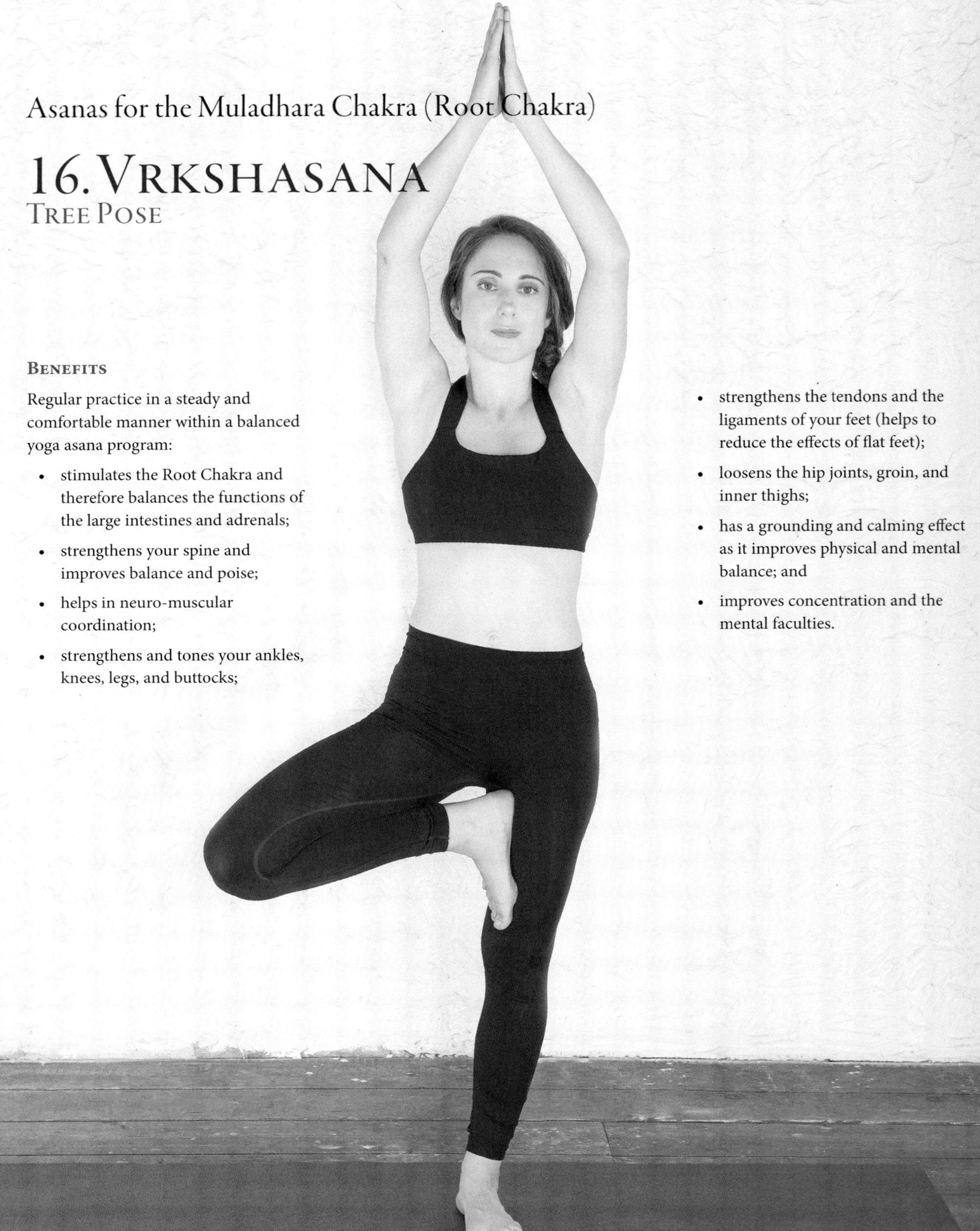

Benefits

Regular practice in a steady and comfortable manner within a balanced yoga asana program:

- stimulates the Root Chakra and therefore balances the functions of the large intestines and adrenals;
- strengthens your spine and improves balance and poise;
- helps in neuro-muscular coordination;
- strengthens and tones your ankles, knees, legs, and buttocks;
- strengthens the tendons and the ligaments of your feet (helps to reduce the effects of flat feet);
- loosens the hip joints, groin, and inner thighs;
- has a grounding and calming effect as it improves physical and mental balance; and
- improves concentration and the mental faculties.

How to come into the pose

Stand straight, with your feet together.

Raise your hands above your head and place your palms together, keeping them in line with your forehead.

Inhale, and raise your right foot and place it against your left inner thigh.

Keep your focus on a point slightly above eye level (approximately 2 meters away), and breathe evenly.

Coming out of the pose

Gently bring your hands down. Release your right foot to the floor and repeat on the other side.

Alignment cues

Your foot should ideally be placed against the opposite inner thigh.

Your hands are reaching toward the ceiling. Make sure to keep the roots of your thumbs in line with your forehead, not over your head and not in front of your face.

Your elbows are slightly bent, and your shoulders lifted only slightly.

The knee of your upper foot is pointing sideways, rotating the leg at the hip joint without lifting your hip up.

Your spine is in a natural curve. Make sure not to "hang" into the lower back and not to lift the chest.

Duration

Beginners: 30 seconds–1 minute each side

Intermediate: 1–3 minutes each side

Advanced: 3–5 minutes each side

Contraindications & cautions

- Ankle issues
- Knee issues

Modifications

Make sure to rotate the working leg at the hip and place it wherever it reaches along the standing leg. You should not feel strain in the ankle or knee joint. The lifted foot can also be placed along the ankle or lower leg or along the inside of your knee (making sure to place the arch of the foot against the side of your knee, not the heel or ball of your foot).

If you feel strain in your arms or shoulders, keep your hands in the Prayer position in front of your chest instead of reaching them up toward the ceiling.

For anyone who might be in danger of losing balance and falling, it is recommended to practice this pose close to a wall and to take support if necessary.

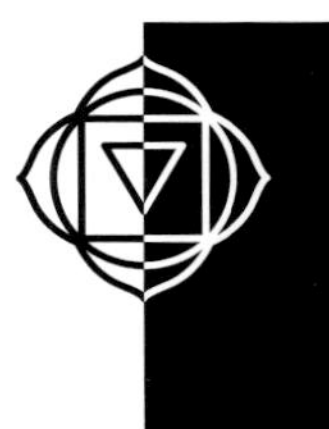

17. Tadasana
Mountain Pose

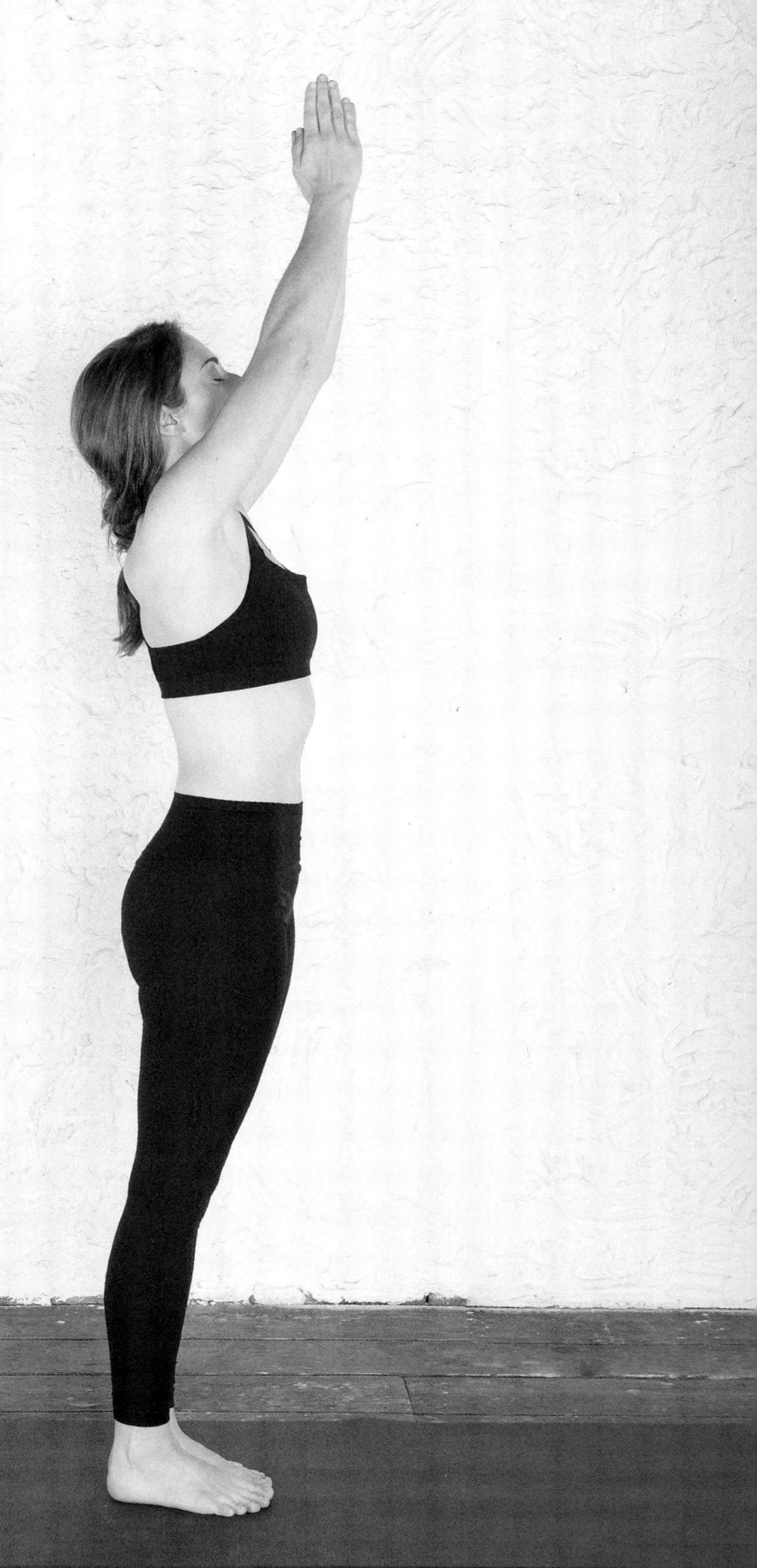

Benefits

Regular practice in a steady and comfortable manner within a balanced yoga asana program:

- stimulates the Muladhara Chakra and therefore balances the functions of your large intestines and adrenals;
- strengthens your spine and improves balance and poise;
- helps in neuro-muscular co-ordination;
- increases strength, power, and mobility in your feet, ankles, thighs, and hips;
- strengthens the tendons and the ligaments of the feet (helping to reduce the effects of flat feet);
- improves overall posture;
- improves the harmony between the right and left sides of your body;
- activates and rejuvenates your entire body;
- harmonizes your body and mind; and
- improves concentration and mental faculties.

How to come into the pose

Stand straight, with the toes and heels of your feet together.

Extend your arms to the ceiling, palms together, keeping your hands in line with your forehead.

Look up in between your palms and close your eyes.

Coming out of the pose

Gently bring your palms in front of your chest and open your eyes.

Alignment cues

Both feet are together, toes and heels touching each other.

Arms are above your head, in line with your forehead.

Elbows are slightly bent, shoulders lifted only slightly.

Chin is slightly lifted, without dropping your head backward.

Eyes are closed and the entire focus is on standing as still and stably as possible, avoiding any weight shift and movement.

Duration

Beginners: 30–60 seconds

Intermediate: 1–2 minutes

Advanced: 2–4 minutes

Contraindications & cautions

There are no general contraindications for this pose. This pose, even though it looks simple, becomes heavy after 30 seconds. If you feel dizzy or start to sweat heavily, release the pose.

Modifications

If closing your eyes provokes a sense of dizziness or struggle for balance, keep your eyes open and simply look at the eye-shaped space in between your palms.

If looking up results in tension or pain in your neck or shoulders, look straight forward and close your eyes.

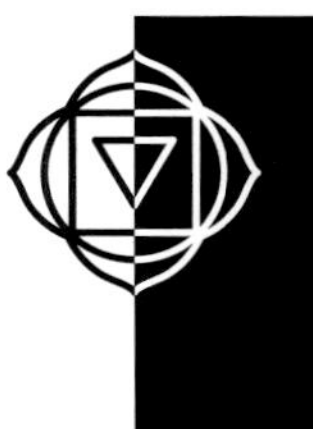

Overview I: The Basic Sequence

1	Initial Relaxation	5 min.
2	(Chanting Om)	
3	Kapalbhati Skull-Shining Breath	3 rounds (5 min.)
4	Anulom Vilom Alternate Nostril Breathing	5 min.
5	Shavasana Corpse Pose	30–45 sec.
6	Surya Namaskara Sun Salutation	6–8 rounds (10 min.)
7	Shavasana Corpse Pose	1 min.
8	Leg Raises	6–10 rep.
9	Shashankasana Child's Pose	30–45 sec.
10	Dolphin	10 rep.
11	Shashankasana Child's Pose	30–45 sec.
12	Shirshasana Headstand Pose	1 min.
13	Shashankasana Child's Pose	30–45 sec.
14	Salamba Sarvangasana Shoulderstand Pose	1 min.
15	Halasana Plough Pose	30 sec.
16	Ardha Setu Bandhasana Half Bridge Pose	30 sec.
17	Pawanmuktasana Air Release Pose	30–45 sec.
18	Matsyasana Fish Pose	30 sec.
19	Shavasana Corpse Pose	30–45 sec.
20	Sukha Gomukhasana Easy Cow Face Pose	1 min. each side
21	Paschimottanasana Seated Forward Bend Pose	1 min.
22	Purvottanasana Upward Plank Pose	10 sec.
23	Makarasana Crocodile Pose	30–45 sec.
24	Bhujangasana Cobra Pose	30–60 sec.
25	Makarasana Crocodile Pose	30–45 sec.
26	Shalabhasana Locust Pose	10–20 sec.
27	Makarasana Crocodile Pose	30–45 sec.
28	Dhanurasana Bow Pose	10–20 sec.
29	Shashankasana Child's Pose	30–45 sec.
30	Ardha Matsyendrasana Half Spinal Twist	30 sec. each side
31	Sukha Kakasana Easy Crow Pose	30 sec.
32	Trikonasana Triangle Pose	30 sec. each side
33	Vrkshasana Tree Pose	1 min. each side
34	Tadasana Mountain Pose	1 min.
35	Final Relaxation	15 min.
36	(Chanting Om Shanti)	

* The durations mentioned do not take into account the time needed for explanation, instructions, and getting into the pose. The timings as displayed above, plus approximately 10–15 minutes extra, are suitable for a 90-minute basic Hatha Yoga class.

Part V

Mastering Sequencing: Creating Customized Sequences

The value of regularity in your yoga routine cannot be over-emphasized. Regularity compounds growth from class to class, session to session. This includes regularity in the time of your practice, and in the sequence of asanas. Such regularity maximizes yoga's physical and mental benefits. If, on the other hand, the session is different every time, your muscle memory builds up more slowly. As a result, you will see less progress. Also, in learning a new routine, your attention will be focused outwardly when it should be anchored deeply within your poses and the gaps between them.

Whenever we approach the topic of creating variation in sequencing we rely on the five fundamental building blocks (page 52) and the basic sequence (page 112) as a strong foundation.

Swami Sivananda created the famous Rishikesh sequence. This foundation provides the basis of our sequence. This flow of poses stimulates and balances the internal body. At the same time, its succession of forward and backward bends, inversions and upright positions, strengthening and stretching movements, twisting and side-bending stretches, and balancing and relaxation phases relaxes, strengthens, and revitalizes the physical body.

When creating a new yoga sequence, initially you should replace only two to three asanas of the basic sequence, and sometimes a warming-up exercise. As you become more adept and better understand the principles, you can start to be more creative and to vary more asanas. You can also start to design sequences toward a certain asana, goal, or theme. As you start to vary your sessions, remember that even when working toward a goal—such as a certain advanced asana, or hip opening, or balancing—a maximum of 40 percent of the asanas and time should be dedicated to the goal. The remaining 60 percent should ensure that the practice stays balanced in terms of chakras, but also on a muscular level (for instance, proper warm-up and balanced forward and backward bends, inversions and upright poses, strengthening and stretching movements, twisting and side-bending stretches, balancing and relaxation).

The easiest way to sequencing is to always keep the structure of the basic sequence by replacing asanas with their variations as categorized in the following chapters. So even if you want to focus on one body part (for example, the hamstrings) you should still keep the structure of the basic sequence. You can, though, decrease the number of postures or duration of postures so that you will have more time to work toward the class goal.

A detailed categorization will follow in the chapters to come, where you will find the chakra categories again, starting with the Crown Chakra and moving downward toward the Root Chakra. In every chakra section there are subsections in which we have provided at least 2 and up to 20 variations per asana. Just before you get started on that, you can also have a look at the following table, where you will find an overview of a more generalized structure of a holistic Hatha Yoga class.

Overview II: General Structure

1	Initial Relaxation (Chanting Om)	5 min.
2	Breathing exercises	10 min.
3	Sun Salutation	10 min.
4	Specific warm-up (e.g. abdominals, upper-body strength)	10 min.
5	Crown & Third Eye Chakra: Headstand variations	5 min.
6	Throat Chakra: Throat squeeze postures	5 min.
7	Heart Chakra: Chest openers, lying on the back or seated	5 min.
8	Solar Plexus Chakra: Seated forward bends and hip openers	5 min.
9	Solar Plexus Chakra: Prone backbends and seated twists	10 min.
10	Sacral Chakra: Hand-balancing postures, squatting postures, standing forward and side-folding postures	5 min.
11	Root Chakra: Standing postures	5 min.
12	Final Relaxation (Chanting Om Shanti)	15 min.

Chapter 11

Warming-Up Variations

Surya Namaskara Variation
Easy Sun Salute

The following variation of the Sun Salutation can be done and applied by anyone with restricted movement, whether from injury or a chronic condition, old age or pregnancy.

Basic Instructions

Starting position: Stand straight, with your spine erect and shoulders relaxed. Your feet are shoulder-width apart. Your knees are straight but not hyperextended. Your arms are relaxed next to your body.

1. **Breathe in and out, bringing your palms together in front of your chest.**

   Shoulders and elbows are relaxed. Knees are straight but relaxed. Back of your neck is long. Reach up with the crown of your head toward the ceiling.

2. **Breathe in and reach your arms up toward the ceiling.**

   Your arms are alongside your ears. Look straight forward, with the back of your neck elongated. Keep your spine's natural curve. Do not arch your lower back or tuck your tailbone under.

3. **Breathe out, reach forward and out, placing your palms on the floor, in front of or in between your feet.**

   Knees are slightly bent. Look in between your knees, with the crown of your head reaching toward the floor.

4. **Keeping your hands there, breathe in and bring your right knee behind you on the floor.**

   Your knee is resting below your pelvis on the floor. Look forward, opening your chest and keeping the back of your neck elongated.

5. **Breathe out and bring your left knee behind you to the floor.**

   Your knee is resting below your pelvis, on the floor. Look to the floor, with the back of your neck elongated. Keep your arms perpendicular to the floor, with your hands directly under your shoulders and flat on the floor. Your knees are hip-width apart.

6. **Breathe in, push your belly button toward the floor, raise your chin, and lift your tailbone.**

   Your elbows are straight and shoulders are away from your ears.

7. **Breathe out and round your spine toward the ceiling.**

   Keep your hands and knees in their original positions. Release your head toward the floor, but avoid forcing your chin toward your chest.

8. **Breathe in and bring your right foot forward outside your right hand.**

   Your left knee remains on the floor. Look forward, open your chest and keep the back of your neck elongated.

9. **Breathe out, keeping your hands where they are, and bring your left foot forward outside your left hand.**

   Your knees are slightly bent. Look in between your knees, with the crown of your head reaching toward the floor.

10. **Breathe in and reach your hands forward and up to the ceiling.**

    Your arms are alongside your ears. Look straight forward, with the back of your neck elongated. Keep your spine's natural curve. Do not arch your lower back or tuck your tailbone under.

11. **Breathe out, bringing your hands in front of your chest, palms together.**

    This completes half a round. Repeat to the left (left leg stepping first back and forward) to complete one full round of Sun Salutation. Perform 4–8 rounds, then rest in Corpse Pose.

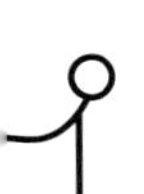
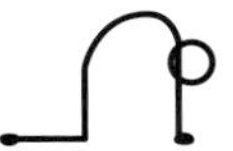
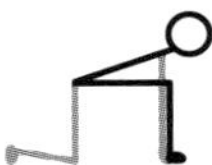
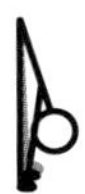

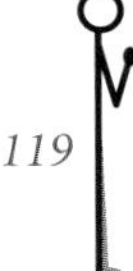

Double Leg Raises Variations

Single Leg Raises

Basic Instructions

Lie on your back, with your feet together and flexed.

Keep your arms by your sides, with your palms facing downward.

Your hands are either tucked in toward your hips or under your hips for extra support.

Keep your back flat on the mat, with the back of your neck elongated and your chin slightly tucked in.

Lift your right leg up until almost perpendicular to the floor and gently lower it down again.

(Lower only as far as you can still keep control in your abdomen and your lower back relatively flat against the floor.) Repeat 6 times to the right and to the left, then rest in Corpse Pose.

Modifications & Adjustments

To decrease the difficulty level of this exercise, you can also keep the static leg bent, with your foot resting on the floor. That will allow you to further relax the lower back during the exercise.

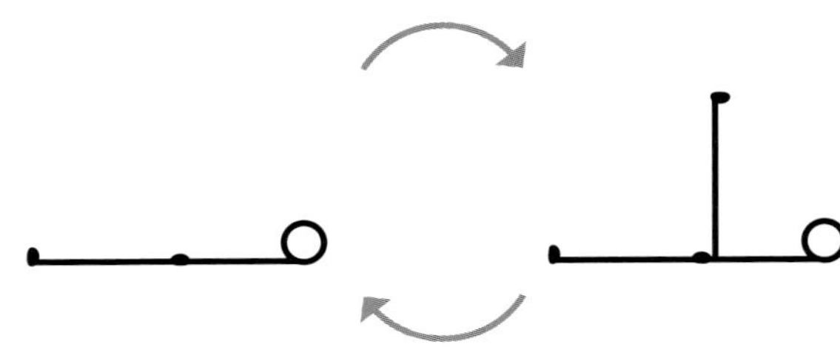

Yogic Bicycle

Basic Instructions

Lie flat on the floor, with your lower back pressed toward the mat.

Interlace your fingers, and place your hands behind your head.

Bring your knees in toward your chest, and lift your shoulder blades off the floor.

Straighten your right leg out to about a 45-degree angle to the floor while turning your upper body toward your left knee.

Bring your right elbow toward the outside of your left knee, making sure your rib cage is moving, and not just your elbows.

Now switch sides, and repeat the same motion on the other side to complete one repetition.

Repeat 6–12 times, then relax in Corpse Pose.

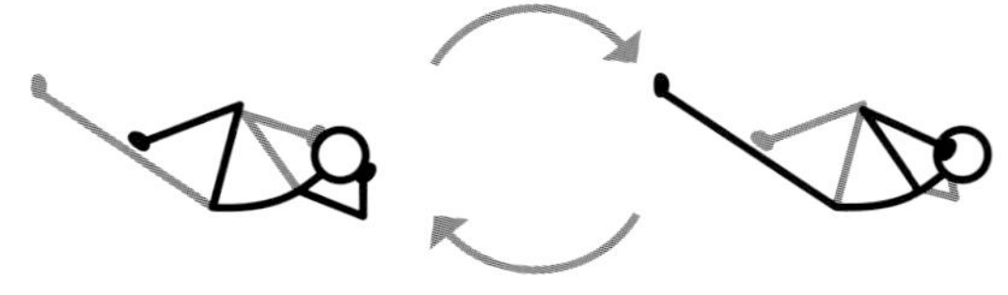

Pilates Splits

Basic Instructions

Lie on your back and lift your upper body off the floor so that your shoulder blades hover.

Lift your left leg off the floor and bring your right leg to 90 degrees.

Use your hands to gently pull your right shin toward your nose.

Keep your upper body lifted as you switch your legs to complete one repetition.

Repeat 6–12 times, then relax in Corpse Pose.

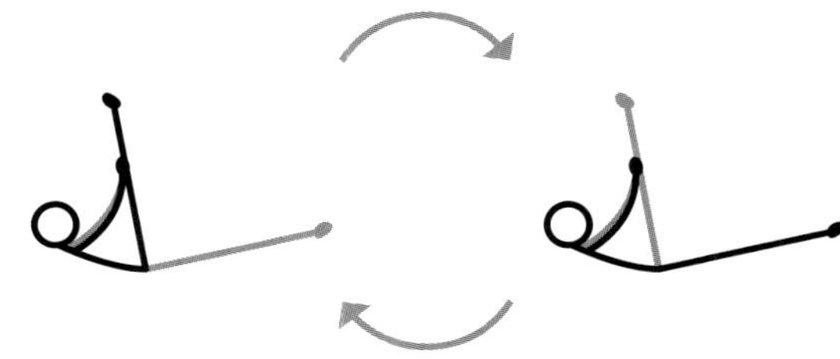

V-Sits

Basic Instructions

Lie on your back and reach your arms overhead, with your palms together and off the floor.

Lift your head and shoulders, lifting your shoulder blades off the floor as well.

Lift your legs off the floor to about a 45-degree angle, and point your feet.

Now sweep your arms sideways and forward and lift your upper body and legs into a V shape, balancing on your sitting bones.

Reach with your hands forward along your knees, keeping your lower back and chest lifted.

Now roll your back down as you sweep your hands sideways back toward the overhead position.

Stop when your back is on the floor, but not your head, shoulders, or legs.

Repeat 6–10 times, then rest in Corpse Pose.

Modifications & Adjustments

If sitting up with straight legs is too intense due to tight hamstrings, you can keep your knees bent. To make this exercise less difficult, catch on to the back of your legs as you sit up.

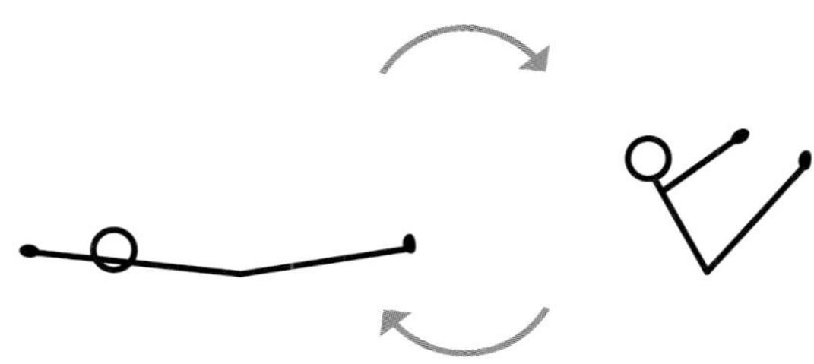

Dolphin Variations
Regular Push-Ups

Basic Instructions

Come onto all fours and place your hands below your shoulders, middle fingers pointing forward.

Straighten your legs and come into a high plank position with your feet hip- or shoulder-width apart.

Ground your toes in the floor and engage your core, glutes, and hamstrings to bring your body into one flat, straight line.

Begin to lower your body—keeping your back flat and eyes focused about a meter in front of you to keep a neutral neck—until your chest almost touches the floor.

Keep your elbows tucked in toward your body.

Keeping your core and entire body engaged, push your body back to the starting position.

Repeat 5–10 times, then rest in Child's Pose.

Modifications & adjustments

Initially you may set your hands wider: mat-width apart. Turn your arms slightly inward and allow your elbows to move sideways. In this way your chest assists the action of your arms, and this is easier for most people.

You can also keep your knees on the floor, with your feet crossed at the ankles. Make sure to keep your body in a straight line here as well. Do not allow your hips to come up.

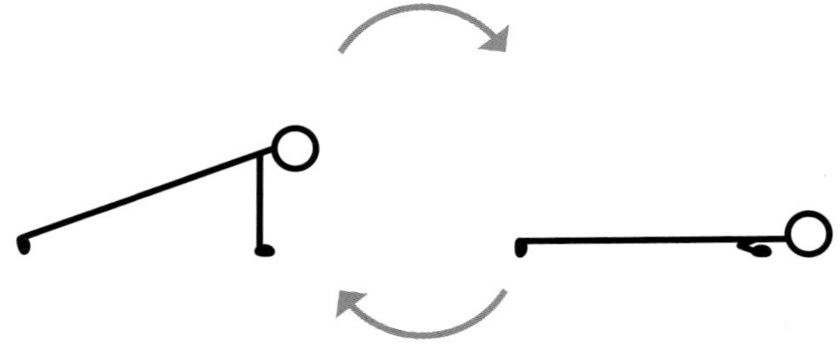

Dand Kriya–Yoga Push-Ups

Basic Instructions

Come into Downward-Facing Dog Pose, with your hands in line with your shoulders and feet hip-width apart.

Now, reaching with your nose down to the floor, lower your body and pull your head toward your hands to then push upward into an Upward-Facing Dog position with your toes curled on the floor.

From there, keeping your arms straight, push your hips up and back and return to the starting position.

Repeat 5–10 times, then rest in Child's Pose.

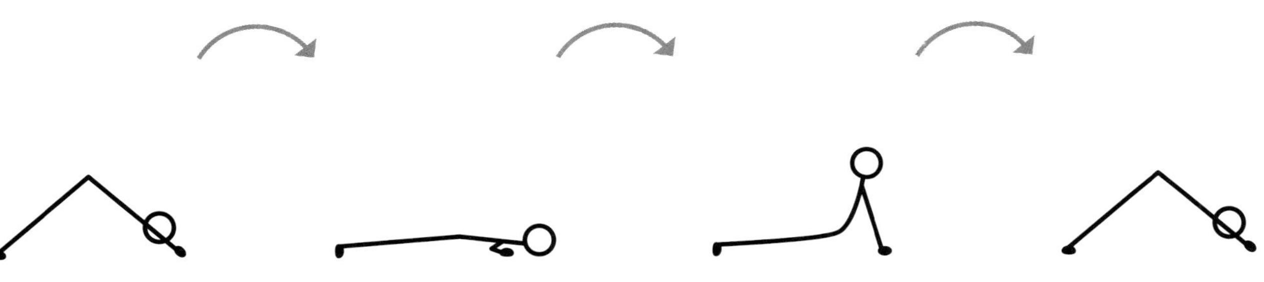

Elbow Push-Ups

Basic Instructions

Come onto all fours and place your hands below your shoulders, middle fingers pointing forward.

Straighten your legs and come into a high plank position with your feet hip- or shoulder-width apart.

Ground your toes into the floor and engage your core, glutes, and hamstrings to bring your body into one flat, straight line.

Lift your right hand off the floor and place your right forearm on the floor on the same spot where your hand just was.

Do the same with your left arm.

Now lift your right forearm off the floor and place your palm back on the floor.

Follow again with your left arm.

Repeat 15–20 times, then rest in Child's Pose.

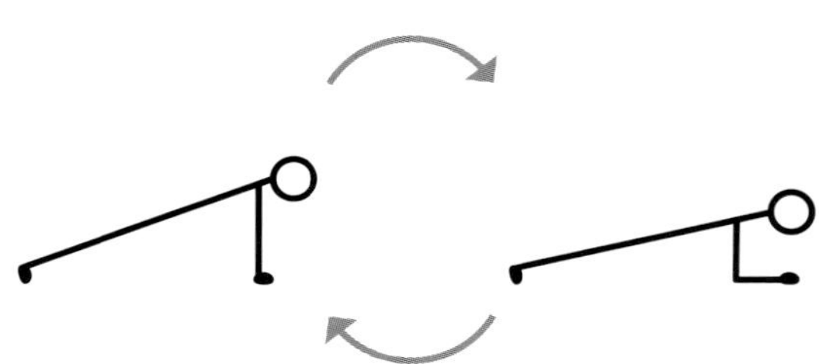

Spiderman Push-Ups

Basic Instructions

Start in Downward-Facing Dog Pose, with your hands in line with your shoulders and feet hip-width apart.

Look forward and bring your right knee to your right elbow or upper arm and lower your entire body down into a low plank position.

Bend your left elbow as well and hug it in to your waist.

Now straighten your arms, place your right foot back on the floor, and raise your hips up into the starting position.

Repeat to your left to complete one round.

Do 5–10 rounds, then rest in Child's Pose.

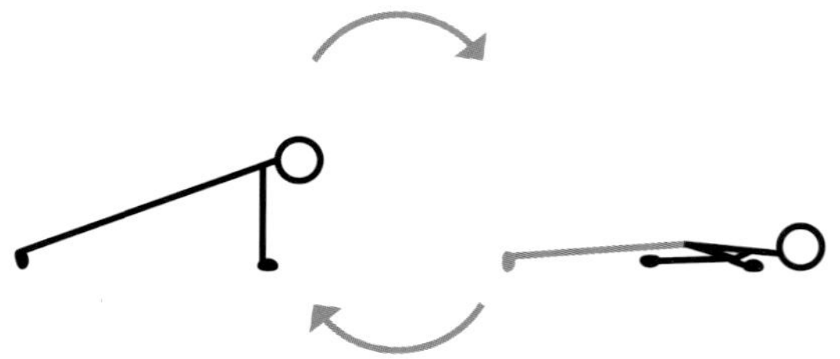

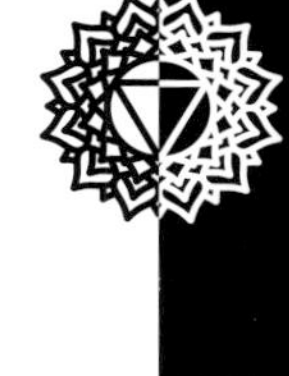

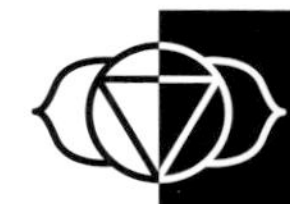

Chapter 12

Variations for the Crown & Third-Eye Chakras

Shirshasana (Headstand) Variations

The following is valid for all the variations to Headstand:

Important alignment cues

Push your body parts (hands, forearms, or elbows) that are supporting your head firmly into the floor and push your shoulders away from your ears so your neck is supported and you have a strong and solid base for your Headstand.

Modifications & adjustments

When practicing on a hard surface and especially if holding the pose for a long duration, place a blanket under your head and arms for extra cushioning.

Counter-pose

Before and after performing any variation of Headstand, stay in Child's Pose for 20–30 seconds. After long holds of Headstand, you might even increase that duration to 60 seconds. This helps to regulate the blood pressure toward the head and reduce feelings of dizziness. After holds of 5 minutes or more, after doing Child's Pose for about 60 seconds, also include Camel Pose for 20–40 seconds.

Sukha Shirshasana
Easy Headstand (Preparatory Pose)

How to come into the pose

Sit on your knees, with your hips resting on your heels, and hold your elbows to measure the ideal distance.

Then bring your arms to the floor under your shoulders.

Place your forearms on the floor and interlock your fingers.

Place the top of your head on the floor, with the back of your head in your cupped hands.

Curl your toes, straighten your legs, and walk as close toward your chest as possible.

Keeping your feet on the ground, hold the pose steadily for as long as comfortable, and breathe evenly.

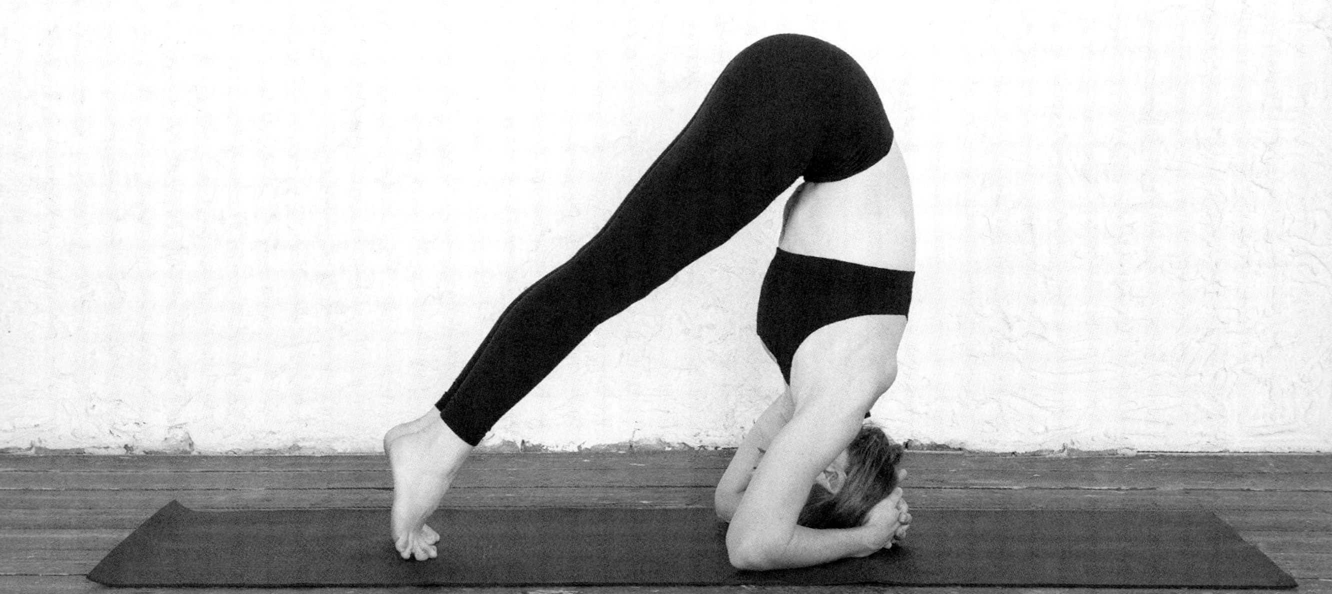

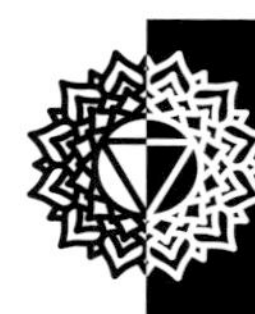

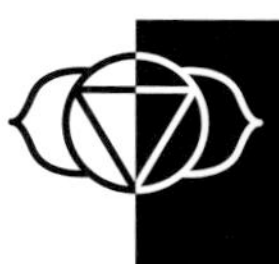

Next pose

Rest in Child's Pose for 30–45 seconds, then continue with Shoulderstand or a variation thereof.

Alignment cues

Push your elbows firmly into the floor and push your shoulders away from your ears.

Aim to shift your weight as much as possible to your head and elbows, while keeping your feet on the floor (heels may be lifted off the floor).

Contraindications & cautions

The same contraindications and cautions apply as in Headstand.

Modifications & adjustments

This variation of Headstand can be straining on your neck if your back is too rounded. This is usually the case for people whose hamstrings or lower back is tight. In that case, focus on keeping your neck elongated, drawing your shoulder blades away from your ears and toward your waist. Also hold for a shorter duration. If this is too difficult still, you can use a block under your feet to elevate your hips higher up over your shoulders and to decrease roundness in your back.

Eka Pada Shirshasana
One-Legged Headstand

How to come into the pose

Sit on your knees, with your hips resting on your heels.

Hold your elbows, place your forearms on the floor, and interlock your fingers.

Place the top of your head on the floor, with the back of your head in your cupped hands.

Curl your toes, straighten your legs, and walk toward your chest, aiming to bring your hips over your shoulders.

While pushing your left foot into the floor, lift your right leg up to the ceiling.

Hold the pose steadily as long as comfortable and breathe evenly.

Take a short rest in Child's Pose, then repeat on the other side.

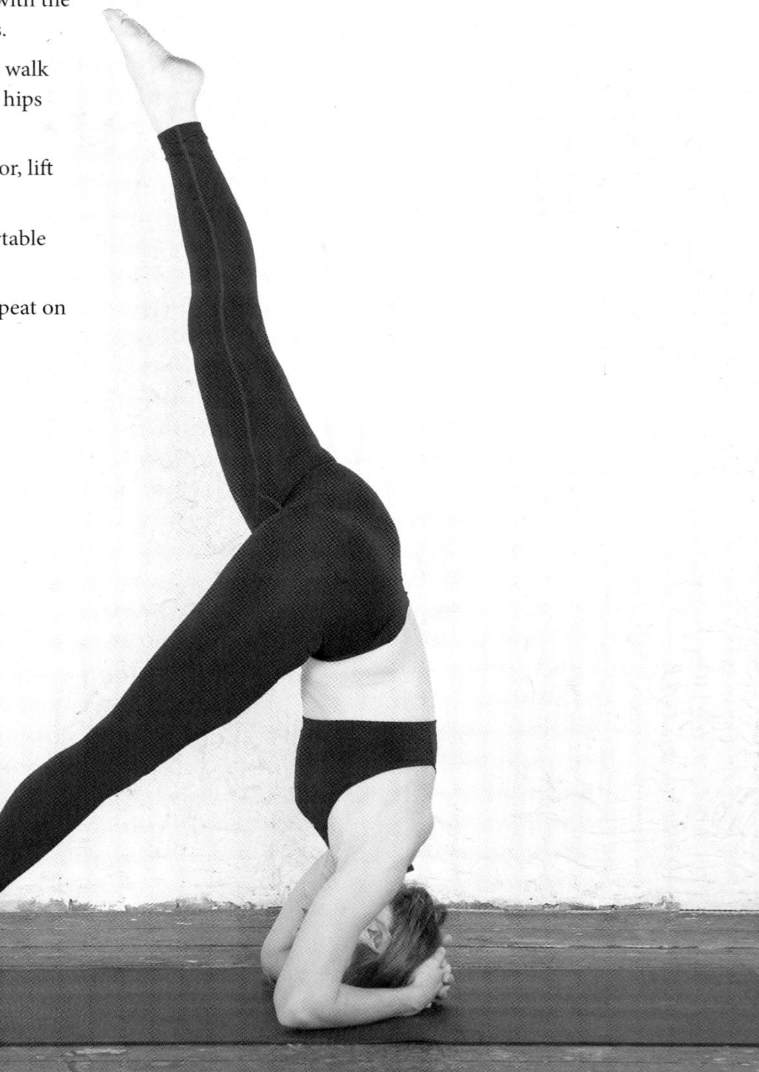

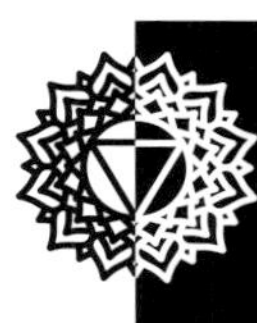

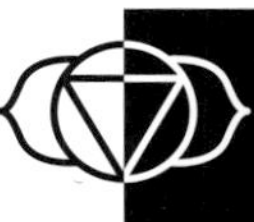

Next pose

Rest in Child's Pose for 30–45 seconds, then continue with Shoulderstand or a variation thereof.

Alignment cues

Push your elbows firmly into the floor and your shoulders away from your ears.

Shift your weight as much as possible to your head and elbows.

Use your foot on the floor as mere support, placing as little weight as possible on that foot.

Your foot reaching up toward the ceiling is relaxed, ideally, but can be flexed or pointed for extra opposition.

Contraindications & cautions

The same contraindications and cautions apply as in Headstand.

Modifications & adjustments

This variation of Headstand can be straining on your neck if your back is too rounded. This is usually the case with people whose hamstrings or hips are tight. In that case, focus on keeping your neck elongated, drawing your shoulder blades away from your ears toward your waist. Also hold for a shorter duration. If this is too difficult still, you can use a block under your foot to elevate your hips higher up over your shoulders and to decrease roundness in your back.

Ardha Shirshasana
Half Headstand

How to come into the pose

Sit on your knees, with your hips resting on your heels.

Hold your elbows, place your forearms on the floor, and interlock your fingers.

Place the top of your head on the floor, with the back of your head in your cupped hands.

Curl your toes, straighten your legs, and walk toward your chest.

Bring your knees one by one to your chest, lifting your feet off the floor.

Hold the pose steadily as long as comfortable and breathe evenly.

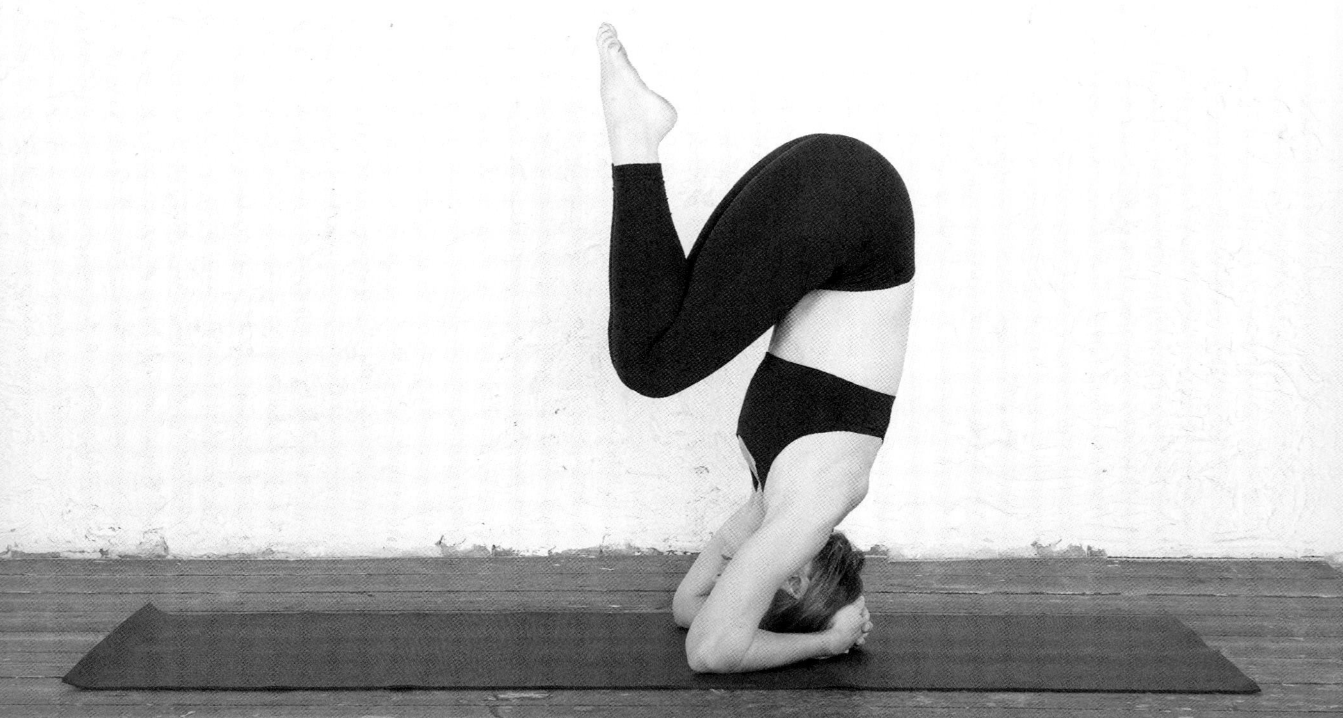

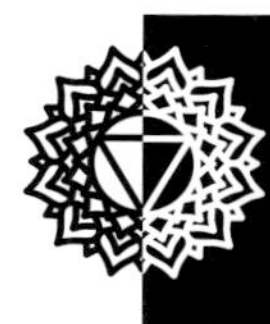

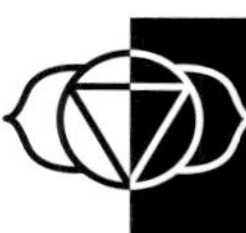

Next pose

Rest in Child's Pose for 30–45 seconds, then continue with Shoulderstand or a variation thereof.

Alignment cues

Keep your hips over your shoulders, with your knees as close as possible to your chest.

Push your elbows firmly into the floor and push your shoulders away from your ears.

If your back is rounded, lift your knees to hip level.

Contraindications & cautions

The same contraindications and cautions apply as in Headstand.

Modifications & adjustments

If you cannot bring both knees into your chest, you can alternate bringing your right knee and your left knee separately to your chest. The closer your knees are drawn into your chest the more difficult the pose is. If you find it too difficult or feel strain in your neck, keep your knees bent but lift them slightly upward. (You can go as far as bringing your knees in line with your pelvis.)

Vistrit Pada Shirshasana
Headstand with Leg Variations

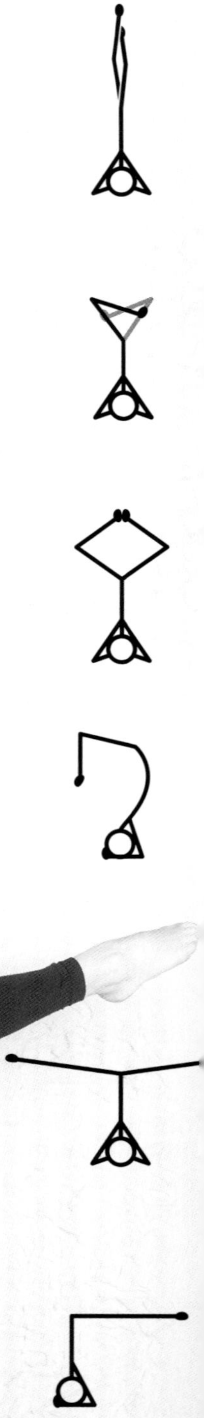

How to come into the pose

Come into a stable and comfortable Headstand.

Create a firm foundation with your elbows, which keeps the movement in your upper body at a minimum, then move into one of the following leg variations.

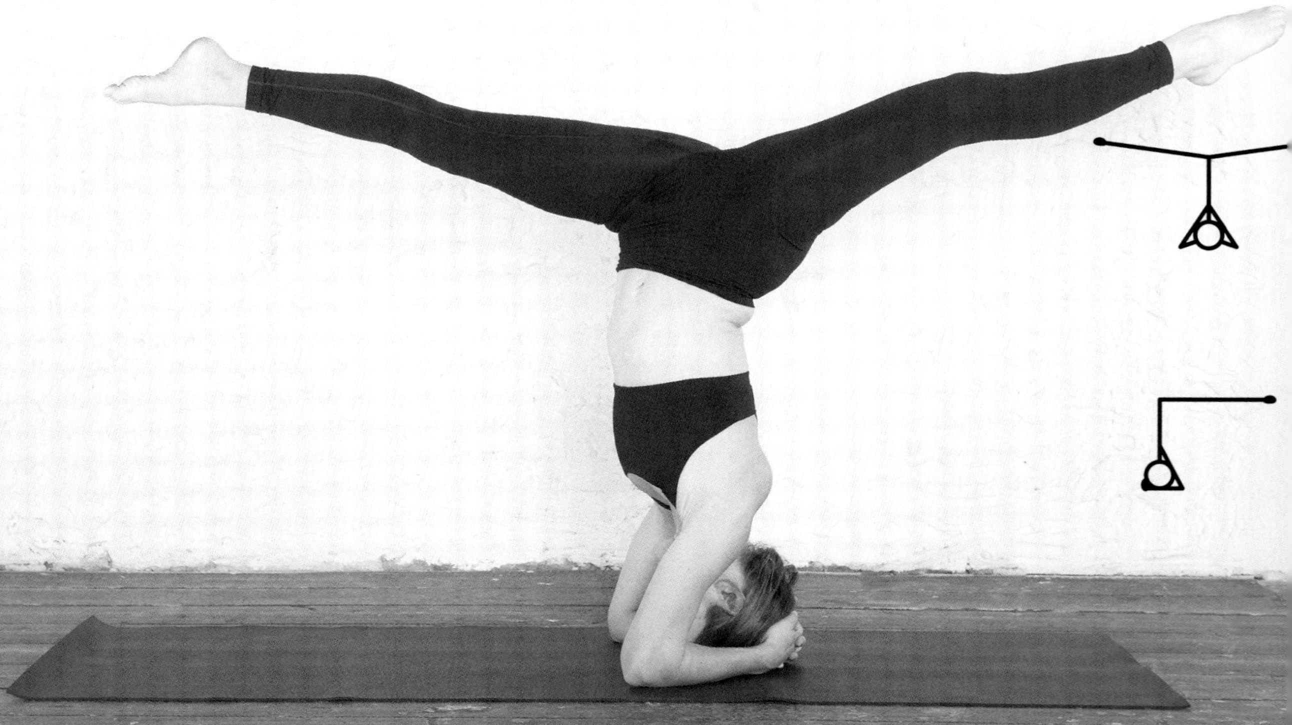

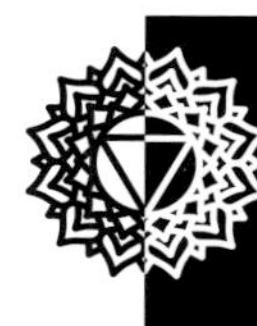

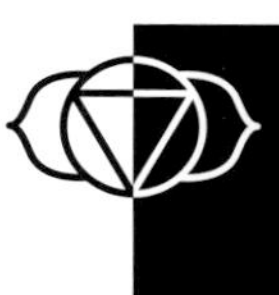

Next pose

Rest in Child's Pose for 30–45 seconds, then continue with Shoulderstand or a variation thereof.

Alignment cues

The movement happens in your legs only.

Your arms, shoulders, and head stay in the same position.

After each leg variation, come back into the basic Headstand before continuing with another variation.

Contraindications & cautions

The same contraindications and cautions apply as in Headstand.

Modifications & adjustments

These variations should be practiced only after you are comfortable and stable for at least 1 minute in the basic version of Headstand and can enter and exit the pose with control.

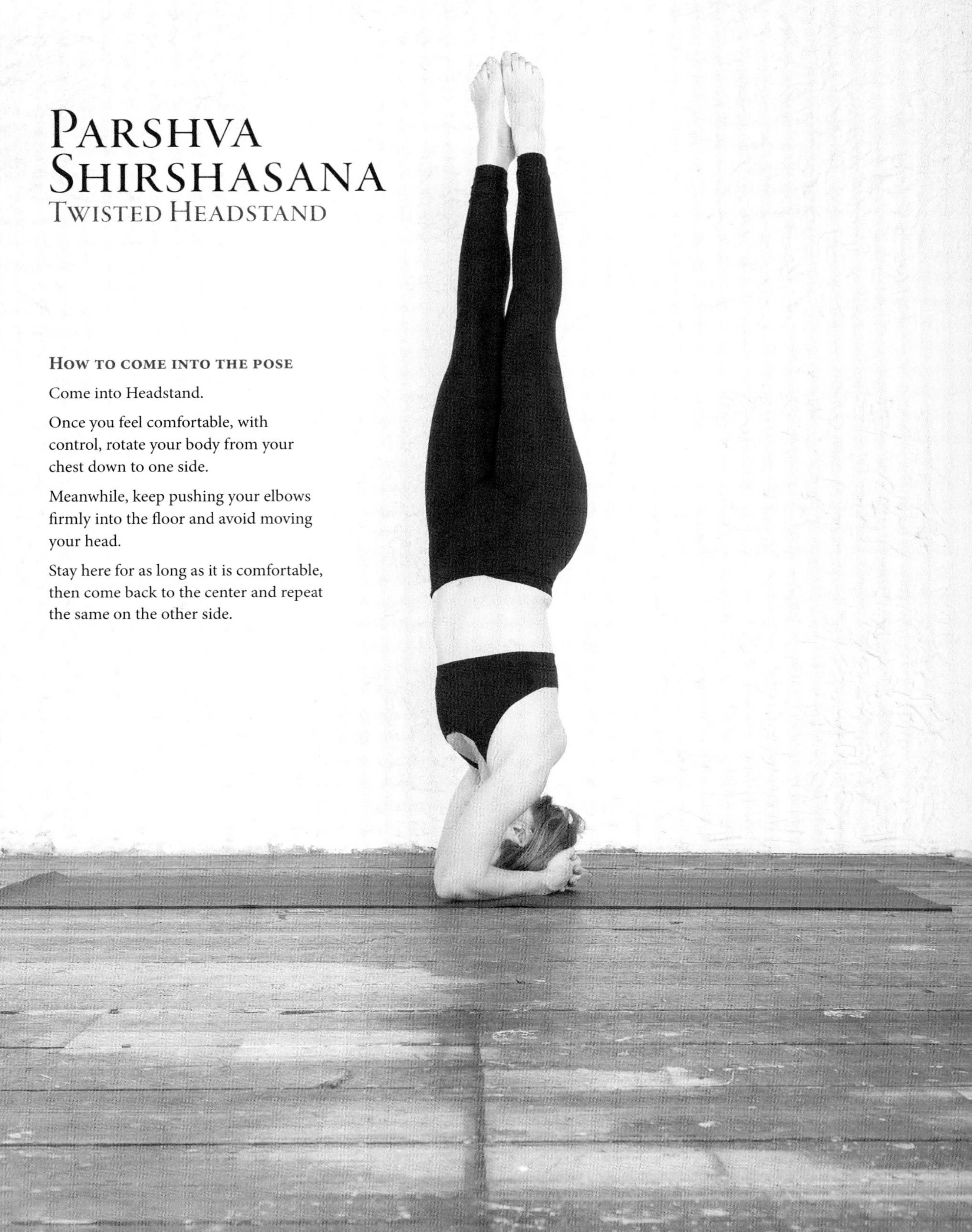

Parshva Shirshasana

Twisted Headstand

How to come into the pose

Come into Headstand.

Once you feel comfortable, with control, rotate your body from your chest down to one side.

Meanwhile, keep pushing your elbows firmly into the floor and avoid moving your head.

Stay here for as long as it is comfortable, then come back to the center and repeat the same on the other side.

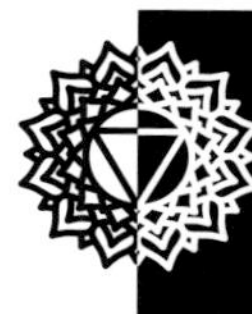

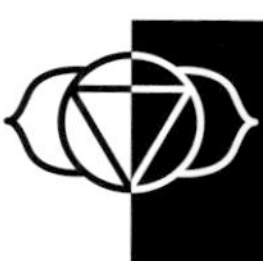

Next pose

Rest in Child's Pose for 30–45 seconds, then continue with Shoulderstand or a variation thereof.

Alignment cues

The rotation starts from the core and hips.

Shoulders, elbows, and head should remain in the neutral position.

Contraindications & cautions

The same contraindications and cautions apply as in Headstand.

Modifications & adjustments

These variations should be practiced only after you are comfortable and stable for at least 1 minute in the basic version of Headstand and can enter and exit the pose with control. This pose can be done with straight legs, as well as with leg variations as explained in Headstand with Leg Variations (to increase the level of complexity).

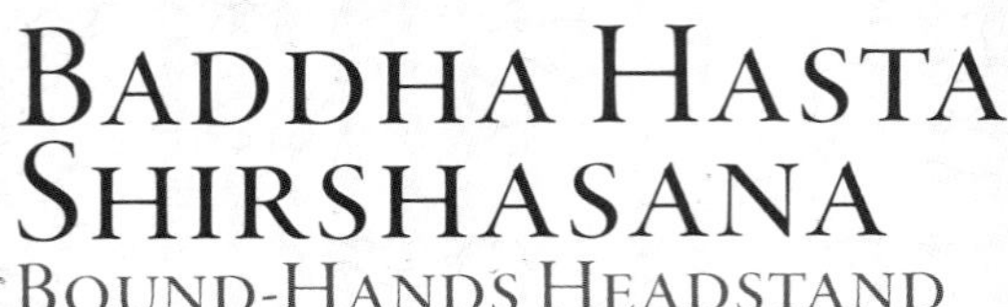

Baddha Hasta Shirshasana

Bound-Hands Headstand

How to come into the pose

Sit on your knees, with your hips resting on your heels.

Tightly hold your opposite upper arms (just above your elbows) and place your forearms on the floor.

Place your forehead against your forearms and place the top of your head on the floor.

Press your elbows and forearms firmly into the floor and bring your shoulders away from your ears.

Curl your toes, straighten your legs, and walk toward your chest, aiming to bring your hips above your shoulders.

Keeping your legs straight or slightly bent, lift them up toward the ceiling.

Hold the pose steadily as long as comfortable and breathe evenly.

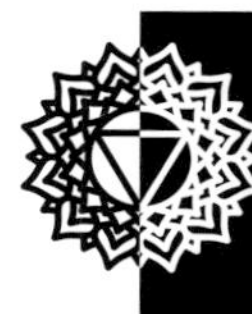

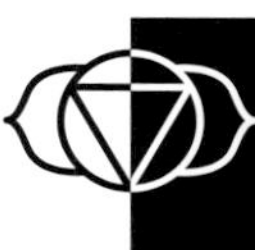

Next pose

Rest in Child's Pose for 30–45 seconds, then continue with Shoulderstand or a variation thereof.

Alignment cues

In this variation there is more weight on your head and neck.

Keep pressing your shoulders away from your ears and press your forearms firmly into the floor so your neck and shoulders are more supported.

To avoid toppling over backward (because there is no support at the back of your head), keep your legs slightly in front of your hips rather than straight above your head.

Contraindications & cautions

The same contraindications and cautions apply as in Headstand.

Modifications & adjustments

This variation should be practiced only once you are comfortable and stable for at least 2 minutes in the basic version of Headstand and can enter and exit the pose with control (ideally with straight legs).

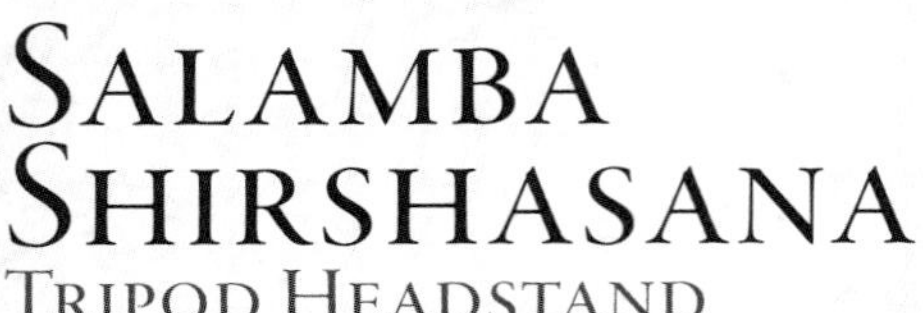

Salamba Shirshasana
Tripod Headstand

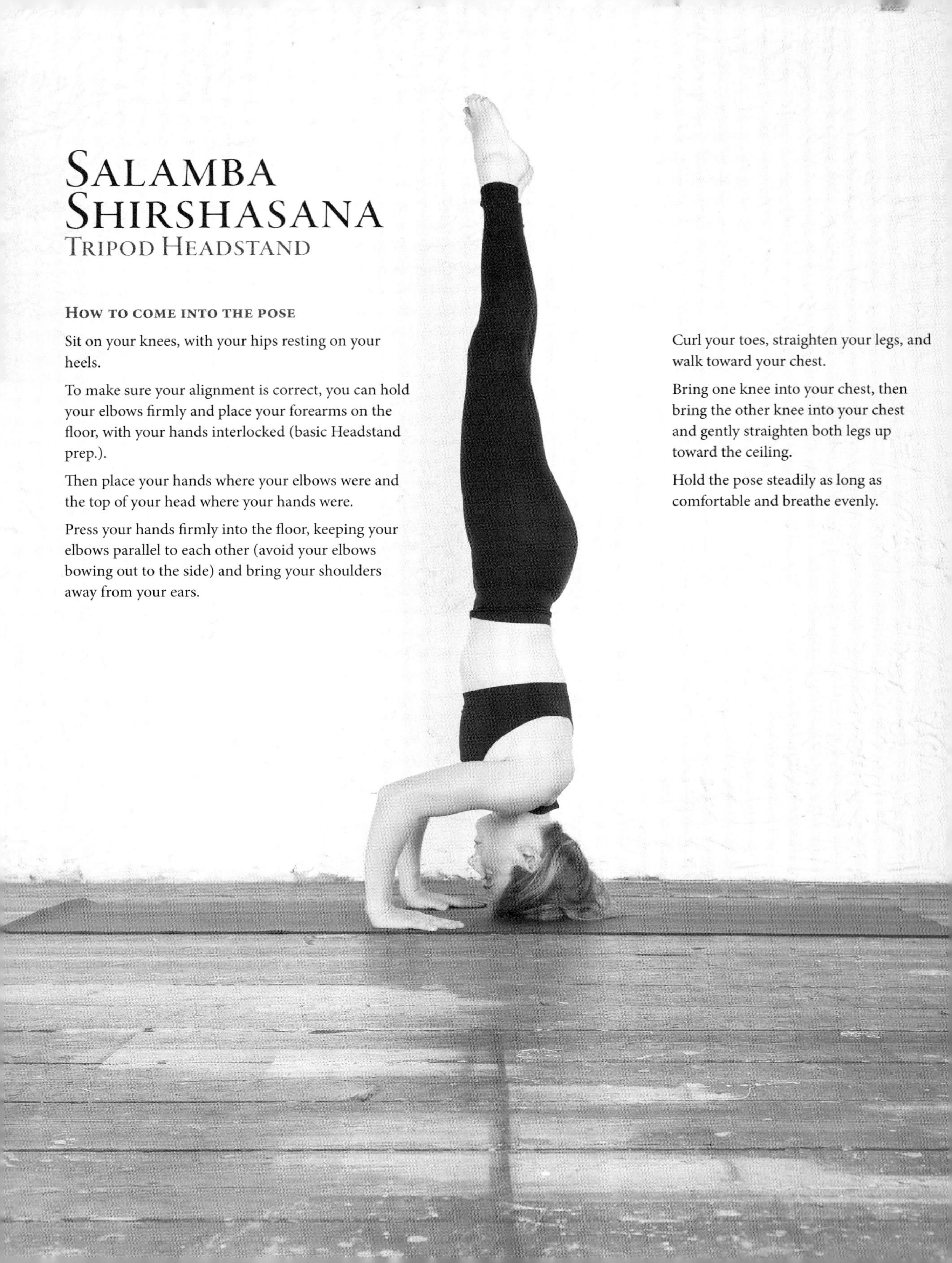

How to come into the pose

Sit on your knees, with your hips resting on your heels.

To make sure your alignment is correct, you can hold your elbows firmly and place your forearms on the floor, with your hands interlocked (basic Headstand prep.).

Then place your hands where your elbows were and the top of your head where your hands were.

Press your hands firmly into the floor, keeping your elbows parallel to each other (avoid your elbows bowing out to the side) and bring your shoulders away from your ears.

Curl your toes, straighten your legs, and walk toward your chest.

Bring one knee into your chest, then bring the other knee into your chest and gently straighten both legs up toward the ceiling.

Hold the pose steadily as long as comfortable and breathe evenly.

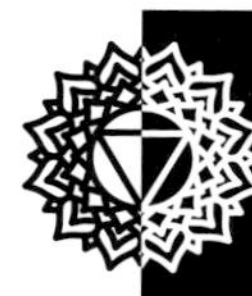

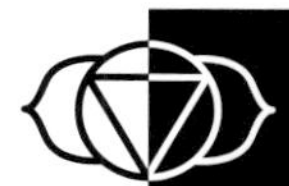

Next pose

Rest in Child's Pose for 30–45 seconds, then continue with Shoulderstand or a variation thereof.

Alignment cues

Your hands should be shoulder-width apart from each other, fingertips pointing to the front of your mat.

Make an equilateral triangle between your head and hands. Your head should not be too close to or too far from your hands.

If you have the right distance, your upper arms and lower arms will form a 90-degree angle when you are in the pose.

Keep drawing your shoulders away from your ears and keep your neck elongated.

For more stability and to lessen the weight on your head, initially you can keep your legs slightly in front of your hips rather than straight above your head.

Contraindications & cautions

The same contraindications and cautions apply as in Headstand.

Modifications & adjustments

Often, beginners find this variation of Headstand easier. However, because there is more weight on your head, this pose is not suitable for long holds until you have progressed to an advanced level. Therefore, this variation should be practiced only once you are comfortable and stable for at least 2 minutes in the basic version of Headstand and can enter and exit the pose with control (ideally with straight legs).

Variation

A challenging variation that trains coordination and core awareness is coming into Tripod Headstand directly from Crow Pose.

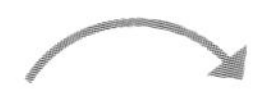

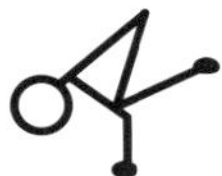

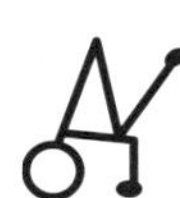

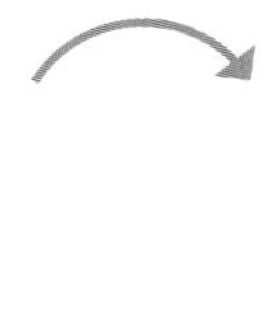

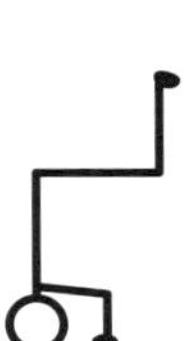

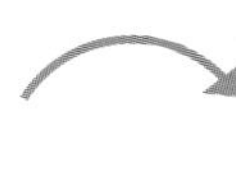

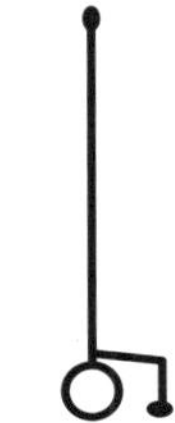

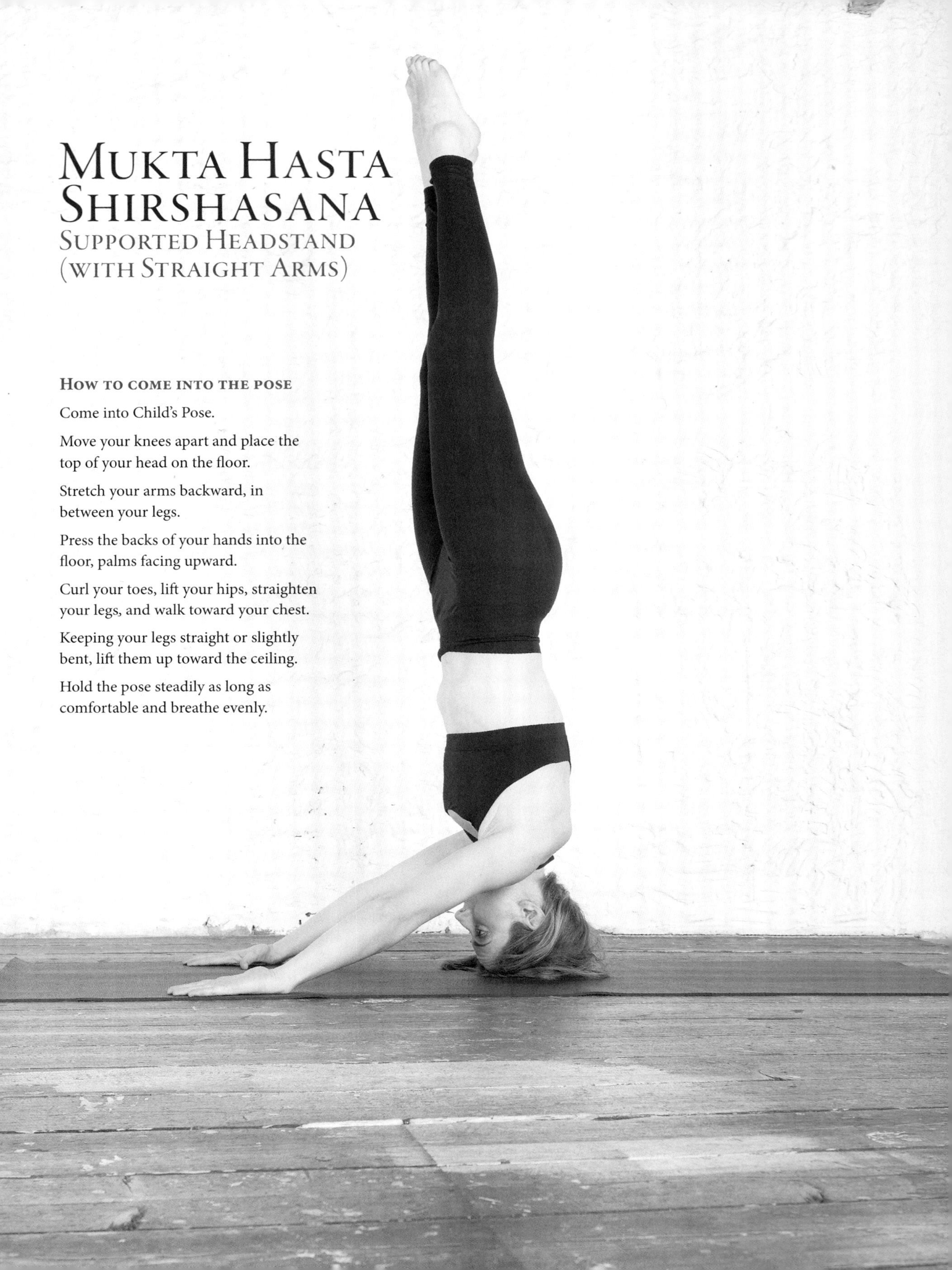

Mukta Hasta Shirshasana

Supported Headstand (with Straight Arms)

How to come into the pose

Come into Child's Pose.

Move your knees apart and place the top of your head on the floor.

Stretch your arms backward, in between your legs.

Press the backs of your hands into the floor, palms facing upward.

Curl your toes, lift your hips, straighten your legs, and walk toward your chest.

Keeping your legs straight or slightly bent, lift them up toward the ceiling.

Hold the pose steadily as long as comfortable and breathe evenly.

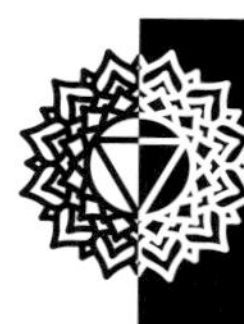

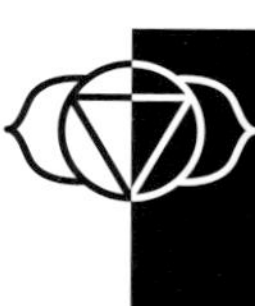

Next pose

Rest in Child's Pose for 30–45 seconds, then continue with Shoulderstand or a variation thereof.

Alignment cues

Your arms are straight, and the backs of your hands are firmly pressing into the floor.

Fingers can be spread out wide for extra stability.

Hands are at least shoulder-width apart.

Keep your shoulder blades drawn away from your ears toward your waist and your neck elongated.

To avoid toppling over backward (because there is no support at the back of your head), keep your legs slightly in front of your hips rather than straight above your head.

Contraindications & cautions

The same contraindications and cautions apply as in Headstand.

Modifications & adjustments

This variation should be practiced only after you are comfortable and stable for at least 2 minutes in the basic version of Headstand and can enter and exit the pose with control (ideally with straight legs).

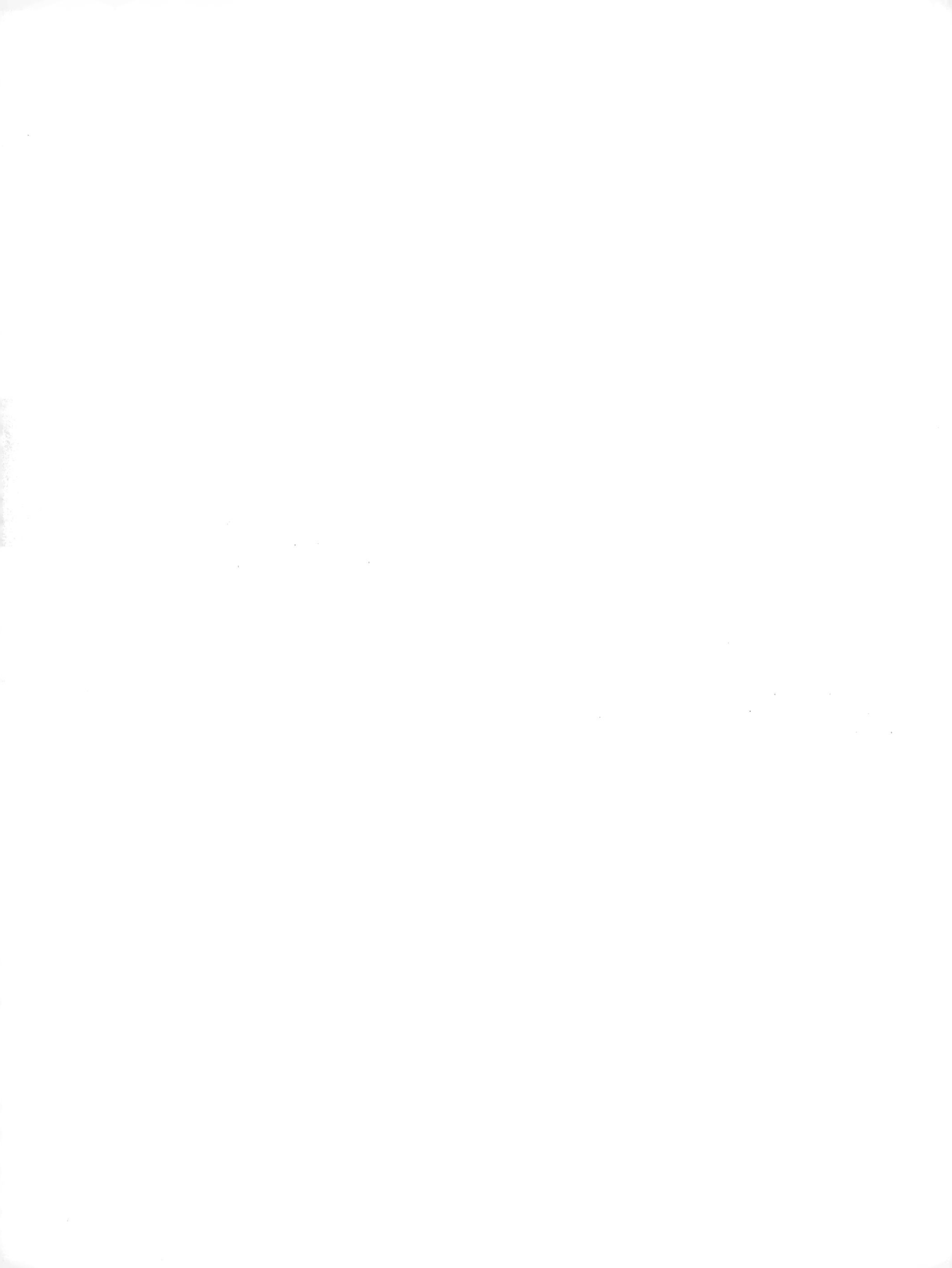

Chapter 13

Variations for the Throat Chakra

Sarvangasana (Shoulderstand) Variations

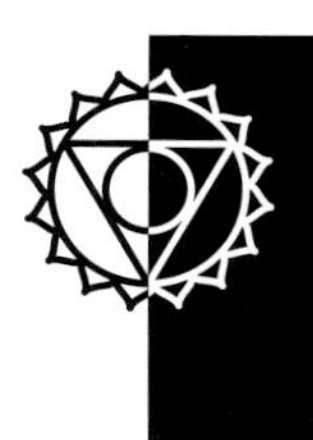

The following is valid for all the variations to Shoulderstand Pose:

Important alignment cues

Although the aim is to keep the ankles, hips, and shoulders in one line, that is not possible for every practitioner (in fact few can do this safely, without straining the neck). The primary aim should be to keep 75 percent of your weight on your shoulders and 25 percent of your body's weight on your elbows. Your neck should not bear any body weight. In fact, it should not be pressing into the floor but keeping its natural curve off the floor. To accomplish this, draw your shoulder blades toward each other and press them firmly into the floor.

Modifications & adjustments

If your neck is pressing onto the floor, place a folded blanket under your shoulder girdle, covering the protruding vertebra (C7) at the base of your neck. The rest of your neck and head are off the blanket. This difference in levels between your head and shoulders reduces strain on your neck.

Counter-pose

Classically, Fish Pose is the most beneficial counter-pose for Shoulderstand as well as for Plough Pose, because it provides a counter-stretch to the throat area. As a counter-pose for the lower back (which often feels a bit tight and tired after long holds of Shoulderstand), Half Bridge Pose followed by Fish Pose is our recommendation.

Vistrit Pada Sarvangasana

Shoulderstand with Leg Variations

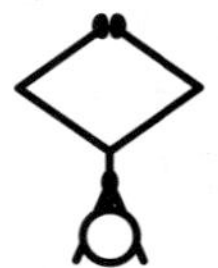

How to come into the pose

Come into Shoulderstand.

Keep your elbows firmly on the floor and your hands on your back in order to maintain the placement of your pelvis, then move into one of the following leg variations.

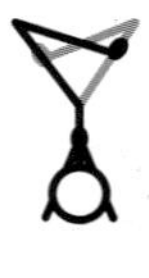

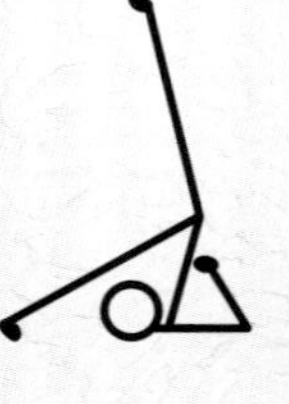

Next pose

Continue with Plough Pose or a variation thereof.

Alignment cues

The movement happens only in your legs, while your shoulders and head stay in a neutral position.

After each leg variation, come back into the center with your legs, before moving into another variation.

Contraindications & cautions

The same contraindications and cautions apply as in the basic Shoulderstand.

Modifications & adjustments

This variation should be practiced only after you are comfortable and stable for at least 1 minute in the basic version of Shoulderstand and can enter and exit the pose with control. To avoid straining the lower back it is important to keep your pelvis right above your shoulders, even as your legs move into different variations and directions.

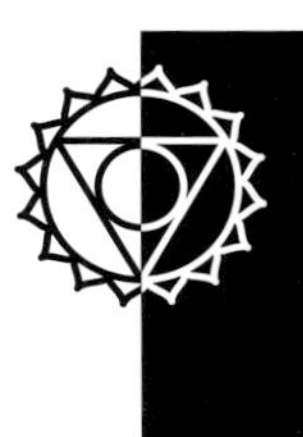

Niralamba Sarvangasana

Unsupported Shoulderstand

How to come into the pose

Come into Shoulderstand.

From there, focus on a point above you on the ceiling, and with control extend your arms toward the ceiling in front of your knees, palms together.

Hold the pose steadily as long as comfortable and breathe evenly.

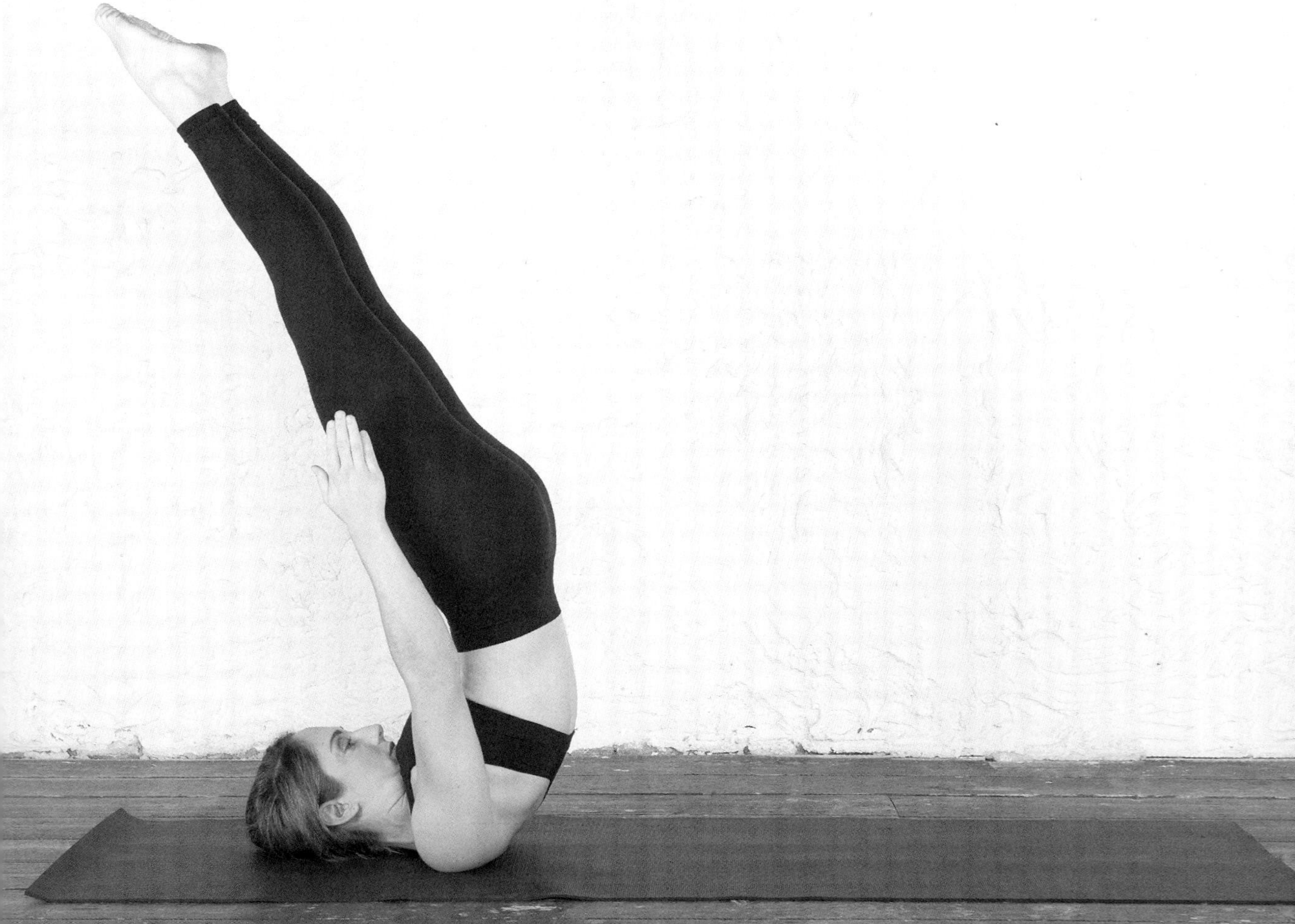

Next pose

Continue with Plough Pose or a variation thereof.

Alignment cues

Hips are engaged and constantly reaching up.

Your hips should be in the same position as in Shoulderstand.

If your hips are sinking, you might be placing too much weight and strain on your neck.

Your palms are together, reaching up toward the ceiling, in front of your legs.

Your feet are together and relaxed.

In this pose your upper back tends to round, and your weight shifts more toward your neck.

Even though your hands are reaching upward, work on keeping your shoulder blades pulled toward each other and your weight, as much as possible, on the shoulder girdle.

Contraindications & cautions

The same contraindications and cautions apply as in Shoulderstand.

Modifications & adjustments

Reaching with your hands up toward your knees might initially be too heavy or difficult to balance. An easier version is to interlock your hands tightly behind your back, on the floor. Make sure to externally rotate your upper arm and draw your shoulder blades in toward each other.

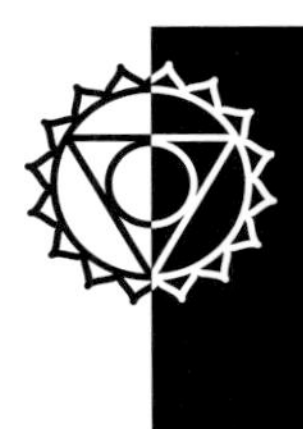

Viparita Karani Mudra
Inverted Pose

How to come into the pose

Come into Shoulderstand.

Place your hands on your lower back.

Keep your legs straight and move your feet as far away as possible from your head, engaging your core as you do so.

Hold the pose steadily as long as comfortable and breathe evenly.

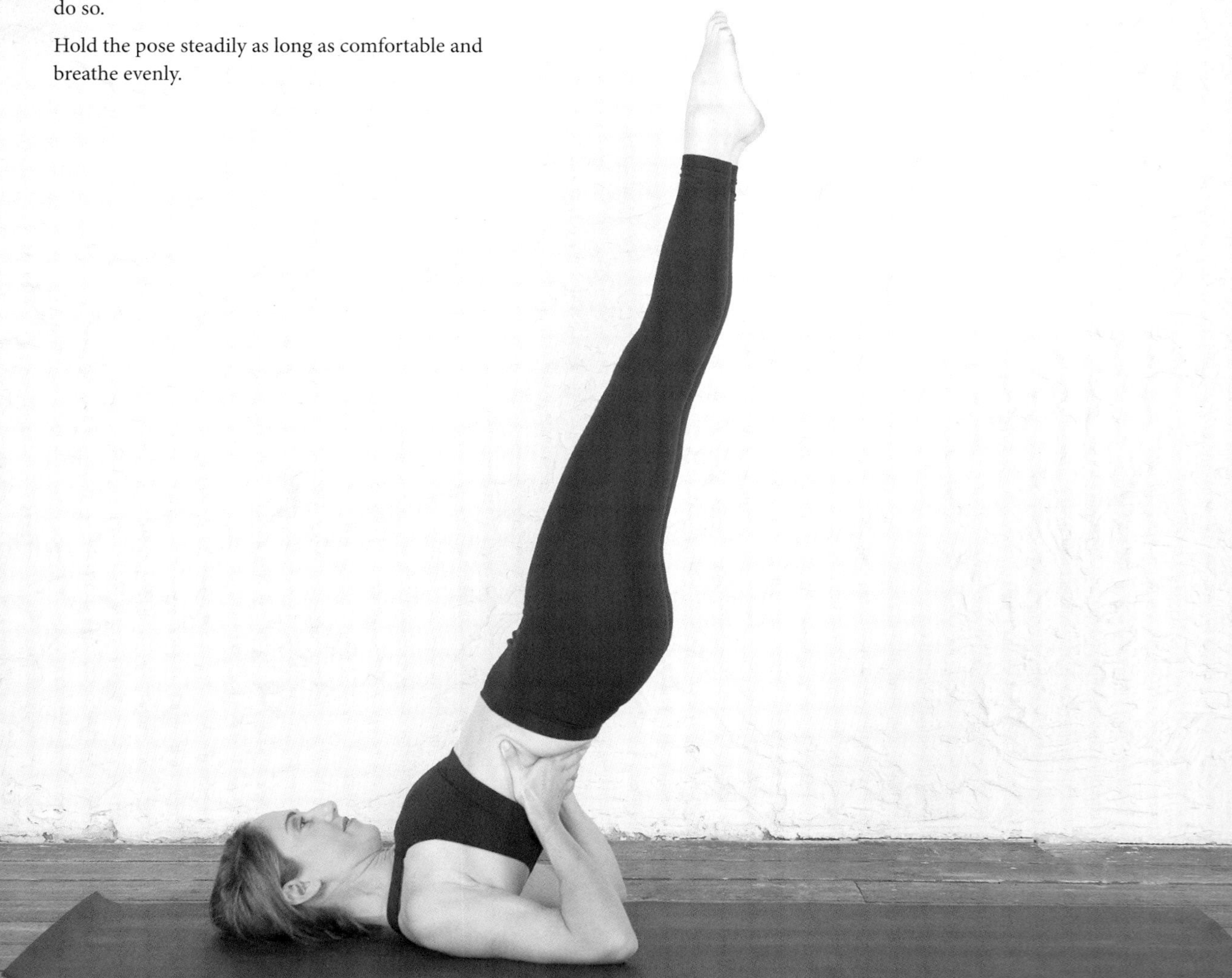

Next pose

Continue with Plough Pose or a variation thereof.

Alignment cues

Engage your core and inner thighs and make your body as stiff as a plank.

Your hands are on your lower back, fingers pointing upward.

Your elbows are drawn toward each other and approximately shoulder-width apart.

The majority of your body weight is resting on your hands.

Your upper body and legs form a straight line.

Shoulders and neck remain on the floor.

Contraindications & cautions

The same contraindications and cautions apply as in Shoulderstand. However, if you have wrist or lower-back issues this pose should be avoided.

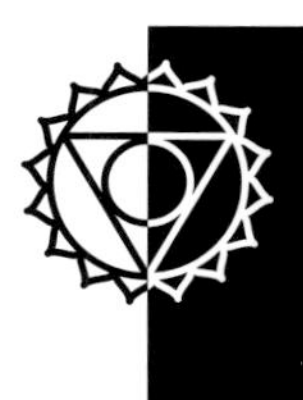

Modifications & adjustments

Your whole body is engaged to hold your legs in place, especially your core. If your core is weak, drop your feet only a little bit away. If your wrists feel sensitive, turn your hands so that your fingers point out toward your sides.

Variations

Sukha Viparita Karani Mudra

Easy Inverted Pose

Come into Shoulderstand. Place your hands against your lower back, with the heels of the palms pointing inward and your fingertips pointing either toward your buttocks or out sideways. Keep your elbows steady on the floor and start to shift the weight onto your hands, allowing your lower back to arch. Aim to keep your legs perpendicular to the ground and the back of your neck long.

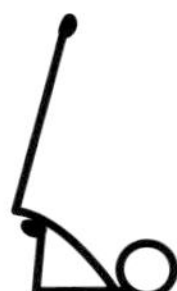

Urdhva Padmasana

Upward Lotus Pose

How to come into the pose

Come into Shoulderstand, with both legs straight and your hands supporting your back.

Bend your left leg away from your body by extending at your hip, then fold your right leg into place.

Take one hand away from your back to assist, if necessary.

Once your right leg is in position, bring your left leg into Lotus, switching hands if necessary to work your legs into a secure and comfortable lotus.

(Caution: Do not use any force and attempt this only if you are experienced in folding safely into Lotus.)

One at a time, take your hands to your knees and push your arms straight.

Create stability in the posture by pressing your knees into your hands and your hands into your knees.

Hold the pose steadily as long as comfortable, breathing evenly.

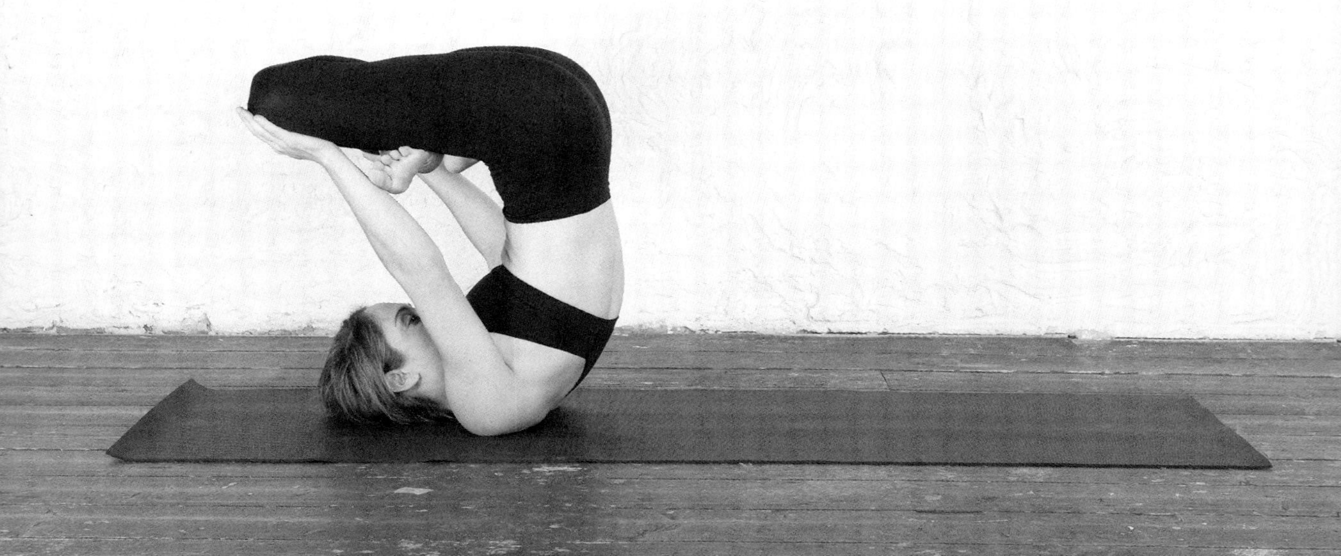

Next pose

Continue with Plough Pose or a variation thereof.

Alignment cues

Your hips are directly over your shoulders; aim to keep your spine elongated.

Lift your sitting bones to facilitate the extension of your spine.

Your hands are pressing up against your knees, while your shoulders are pressing down against the floor.

Your shoulders bear the great majority of your body weight.

Contraindications & cautions

The same contraindications and cautions apply as in Shoulderstand. However, if you have tight hips or knee issues you should practice this pose with the below-mentioned modifications.

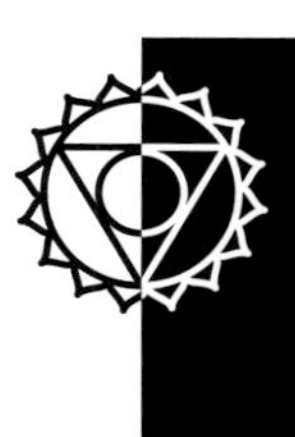

Modifications & adjustments

If you are not able to fold comfortably and without strain into Lotus position here, keep your legs crossed at your calves, as in Easy Sitting Pose (Sukhasana). Then bring your hands to your knees and create the same opposition as described above.

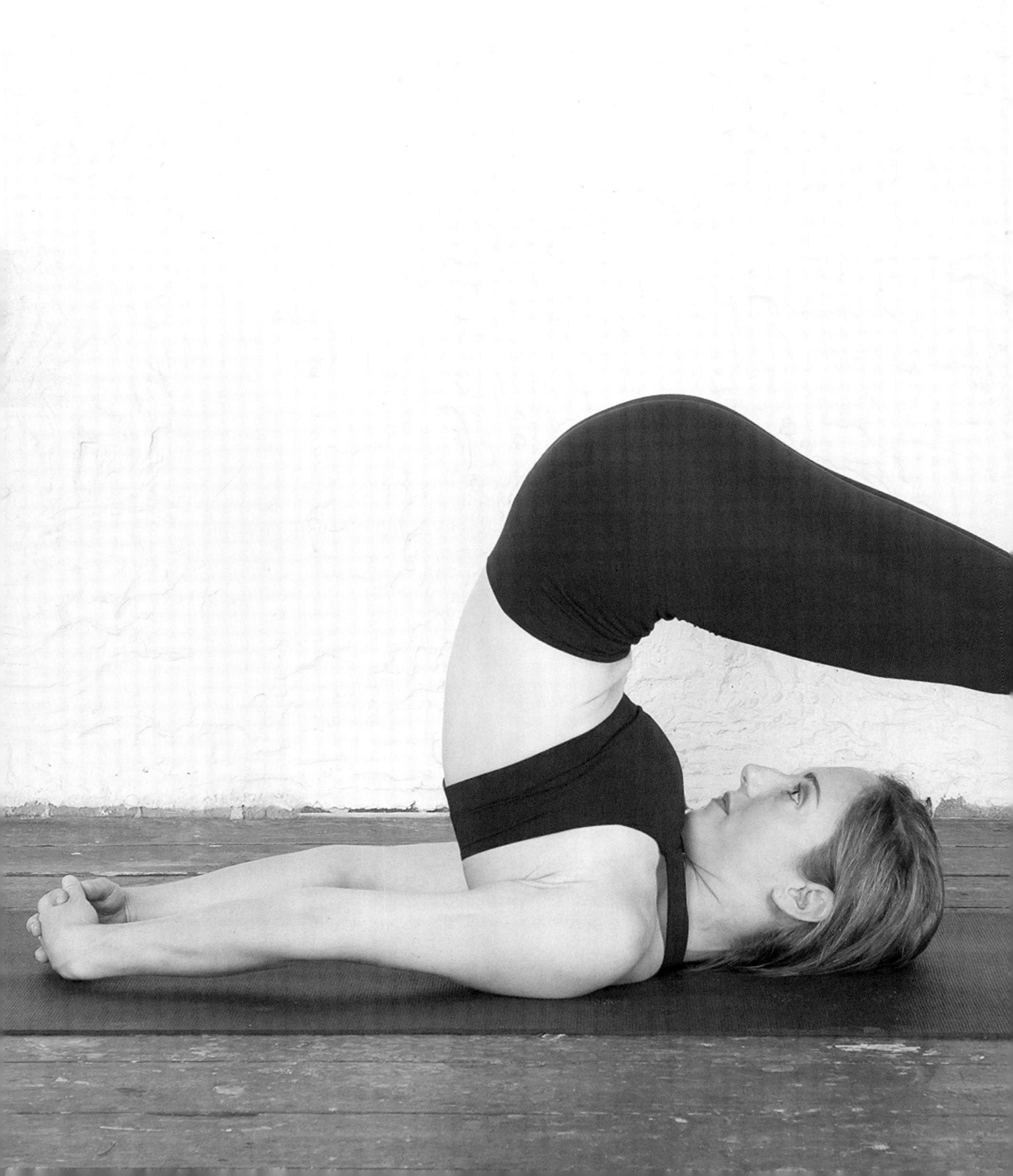

Halasana (Plough Pose) Variations

The following is valid for all variations to Plough Pose:

Important alignment cues

Your hips should be right over your shoulders or slightly back. Do not aim to bring your hips over your head, because that places too much pressure on your neck. Your neck should not bear any body weight. In fact, ideally it should not be pressing into the floor but maintaining its natural curve. To accomplish this, draw your shoulder blades toward each other, and press the tops of your shoulders firmly into the floor.

Modifications & adjustments

If your neck is pressing into the floor, place a folded blanket under your shoulder girdle, covering the protruding vertebra (C7) at the base of your neck. The rest of your neck and head are off the blanket. If your feet do not reach the floor, use a block or the wall to rest them on. In that case also keep your hands on your lower back for support.

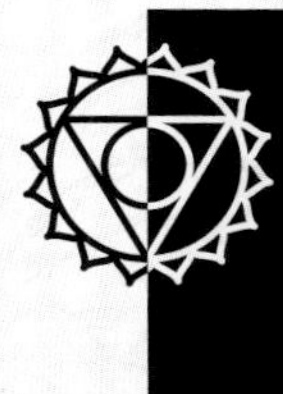

Counter-pose

Fish Pose is the most beneficial counter-pose for Plough Pose and its variations because it provides a counter-stretch to the throat area. As a counter-pose for the lower back (which often feels a bit tight and tired after long holds of Plough Pose), starting with Half Bridge Pose followed by Fish Pose is our recommendation.

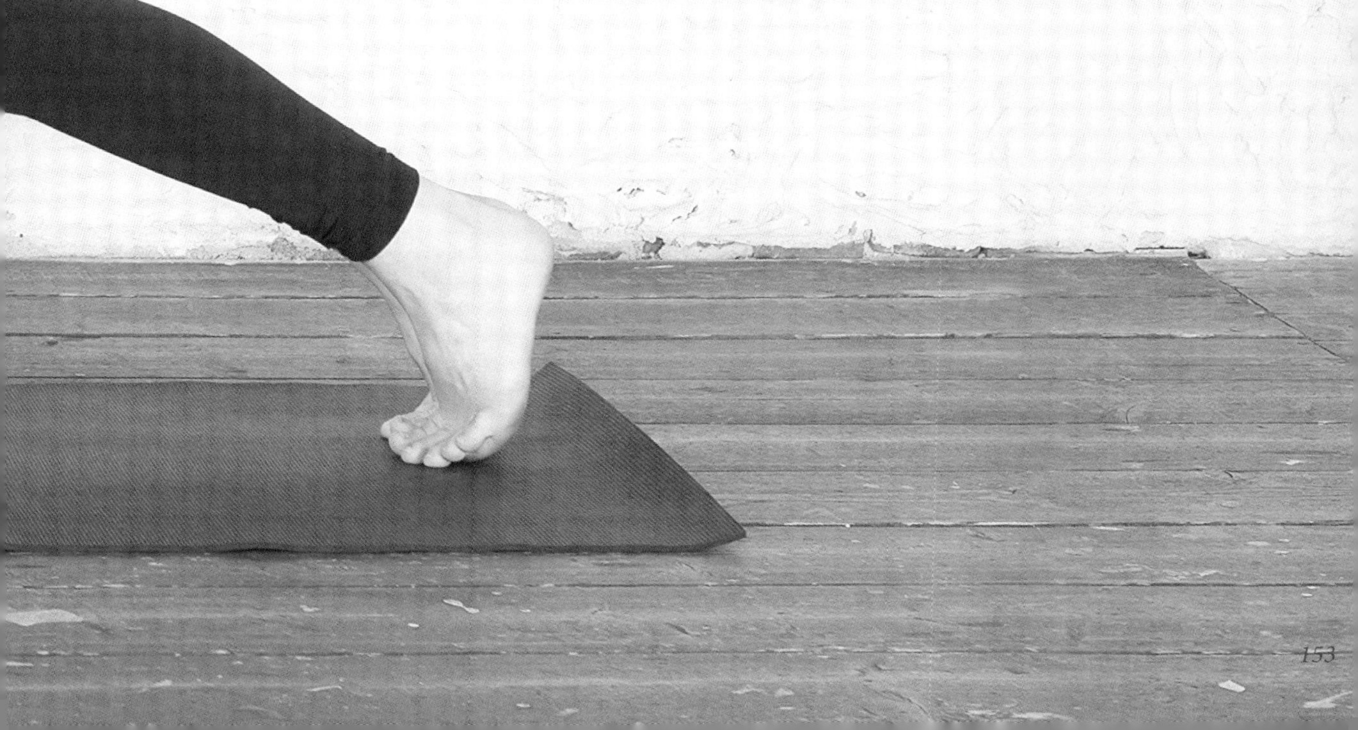

Karnapidasana I
Ear Pressure Pose

How to come into the pose

Come into Plough Pose, with your hands supporting your lower back.

Open your feet hip-width apart.

Point your feet, bend your knees, and allow your knees to drop down toward the floor, with your right knee next to your right ear and your left knee next to your left ear.

Bring your big toes together and let the weight of your legs pull your knees toward the floor (do not force them downward).

If your knees touch the floor, interlock your hands behind your back.

Hold the pose steadily as long as comfortable and breathe evenly.

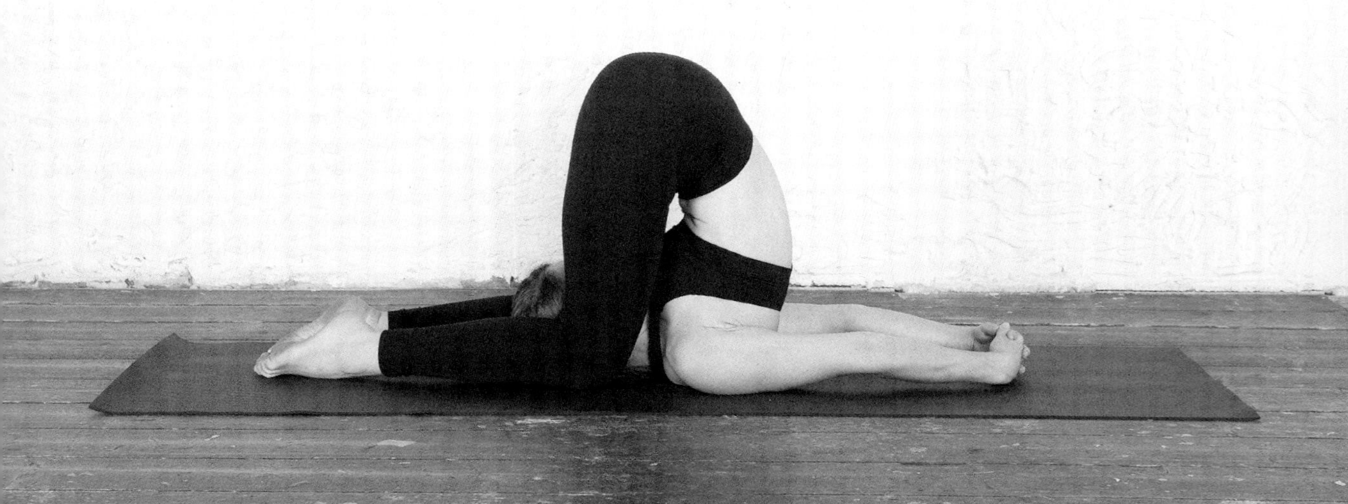

Next pose

Continue with Half Bridge Pose or a variation thereof.

Alignment cues

Your back is slightly rounded.

Your knees are dropped next to your ears, big toes touching each other, with your feet pointed.

Your hands are supporting your lower back or can be interlocked behind your back.

Your shoulders bear the great majority of your body weight, and your shoulder blades are drawn toward each other.

There should be a small gap between the floor and your neck.

Contraindications & cautions

The same contraindications and cautions apply as in Plough Pose.

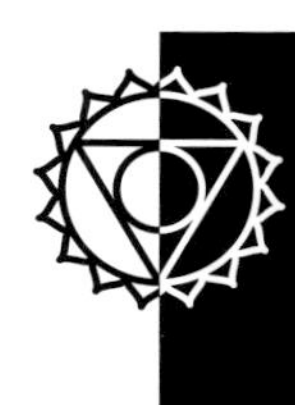

Modifications & adjustments

If your feet do not reach the floor, support them on a block or against the wall. Do not let them dangle in the air, because that can strain your lower back and neck.

Variations

Karnapidasana II

From Plough Pose, walk your feet to your left. Walk as far as possible, making sure that both your shoulders stay on the floor. Feet are flexed and heels are pushing away. From there, point your left foot and drop your left knee next to your right ear.

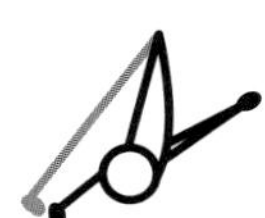

Supta Konasana
Reclining Angle Pose

How to come into the pose

Come into Plough Pose, with your legs straight and hands on your lower back.

Open your feet at least mat-width apart.

Hold on to your big toes.

Hold the pose steadily as long as comfortable and breathe evenly.

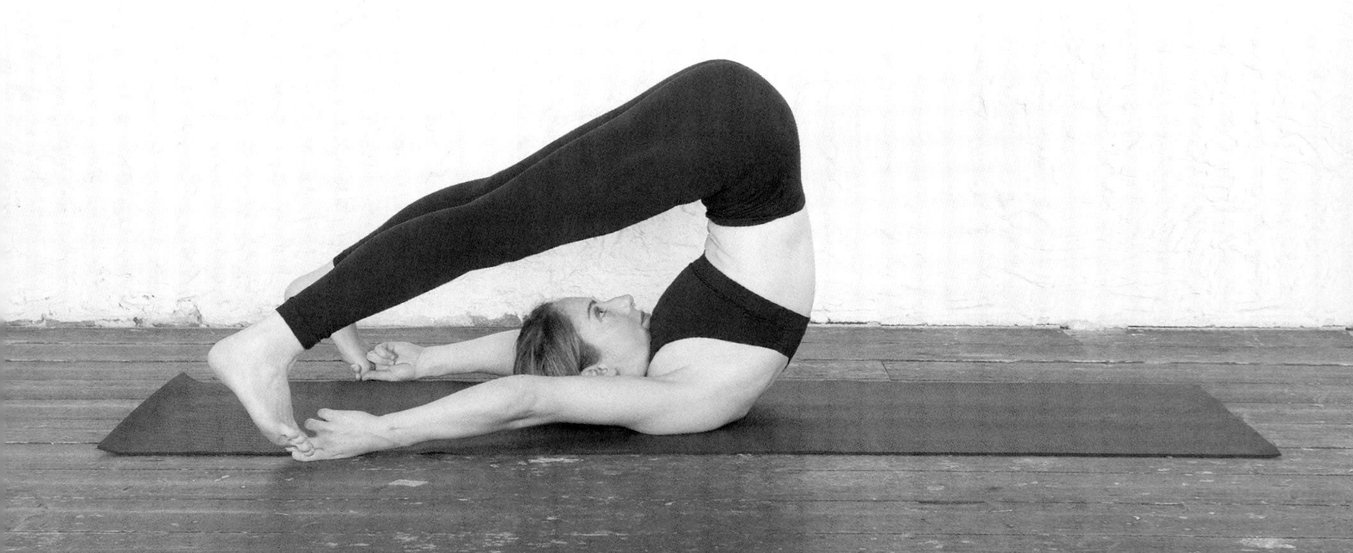

Next pose

Continue with Half Bridge Pose or a variation thereof.

Alignment cues

Legs are straight and at least mat-width apart.

Feet are flexed, with heels pushing away.

Arms are reaching backward and sideways, with your hands holding on to your big toes.

Hips are above your shoulders, with your sitting bones reaching upward, making your back straight.

Your shoulders bear the great majority of your body weight, and your shoulder blades are drawn toward each other.

There should be a small gap between the floor and your neck.

Contraindications & cautions

The same contraindications and cautions apply as in Plough Pose.

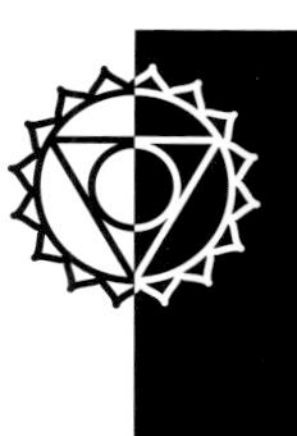

Modifications & adjustments

If due to tight hamstrings your knees remain slightly bent, make sure that you try to keep your spine as straight as possible and your hips above your shoulders.

Supta Urdhva Pada Vajrasana
Sleeping Raised-Foot Thunderbolt Pose

How to come into the pose

Come into Shoulderstand, with both legs straight and your hands supporting your back.

Bend your left leg away from your body by extending at your hip, then fold your right leg into Half Lotus Pose.

Use your opposite hand if necessary to bring your foot into your right position.

(Caution: Do not use any force and attempt this only if you are experienced in folding safely into Half Lotus Pose.) Wrap your right arm around your back and catch hold of your right big toe with your right hand.

With control, lower your left foot to the floor and hold on to your left big toe with your left hand.

Push your left heel away, push your shoulders into the floor.

Hold the pose steadily as long as comfortable and breathe evenly.

To release the pose, lift your left foot halfway up, unwind your right leg, and come into Shoulderstand.

From here either roll down and relax for a moment or proceed straight away to the other side.

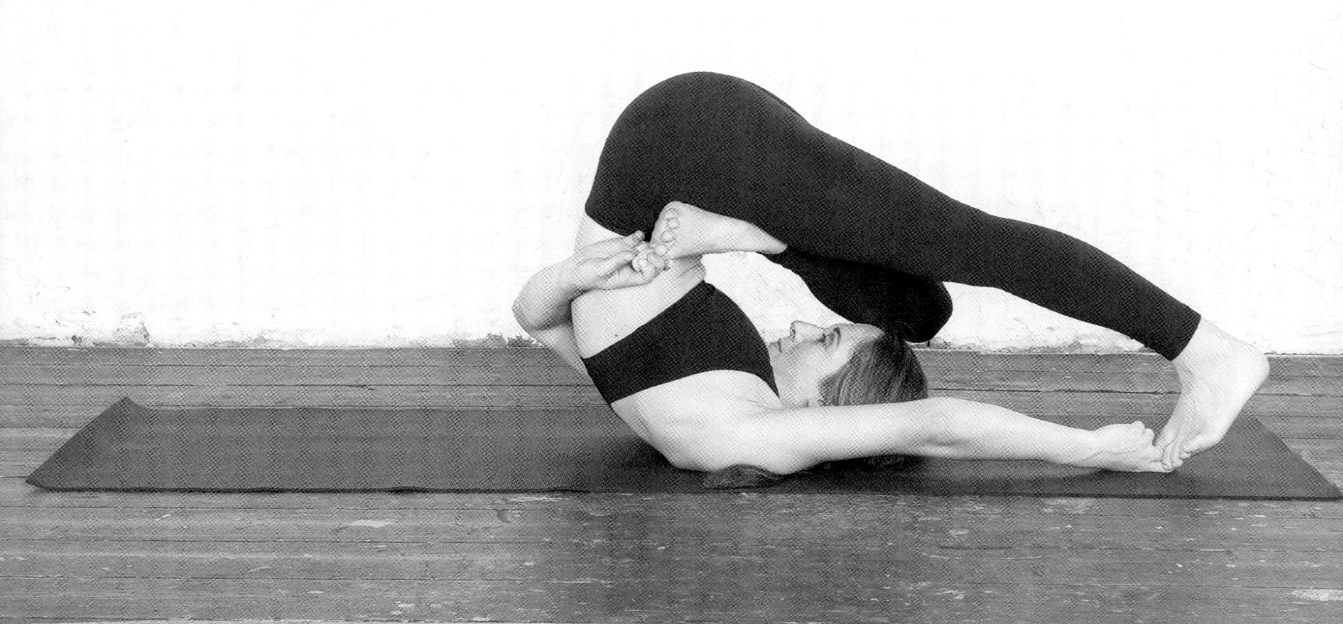

Next pose

Continue with Half Bridge Pose or a variation thereof.

Alignment cues

The foot of your extended leg is flexed, toes resting on the floor or on a support.

Your hips are above your shoulders; your spine is rounded.

Your shoulders bear the great majority of your body weight, and there should be a small gap between the floor and your neck.

Contraindications & cautions

The same contraindications and cautions apply as in Plough Pose. However, if you have tight hips or suffer from issues with your knees, either avoid the pose altogether or try the modified pose, as described next.

Modifications & adjustments

If you are not able to fold comfortably and without strain into Half Lotus Pose here, simply fold your right ankle just above your left knee. If necessary, you can support your left foot with a block or cushion and keep both hands against your back, firmly pressing your shoulders into the floor.

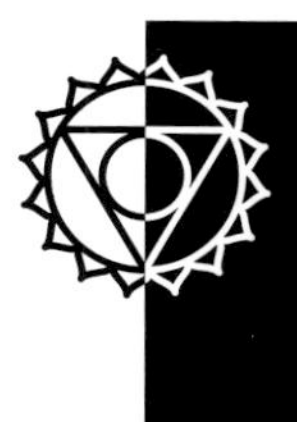

Pindasana
Embryo Pose

How to come into the pose

Come into Shoulderstand, with both legs straight and your hands supporting your back.

Bring your legs into Lotus Pose, by first folding your right leg into place.

Take one hand away from your back to assist, if necessary.

Once your right leg is in position, bring your left leg into Lotus, switching hands if necessary to work your legs into a secure and comfortable Lotus Pose.

(Caution: Do not use any force and attempt this only if you are experienced in folding safely into Lotus Pose.)

Draw your Lotus legs toward your chest and wrap your arms around the outside of your legs, clasping your hands together.

Allow your knees to move down on either side of your head, and let your body curl into an embryo shape.

Hold the pose steadily for as long as is comfortable and breathe evenly.

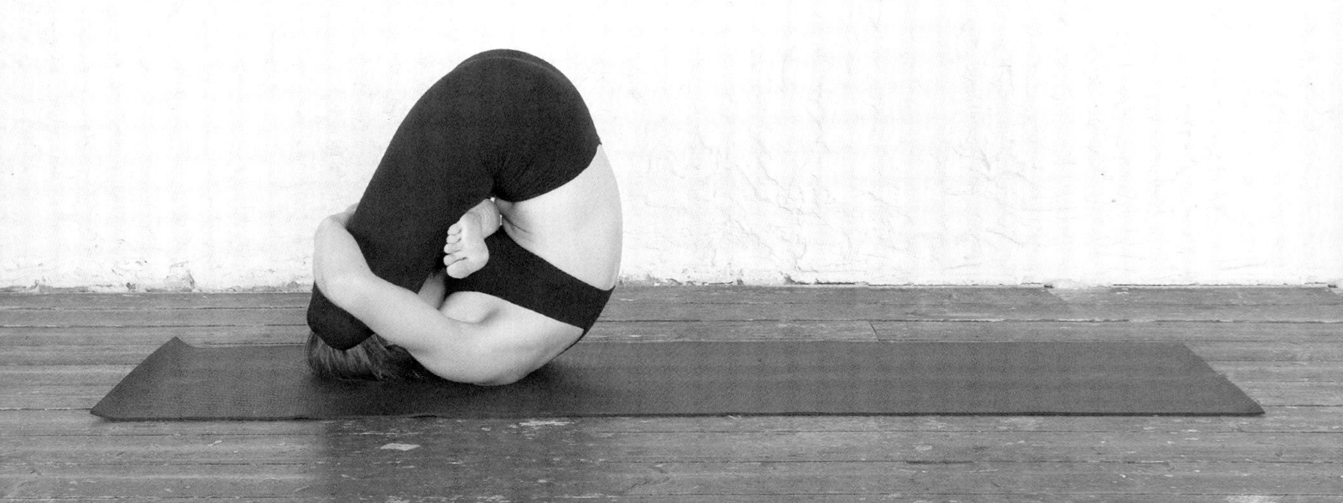

Next pose

Continue with Half Bridge Pose or a variation thereof.

Alignment cues

Your hips are above your shoulders; your spine is rounded.

Your legs are in Lotus position.

Your arms are wrapped around your thighs and hands interlocked.

Your shoulders bear the great majority of your body weight, and there should be a small gap between the floor and your neck.

Contraindications & cautions

The same contraindications and cautions apply as in Plough Pose. However, if you have tight hips or suffer from pain in or injury of your knees, either avoid this pose or try the modified pose as described next.

Modifications & adjustments

If you are not able to fold comfortably and without strain into Lotus Pose here, keep your legs crossed at your calves, as in Easy Sitting Pose, then wrap your arms around your legs and clasp your hands.

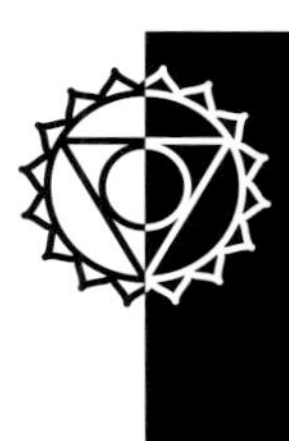

Chapter 14

Variations for the Heart Chakra

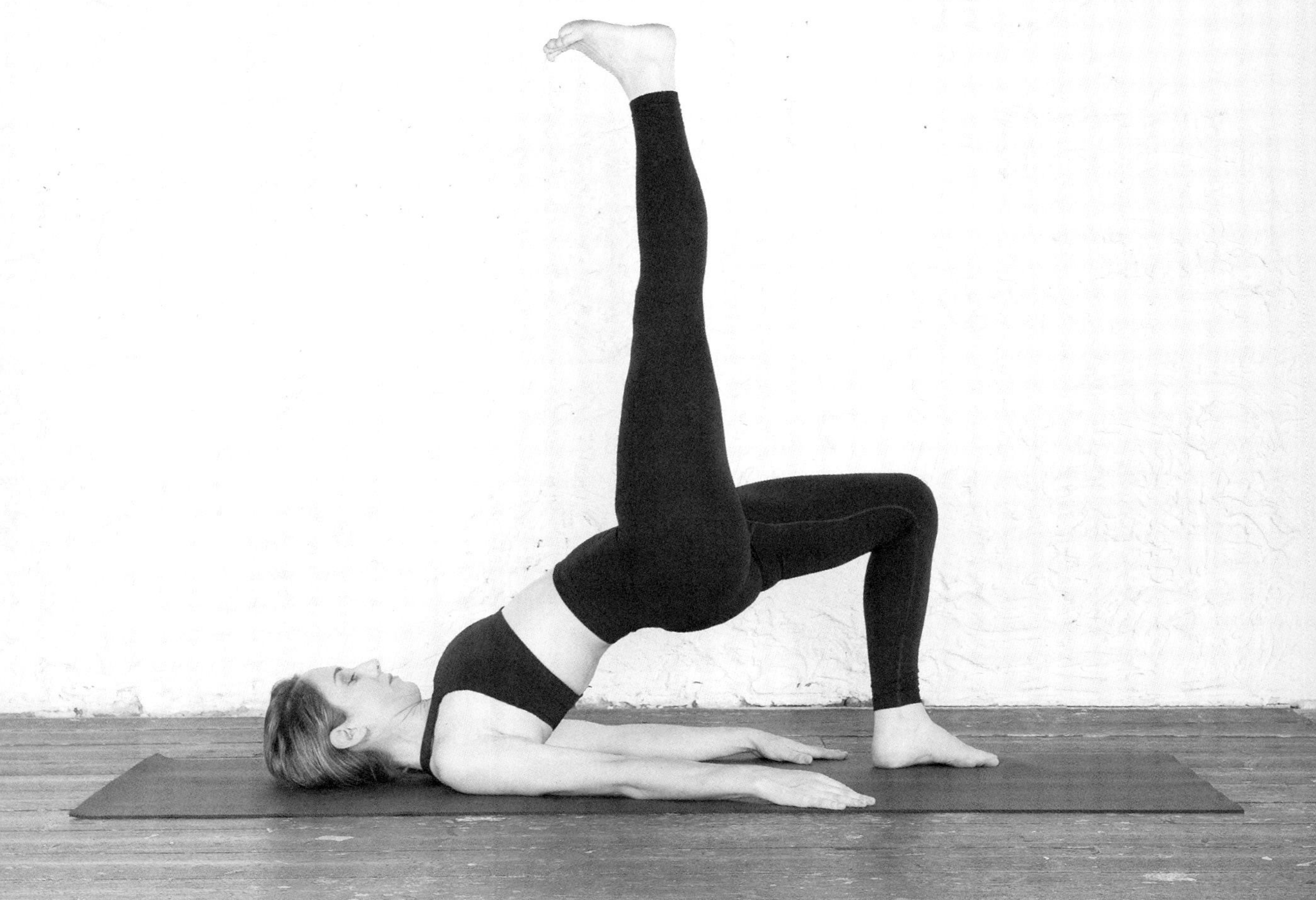

Ardha Setu Bandhasana (Half Bridge Pose) Variations

Eka Pada Ardha Setu Bandhasana

One-Legged Half Bridge Pose

How to come into the pose

Come into Half Bridge Pose, with your hands either pressing into the floor or interlocked.

Lift your right foot off the floor and point your foot straight to the ceiling.

Press your left foot into the floor to lift your hips and your right foot as high up as possible.

Hold the pose steadily as long as comfortable and breathe evenly.

Then release and repeat the same on the other side.

Next pose

Continue with Air-Releasing Pose or a variation thereof.

Alignment cues

Shoulder blades are drawn toward each other.

The aim is to bring your hands toward your heels, chest pushing up and back toward your chin.

Your foot on the floor is right below your knee, and your other leg is reaching as straight as possible up toward the ceiling, with your knee straight and foot flexed or gently pointed.

Contraindications & cautions

There are no general contraindications and cautions to this pose. However, respect your limit of movement and do not push further than that, because that can cause strain in your neck or knees.

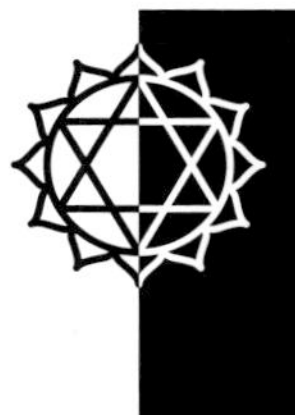

Modifications & adjustments

If you feel tension in your knee or if your big toes are coming off the floor, you can rotate your toes slightly outwards.

Setu Bandhasana
Bridge Pose

How to come into the pose

Come into Half Bridge Pose.

Place your hands on your lower back, with your wrists in and fingers pointing outward.

Bring your legs together, then walk your feet away from your body until your legs are straight and the majority of your body weight is resting on your hands.

Hold the pose steadily as long as comfortable and breathe evenly.

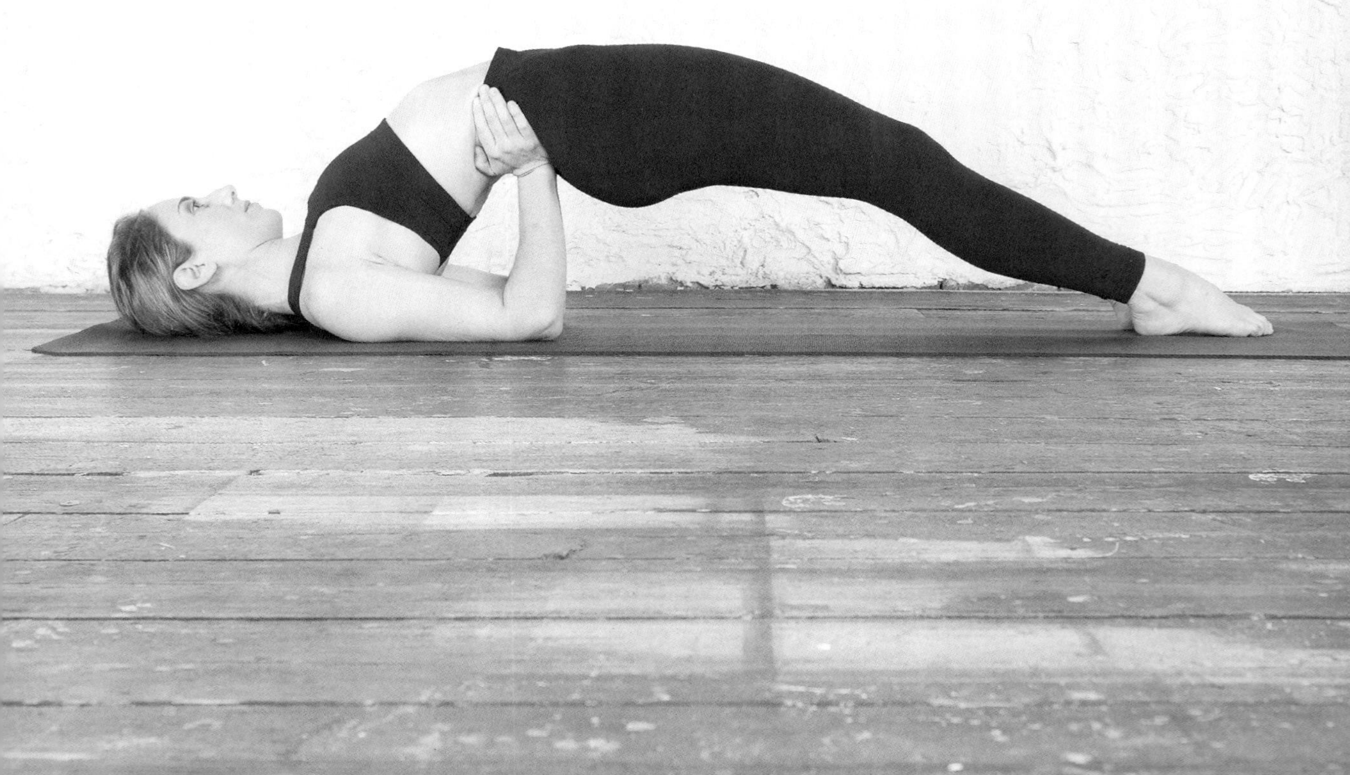

Next pose

Continue with Air-Releasing Pose or a variation thereof.

Alignment cues

Shoulders remain on the floor.

Elbows are under your body, below your wrists.

Legs are straight and feet are together and flat on the floor.

Contraindications & cautions

- Lower-back issues
- Wrist issues
- Arthritis

Modifications & adjustments

This pose requires a certain flexibility in the lower back. If that range is not available, you might find the pose heavy on your wrists, or you will find it difficult to straighten your legs while keeping your shoulders on the floor. In this case, bring your legs together and start to walk your feet away only until still comfortable, allowing your legs to remain slightly bent.

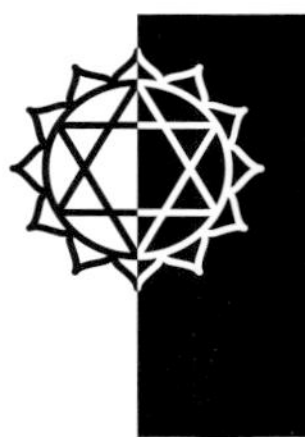

Shirsh Setu Bandhasana
Head Bridge Pose

How to come into the pose

Come into Half Bridge Pose, with your hands on your lower back, with the wrists pointing inward and your fingers pointing outward.

Shift your weight forward (toward your toes) and then place the top of your head on the floor.

Bring your legs together, then walk your feet away from your body until your legs are straight.

Hold the pose steadily as long as comfortable and breathe evenly.

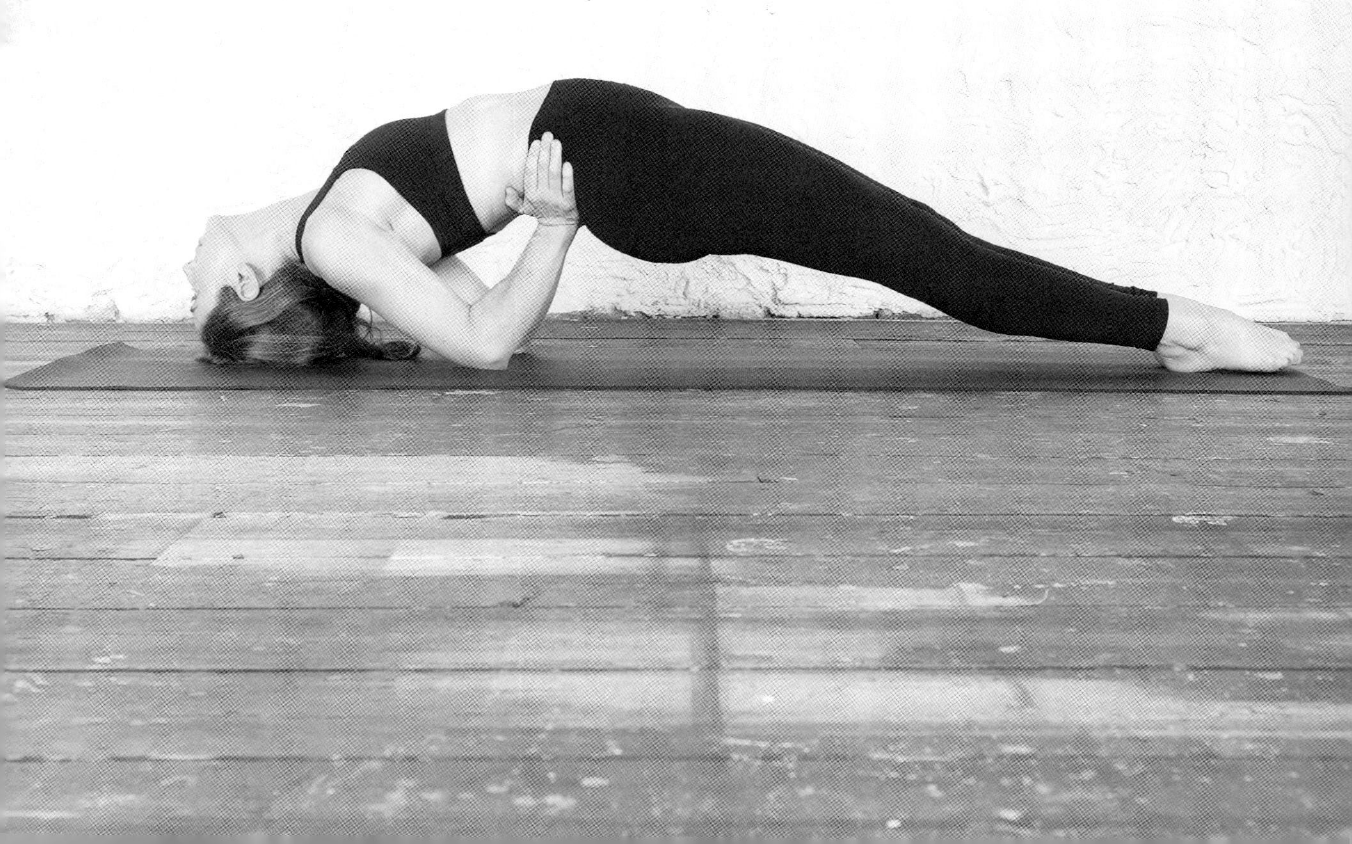

Next pose

Continue with Air-Releasing Pose or a variation thereof.

Alignment cues

Your shoulders are off the floor.

Your weight is divided between your elbows and your head.

Elbows are below your body, in line with your wrists.

Feet are together and flat on the floor.

Contraindications & cautions

- Lower-back issues
- Wrist issues
- Neck issues
- Hypertension
- Arthritis

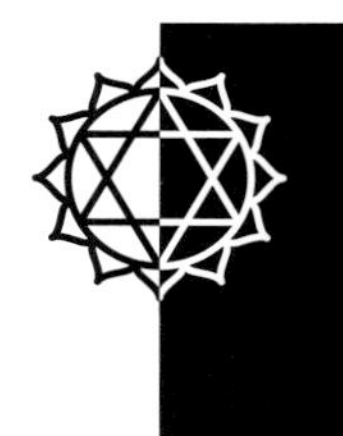

Variations

Shirsh Setu Bandhasana II

Head Bridge Pose II

Lie down on your back, arching your upper back, with your hands next to your ears, and the top of your head on the floor. Bend your knees and turn your toes outward. On the next inhalation push your feet into the floor and straighten your knees. Shift your body weight so your forehead comes to the floor. Bring your palms together and reach your hands diagonally up. To release the pose, place your hands next to your ears and roll back down. (Caution: This pose is heavy on your neck, so initially practice only under supervision of a competent teacher.)

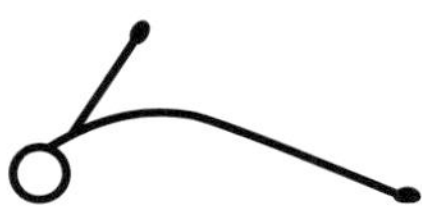

Chakrasana
Wheel Pose

How to come into the pose

Start from a supine position, legs bent and hip-width apart, with feet flat on the floor.

Place your hands next to your ears, with elbows pointing toward the ceiling, arms parallel.

Inhale and push your hands and feet into the floor, lifting your pelvis up toward the ceiling.

Look at a point straight behind you.

Holding the pose steadily as long as comfortable, breathe evenly.

To come out of the pose, bring your chin to your chest and slowly come down on your back again.

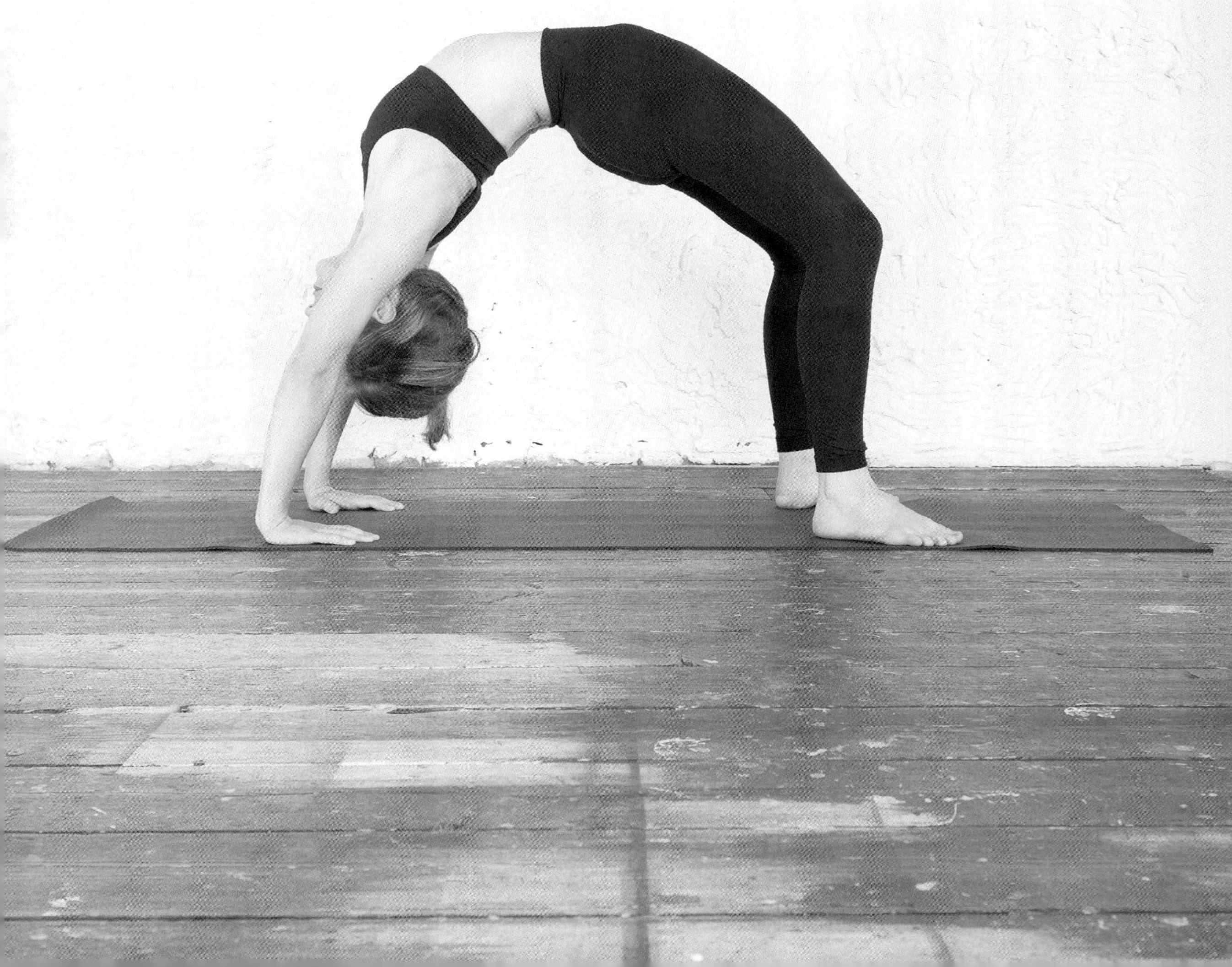

Next pose

Continue with Air-Releasing Pose or a variation thereof.

Alignment cues

Your weight is equally distributed between your feet and hands.

Gaze at a point straight behind you, so your neck can relax.

Your knees are as parallel as possible; heels are on the floor.

Aim to straighten your arms, while keeping them parallel to each other, with the elbows pointing straight backward.

Contraindications & cautions

- Lower-back and shoulder issues
- Wrist pain
- Neck issues
- Arthritis
- Hypertension

Modifications & adjustments

If you have stiff or sensitive wrists, you can elevate them by placing a blanket under the heels of your hands.

If you feel tension in your knees you can turn your toes slightly outward.

Initially you might lack the strength or coordination to push yourself up completely. In that case, start by placing the crown of your head on the floor, while still actively pushing your hands and feet into the floor and lifting your pelvis up. Eventually, as this becomes comfortable, proceed to push up all the way from here.

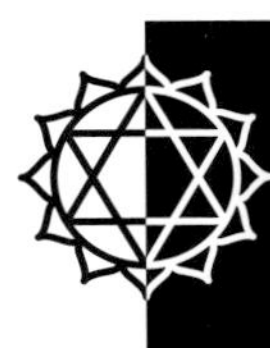

Variations

Eka Pada Chakrasana

ONE-LEGGED WHEEL POSE

Come into Wheel Pose, then proceed to shift your weight toward your left foot. Lift your right leg straight up toward the ceiling. Stay for a few breaths, then repeat on the other side.

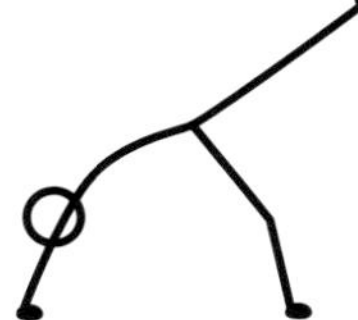

Eka Pada Eka Hasta Chakrasana

ONE-LEG-ONE-HAND WHEEL POSE

From Wheel Pose, shift your weight toward your left foot and hand, then lift your right leg and arm off the floor. Keep your right leg and arm parallel to the floor, focusing on a point behind you to find your balance. Stay for a few breaths and repeat on the other side.

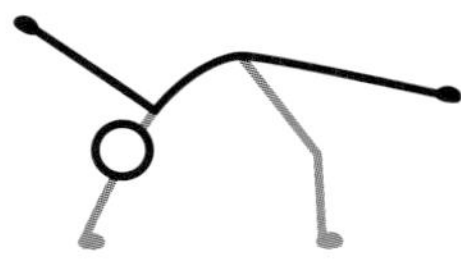

Purna Chakrasana

FULL WHEEL POSE

Come into Wheel Pose. Walk your hands toward your feet as close as possible, until your fingers touch your heels, or if possible you can hold on to your ankles.

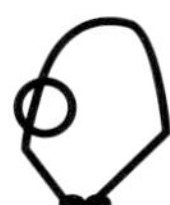

Viparita Dandasana

Inverted Staff Pose

How to come into the pose

Come into Wheel Pose (head can rest on the floor if full Wheel Pose is not accessible).

While keeping your pelvis as high as possible, place the top of your head in between your hands, on the floor.

Interlock your fingers behind your head and place your forearms on the floor, making a triangle of your hands and elbows.

Bring your feet together, keeping your hips lifted and engaged, and walk your feet away from you until your legs are straight.

Hold the pose steadily as long as comfortable and breathe evenly.

To come out of the pose, walk your feet back to just below your knees, place your hands back on the floor next to your ears, tuck your chin into your chest, and slowly come down on your back again.

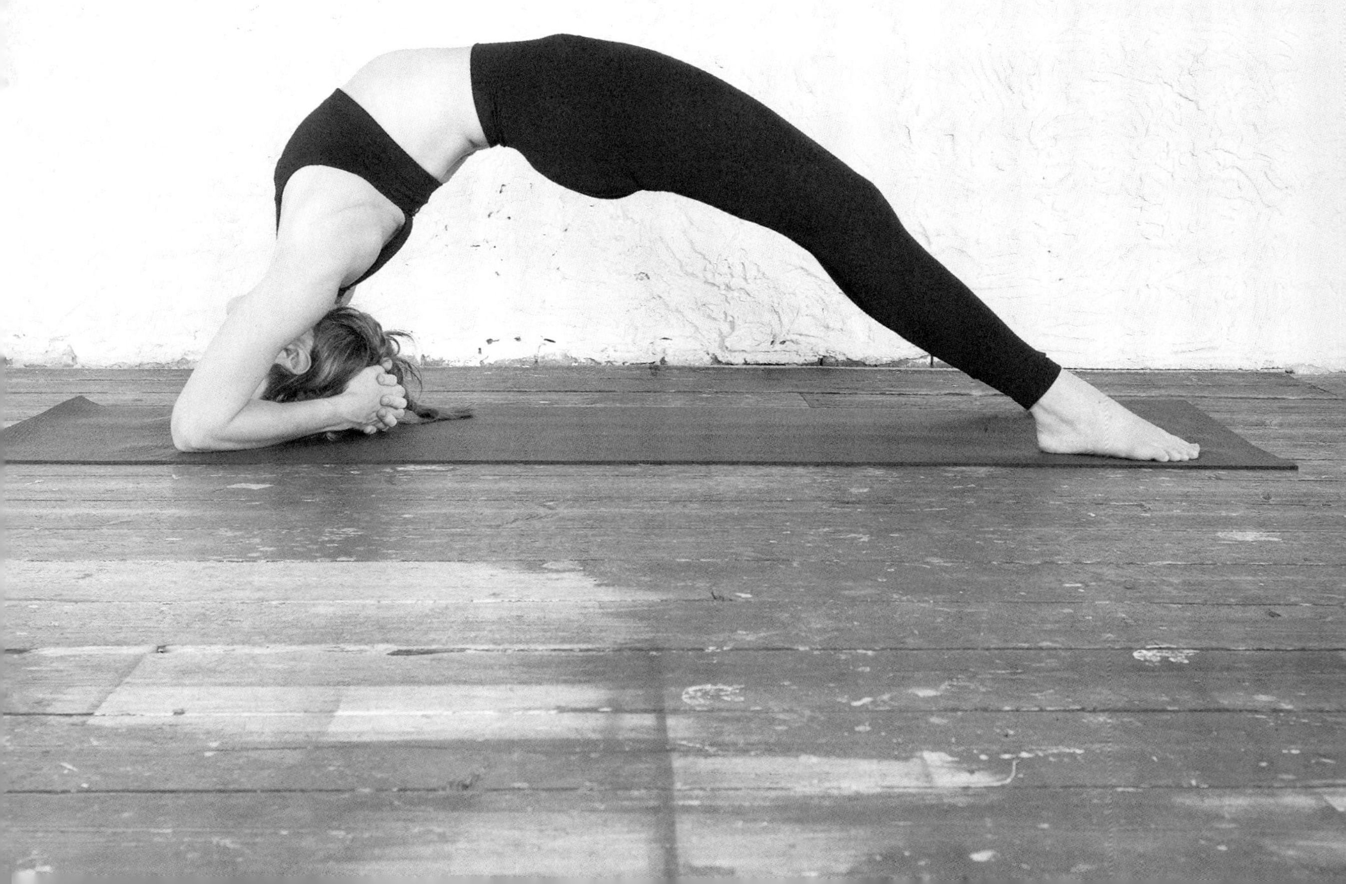

Next pose

Continue with Air-Releasing Pose or a variation thereof.

Alignment cues

Hands are clasped around the back of your head, with the top of your head on the floor (same hand position as in basic Headstand).

Legs are straight and together.

Elbows are pushing firmly into the floor; shoulders are pushed away from the ears and toward your waist.

Contraindications & cautions

- Lower-back and shoulder issues
- Neck issues
- Arthritis
- High blood pressure

Modifications & adjustments

If you feel tension in the quadriceps or knees when straightening your legs and keeping the feet together, you can open your feet hip-width apart.

If you struggle to keep the feet flat on the floor, you can turn your toes slightly outward.

If you feel tension or lack of mobility in the lower back, you can keep your legs slightly bent and hip-width apart.

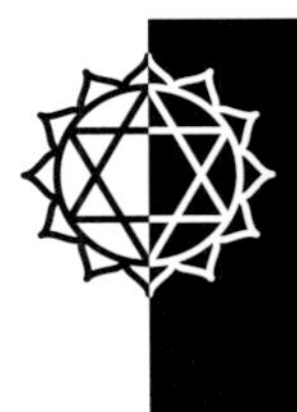

Variations

Eka Pada Viparita Dandasana

Start to come into Inverted Staff Pose, but keep your knees bent and hip-width apart. Then proceed to shift your weight toward your left foot. Lift your right leg straight up toward the ceiling. Stay for a few breaths, then repeat on the other side.

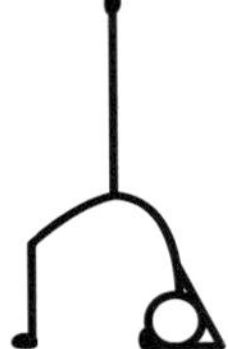

Pawanmuktasana (Air-Releasing Pose) Variations

GARBHASANA
WOMB POSE

HOW TO COME INTO THE POSE

Begin by lying on your back, with your legs extended and your arms resting alongside your body.

Bend your knees, placing the soles of your feet flat on the floor.

Separate your feet so they are hip-width apart.

Your thighs should be parallel to each other.

Straighten your right leg upward, extending your heel toward the ceiling.

Then bend your right knee and cross your right ankle over your left knee.

Then flex your right foot, actively pressing through your heel.

On an exhalation, draw your left knee in toward your chest.

Slide your right hand and forearm through the space between your legs and clasp both hands around your left knee cap.

Gently pull your knee to your chest and lift your head upward off the floor, reaching with your nose toward your left knee.

Hold the pose steadily as long as comfortable and breathe evenly.

To release the pose, place your head back on the floor, release the grip of your knee, and unwind your legs.

Then repeat on the other side.

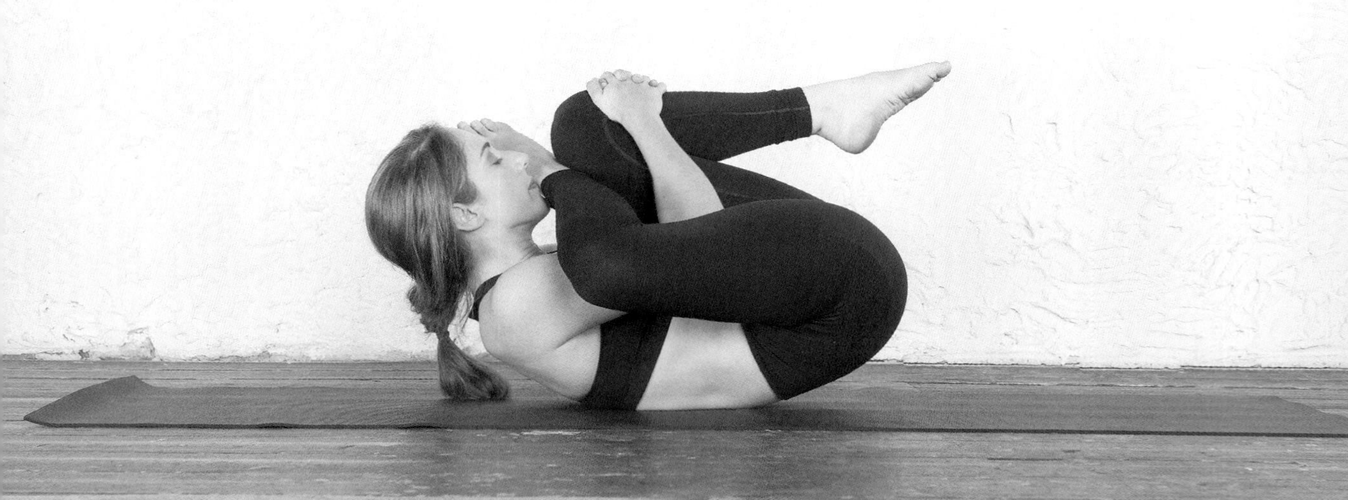

Next pose

Continue with Fish Pose or a variation thereof.

Alignment cues

Pull your knee in only until you feel the stretch in your buttocks.

You should not feel any strain in your knee.

Make sure to not sickle your foot that is crossing over. Keep it flexed and push out through the heel.

Lower and middle back are resting on the floor.

Tailbone and upper back can be lifted off the floor in an effort to bring the nose and knees closer together.

Contraindications & cautions

The same contraindications and cautions apply as in Air-Releasing Pose. However, be cautious with this pose if you have knee issues.

Modifications & adjustments

Keep your head on the floor if you have neck or shoulder pain. If due to tight hips you cannot pull your knee close to your chest, use a strap to bridge the gap and allow your upper back and head to rest on the floor or on a cushion.

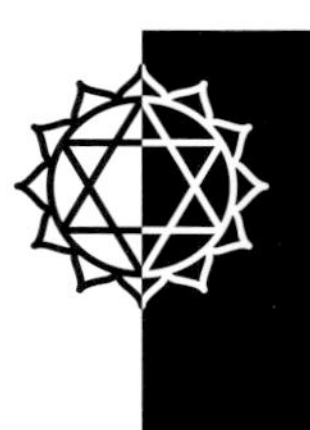

Ananda Balasana
Happy Baby Pose

How to come into the pose

Lie on your back and hug your knees to your chest.

Move your knees apart and hold on to the bottom of your heels from the inside.

Now gently push your feet up toward the ceiling, so that your shins come perpendicular to the floor.

From here gently pull your feet downward, bringing your knees closer to the floor.

Hold the pose steadily as long as comfortable and breathe evenly.

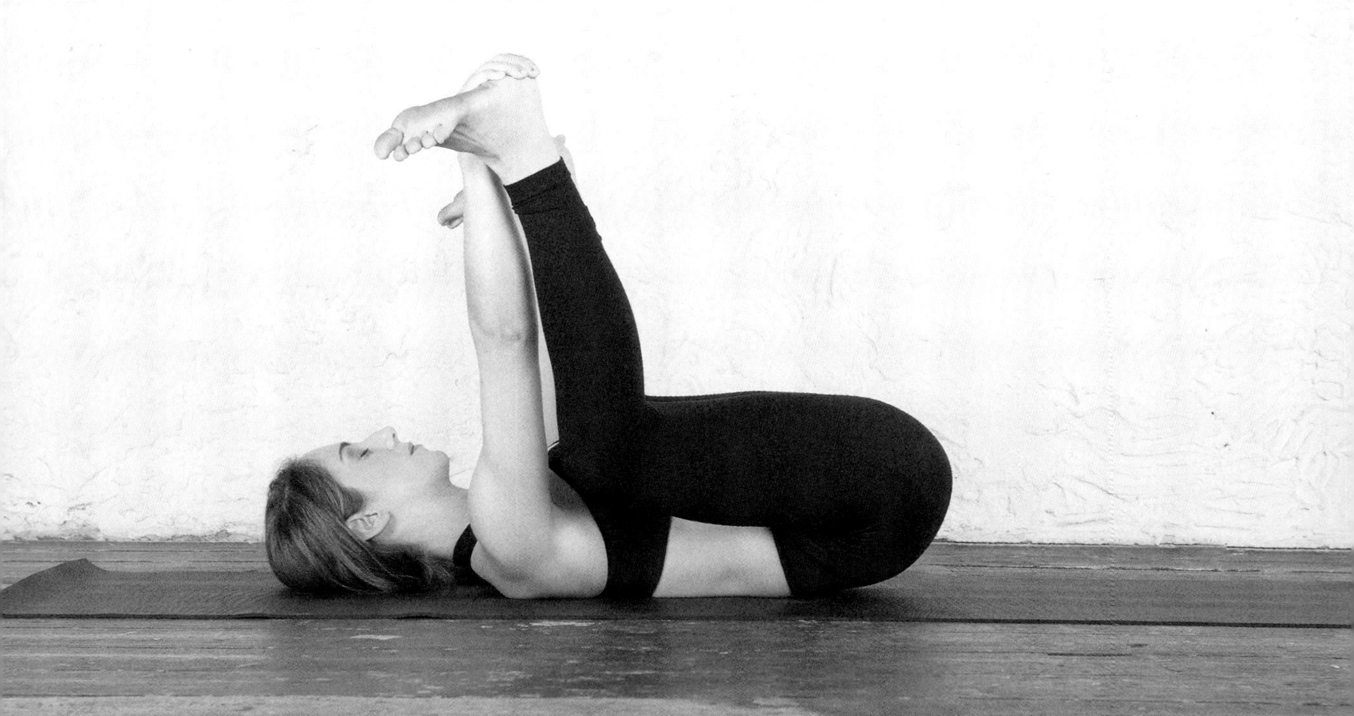

Next pose

Continue with Fish Pose or a variation thereof.

Alignment cues

Your entire back is resting on the floor.

Knees are slightly more than shoulder-width apart

Contraindications & cautions

The same contraindications and cautions apply as in Air-Releasing Pose. Also be cautious with this pose if you have groin or hamstring issues.

Modifications & adjustments

If the top of your head comes off the floor in the effort to hold on to the soles of your feet, modify and hold on to your shins or knees instead, or rest your head on a cushion.

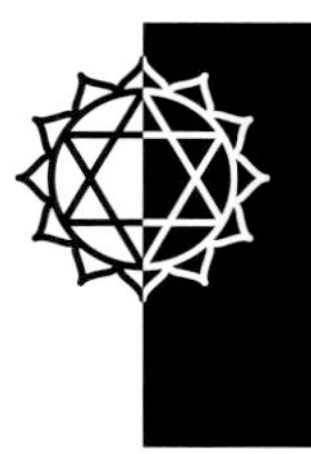

Matsyasana (Fish Pose) Variations

PADMA MATSYASANA

FISH IN LOTUS POSE

HOW TO COME INTO THE POSE

From a seated position, fold your legs into Lotus Pose.

Gently lower yourself down to your back.

Push your elbows into the floor, lift your chest to the ceiling and place the top of your head on the floor.

Hold on to your big toes (right big toe with your right hand and left big toe with your left hand).

Take deep breaths and arch your upper back further with every inhalation.

To come out of the pose, release your toes, place your elbows on the floor, and look up toward your feet.

Gently unwind your legs and release your upper body down to the floor.

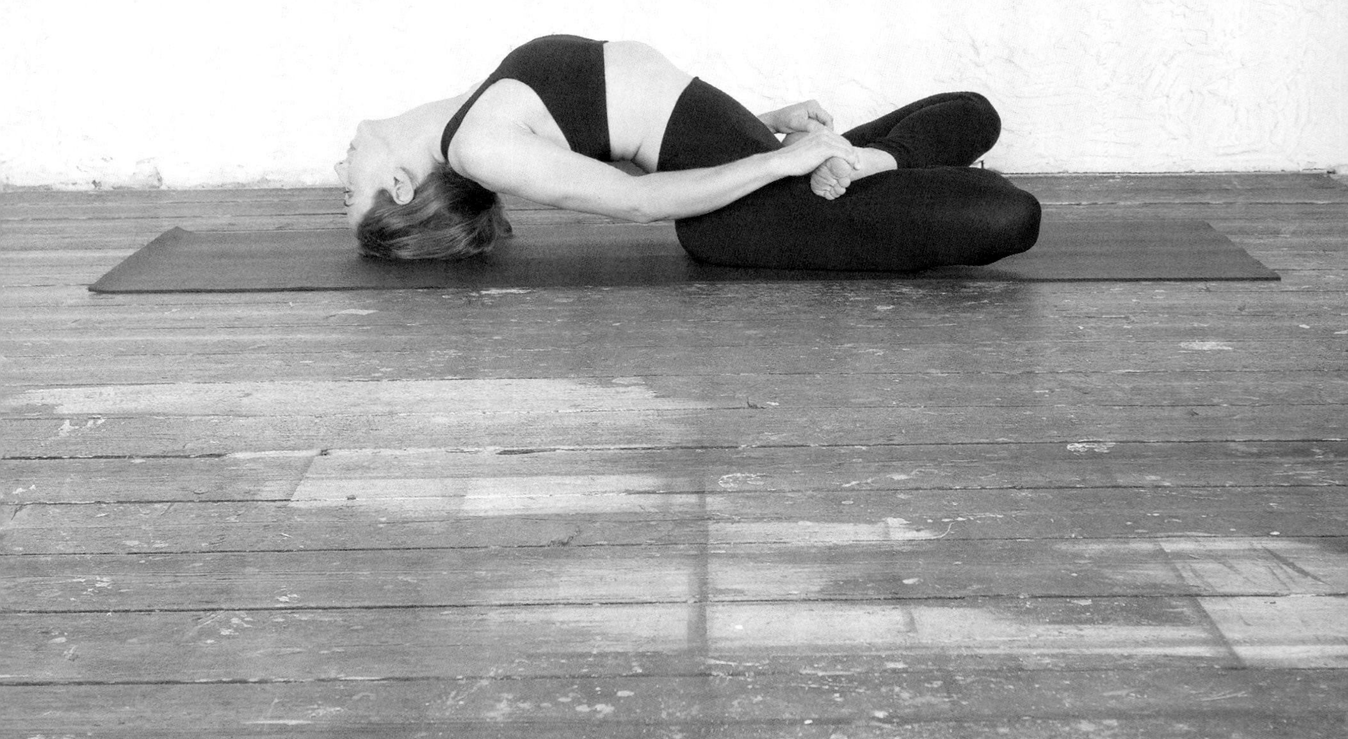

Next pose

Continue with Easy Cow Face Pose or a variation thereof.

Alignment cues

The chest is lifted maximally and the crown of your head is gently pushing against the floor.

Hands are grabbing the feet or big toes, using the opposition to pull the upper body into an arch.

Contraindications & cautions

The same contraindications and cautions apply as in Fish Pose. Also be cautious with this pose if you have tight hips or knee issues.

Modifications & adjustments

If you are not able to fold comfortably and without strain into Lotus Pose, keep your legs crossed at the calves, as in Easy Sitting Pose. Instead of pulling your toes, you can firmly clasp your inner thighs to create the desired opposition.

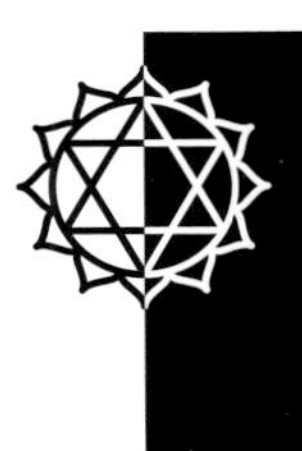

Uttanpadasana
Raised-Leg Pose

How to come into the pose

Come into Fish Pose, but instead of placing your hands underneath your hips, keep them next to your hips.

From Fish Pose, first lift both legs 45 degrees off the floor, feet together and pointed.

Push your head into the floor and lift your arms, reaching with your hands toward your knees.

Keep pushing your chest toward the ceiling and take deep breaths.

To release the pose, place your elbows on the ground and release your legs down to the floor.

Now, shifting your weight toward your elbows, gently tuck your chin toward your chest and relax the upper body to the ground.

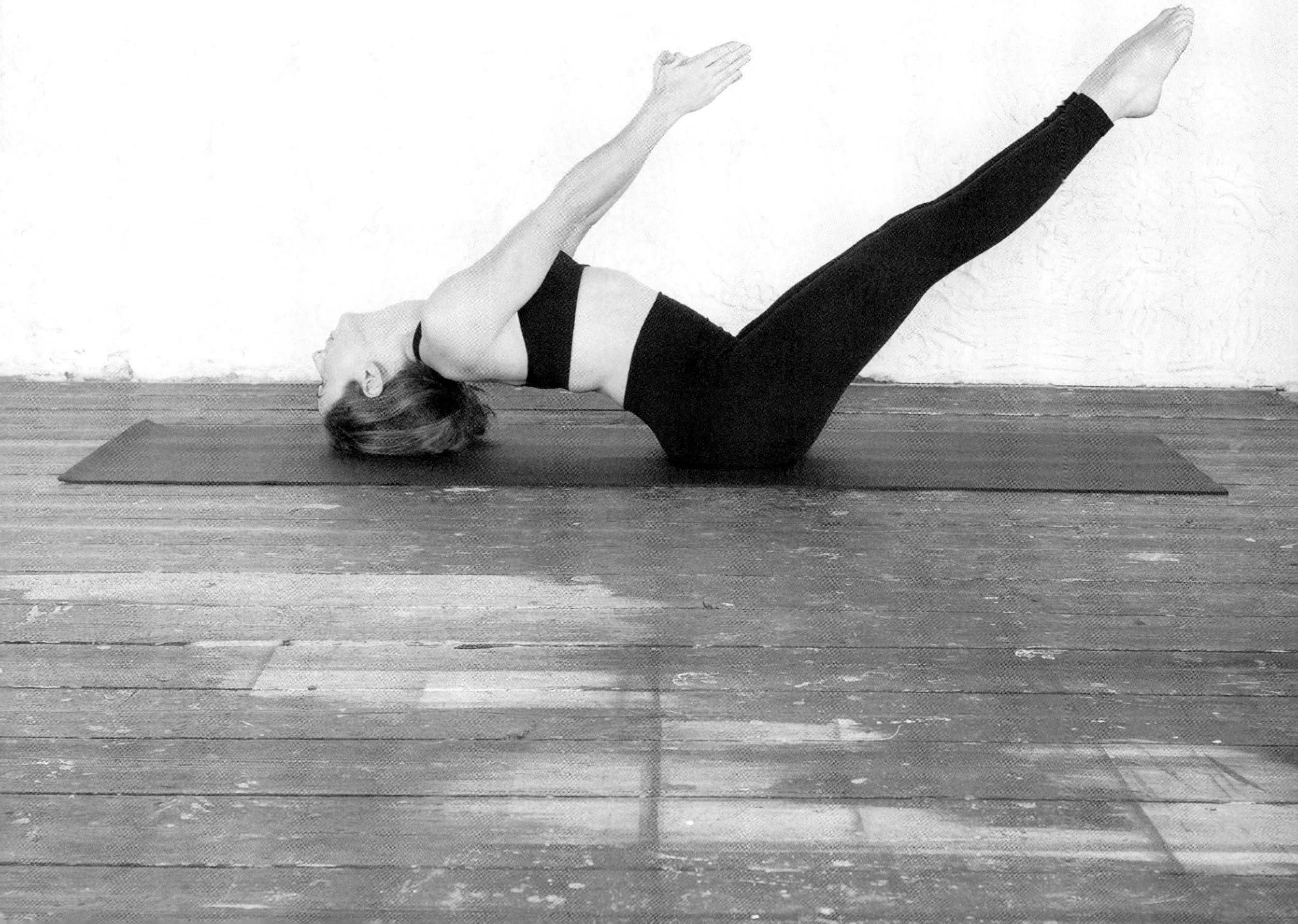

Next pose

Continue with Easy Cow Face Pose or a variation thereof.

Alignment cues

Weight is resting on your hips and head.

Feet are together and pointed at an approximately 45-degree angle to the floor.

Hands are reaching toward your knees, palms together.

Your back is maximally arched and your chest is maximally expanded.

Contraindications & cautions

The same contraindications and cautions apply as in Fish Pose. Also be cautious with this pose if you have lower-back issues.

Modifications & adjustments

To build up to this pose, you can start either by lifting only your legs off the floor, while keeping your elbows as a support on the floor, or by keeping your legs on the floor and lifting only your arms up.

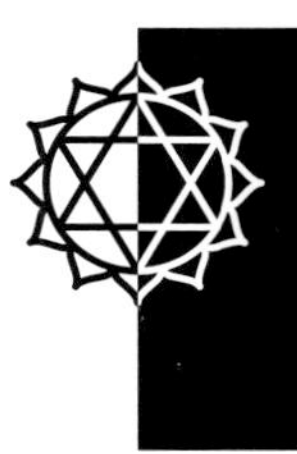

Sukha Gomukhasana (Easy Cow Face Pose) Variations

GOMUKHASANA
CLASSICAL COW FACE POSE

HOW TO COME INTO THE POSE

Sit on your heels, with knees together.

Shift your weight to your right and sit on your right hip.

Cross your left leg over your right, placing your left heel next to your right hip.

Your left knee is on top of your right knee.

Reach out and around with your right hand and place it in between your shoulder blades, as high up as possible (palm facing outward).

Reach up to the ceiling with your left hand, bend your elbow, and clasp your hands behind your back.

Hold the pose steadily as long as comfortable and breathe evenly.

Then release and repeat on the other side.

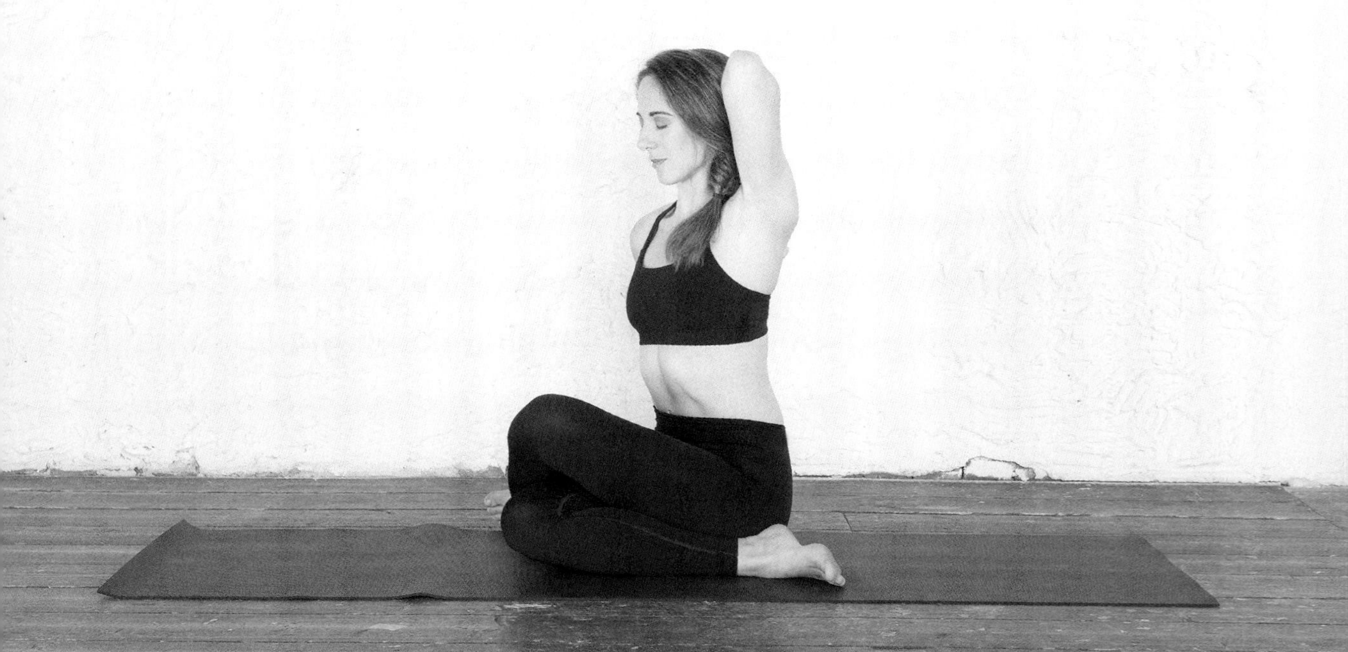

Next pose

Continue with Seated Forward Bend or a variation thereof.

Alignment cues

The same-side knee and elbow are up.

The elbow of your top arm is reaching up toward the ceiling.

Sitting bones should be on the floor; avoid sitting on your opposite heel.

Contraindications & cautions

The same contraindications and cautions apply as in Easy Cow Face Pose. Also be cautious with this pose if you have tight hips or knee issues.

Modifications & adjustments

If you feel uncomfortable in this sitting position (due to tight hips or knee issues), you can practice Easy Cow Face Pose instead.

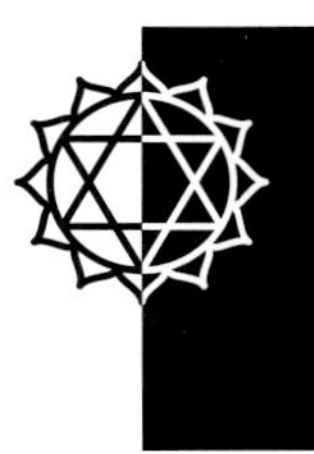

Sidana Garudasana
Seated-Eagle Pose

How to come into the pose

Sit on your heels, with your knees together.

Shift your weight to your right, and sit on your right hip.

Cross your left leg over your right leg, placing your left heel next to your right hip.

Your left knee is on top of your right knee.

Extend your right arm in front of you, at shoulder level.

Cross your left arm under your right and bring your palms together.

Raise your elbows to almost shoulder level and gently press your hands away from your face, bringing the forearms perpendicular to the floor.

Hold the pose steadily as long as comfortable and breathe evenly.

Then release and repeat on the other side.

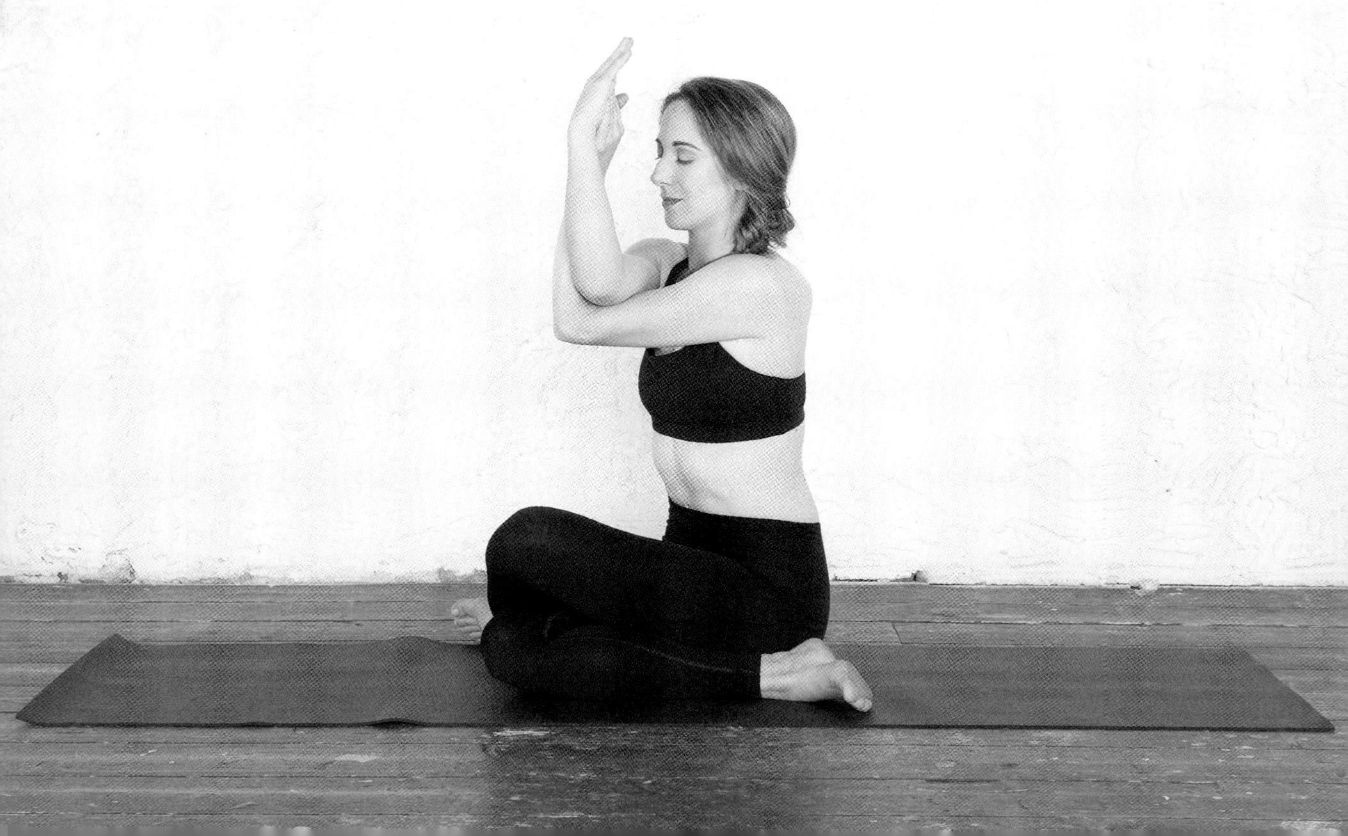

Next pose

Continue with Seated Forward Bend or a variation thereof.

Alignment cues

Elbows are lifted slightly away from the chest.

Shoulders are pushing away from your ears, toward your waist.

Both sitting bones should be on the floor; avoid sitting on your heels.

Contraindications & cautions

The same contraindications and cautions apply as in Easy Cow Face Pose.

Modifications & adjustments

If this pose is challenging due to tightness in the hips or knees, you can support either both or one side with a folded blanket or a block.

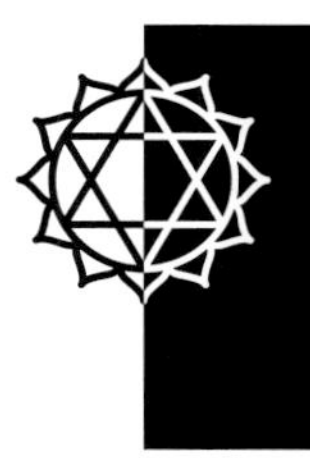

USHTRASANA
CAMEL POSE

HOW TO COME INTO THE POSE

Start from a kneeling position, with your knees hip-width apart and pelvis lifted.

Push your pelvis forward and hold your right heel with your right hand.

Open your chest and bring your left hand to your left heel.

Push your pelvis forward so that it is right above your knees and gently drop your head backward.

Hold the pose steadily as long as comfortable and breathe evenly.

To come out of the pose, bring your hands to your lower back and using your hands as a support, lead with your chest to come all the way up.

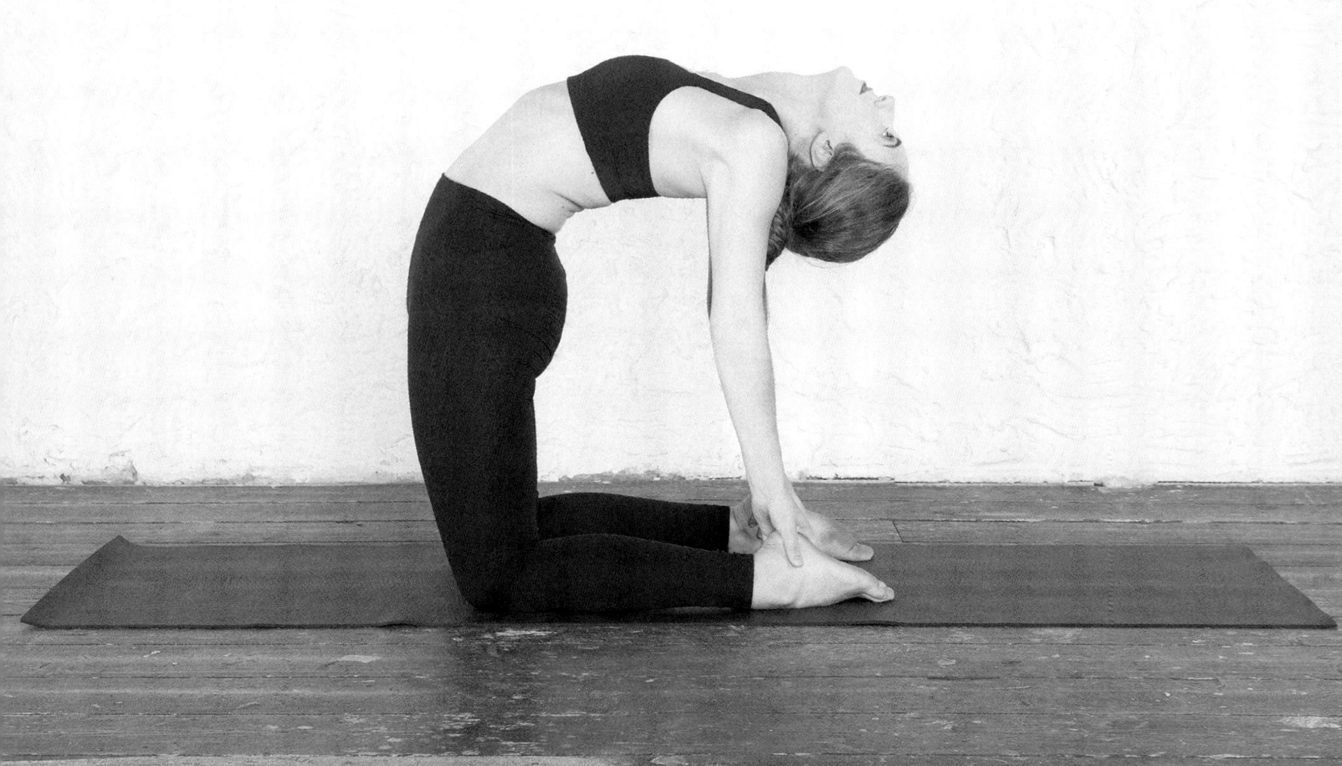

Next pose

Relax in Child's Pose for 30–45 seconds and then continue with Seated Forward Bend or a variation thereof.

Alignment cues

Knees are hip-width or maximum shoulder-width apart; feet are pointed.

Pelvis should be right above your knees.

Chest is expanded, and shoulder blades are drawn toward each other.

Contraindications & cautions

The same contraindications and cautions apply as in Easy Cow Face Pose. Also be cautious with this pose if you have neck issues or hypertension.

Modifications & adjustments

If your pelvis drops behind your knees when reaching toward your heels with your hands, you can place the toes on the floor to lift the heels and then hold on to your heels before gently releasing your head backward.

An even more accessible modification is to place your hands on your lower back, with your fingertips pointing downward. From here, press your elbows toward each other as you push your pelvis forward and look diagonally up, keeping the back of your neck elongated.

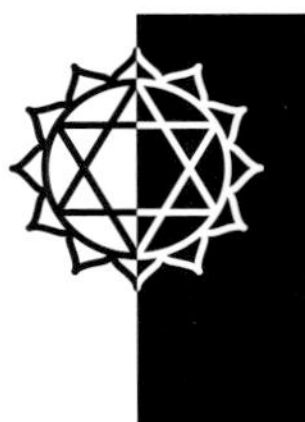

Variations

Purna Ushtrasana

Full Camel Pose

Full Camel Pose requires a truly deep backbend, as well as an open chest and a good rotation in your shoulders. To come into the pose, first start in Camel Pose. From there, reach your hands one by one over your head, arching your back further until your palms touch the floor (fingertips pointing toward your knees). From here, keep pushing your pelvis upward and forward, bending your arms and placing your elbows on the floor. Firmly press your elbows into the floor, hold on to your heels, and look in between your knees.

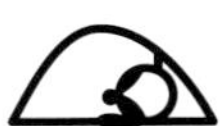

Laghu Vajrasana

Little Thunderbolt Pose

Begin in a kneeling position, with your thighs perpendicular to the floor. Lift your chest to lengthen your spine as you move into Camel Pose. Walk your hands forward to tightly hold on to your thighs. Gently drop your head backward. Firmly ground through your legs, and with control slowly lower your crown to the floor, coming into an even deeper backbend. Keeping your arms straight, walk your hands further down toward your knees.

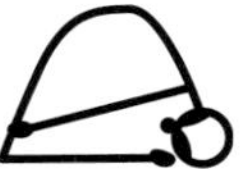

Anahatasana
Melting-Heart Pose

How to come into the pose

Come onto all fours, with your shoulders above your wrists and your hips above your knees.

Walk your hands forward and start to arch your back, reaching with your chest toward the floor.

Keeping the hips above the knees, rest your chin and if possible your chest on the floor.

Hold the pose steadily as long as comfortable and breathe evenly.

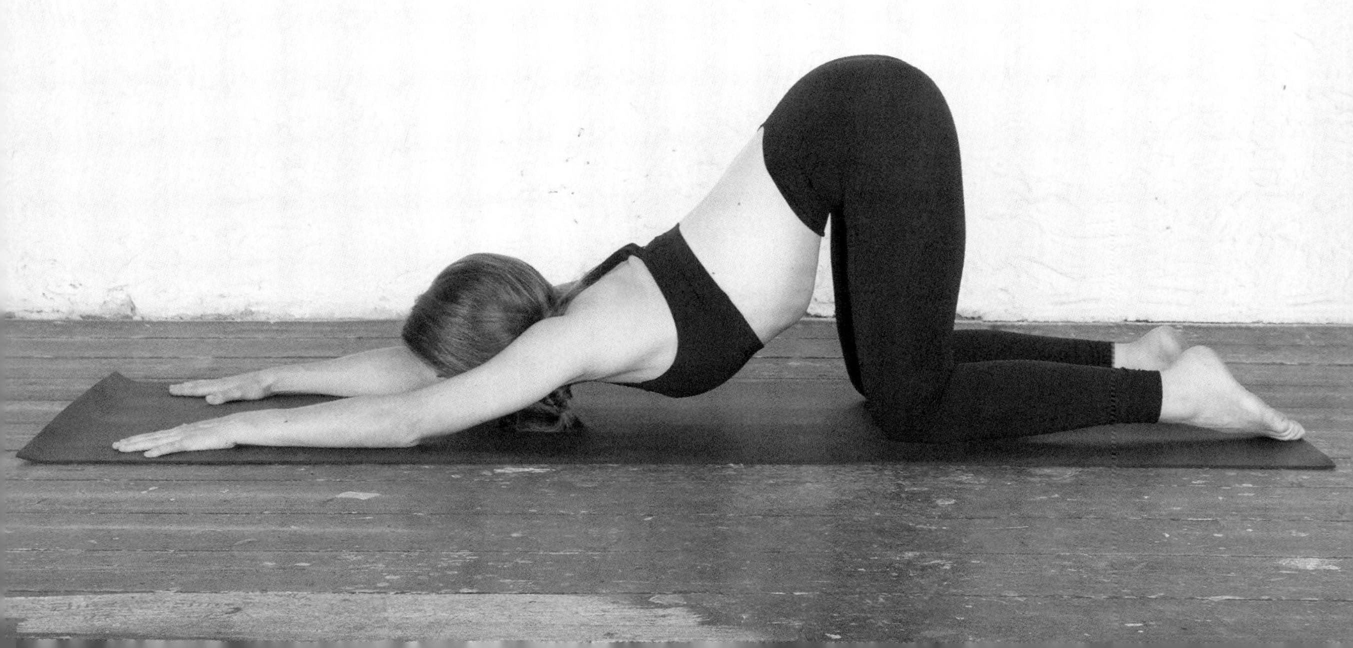

Next pose

Continue with Seated Forward Bend or a variation thereof.

Alignment cues

The hips remain right above the knees.

Press the hands down and stretch through the arms, while keeping your hips above your knees.

Keep your neck elongated, the collarbones wide, and the shoulders relaxed.

Contraindications & cautions

The same contraindications and cautions apply as in Easy Cow Face Pose. Also be cautious with this pose if you have neck issues or hypertension.

Modifications & adjustments

To decrease the intensity of the pose (especially for the neck and upper back), you can rest your forehead on the ground instead of your chin.

If you feel tenderness or pain in your knees from kneeling on the ground, place a folded blanket underneath them for cushioning.

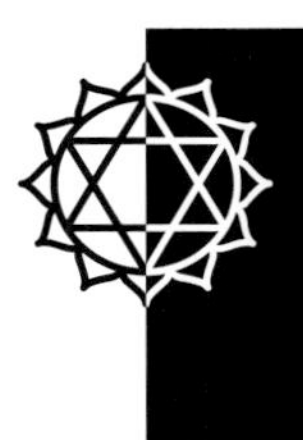

Pashchima Namaskarasana

Seated Reverse Prayer Pose

How to come into the pose

Sit on your knees, with your hips on your heels.

Join the palms of your hands behind your back, fingers reaching upward in Reverse Prayer Pose.

Gently push your hands up between your shoulder blades.

Inhale and open your chest, push your shoulders down and back, and look straight forward.

Hold the pose steadily as long as comfortable and breathe evenly.

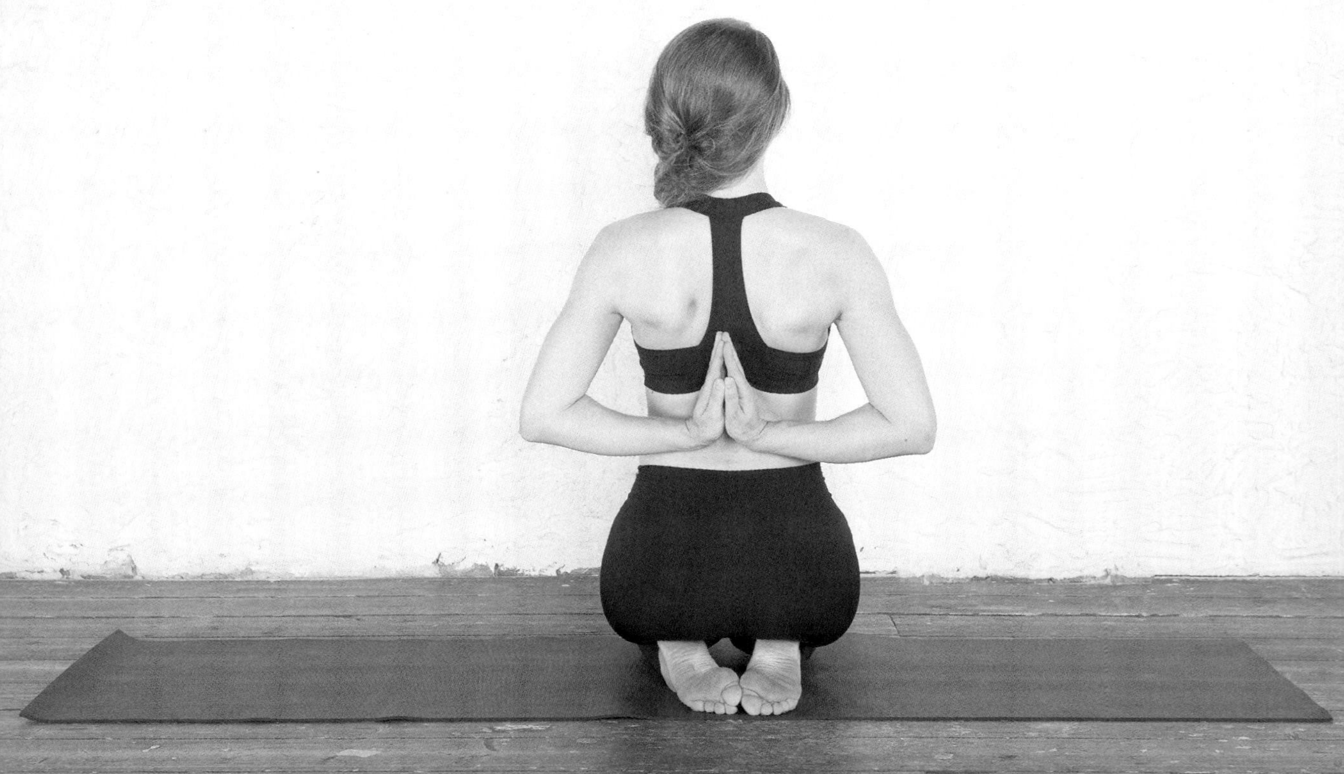

Next pose

Continue with Seated Forward Bend or a variation thereof.

Alignment cues

Spine is erect, the back of your neck elongated.

Hands are as far up in between your shoulder blades as possible.

The focus is on widening the collarbones and rolling the shoulders backward.

Contraindications & cautions

The same contraindications and cautions apply as in Easy Cow Face Pose. Also be cautious with this pose if you have wrist issues.

Modifications & adjustments

If there is too much tension or pain in your shoulders or wrists, you can either hold your elbows or interlock your fingers behind your back and push your hands down and away from you.

If you feel tension in your knees when sitting, place a cushion under your hips.

Classically this pose was performed in Full Lotus Pose. You can also perform this pose in Half Lotus Pose or Easy Sitting Pose or any other seated position where your spine is straight.

To intensify the pose, you can also fold forward, to place your forehead on the floor, after placing your hands in Reverse Prayer Pose or a variation thereof as described above.

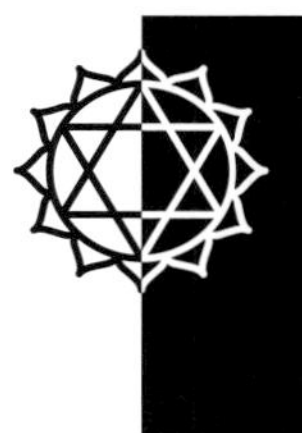

Sukha Gomukhasana (Easy Cow Face Pose) Alternatives

Marjaryasana I & II

Cat Pose I & II

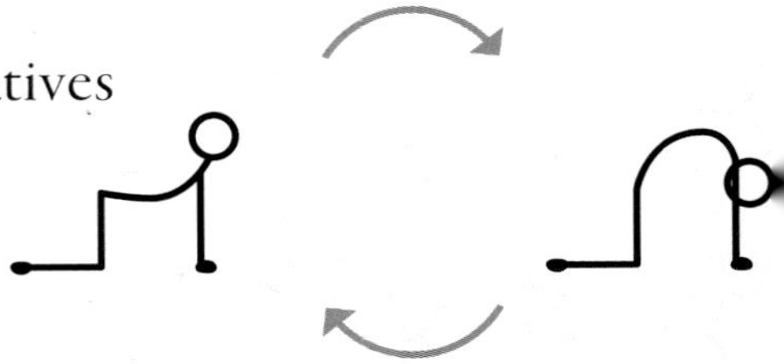

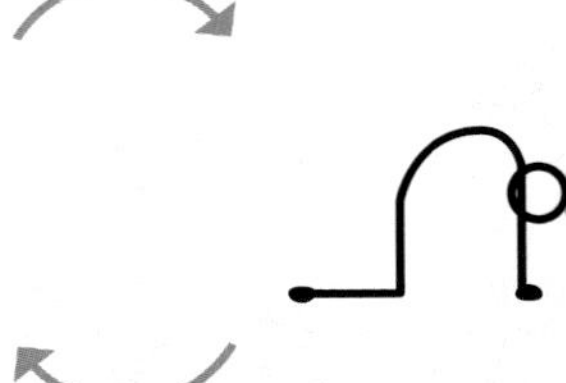

How to come into the pose

Come onto all fours, with your knees right below your hips and your wrists below your shoulders.

As you inhale, arch your back, open the chest, push your belly button toward the floor, and look up (Marjaryasana I).

As you exhale, push your hands and knees into the floor and round your back as much as possible, bringing your chin to your chest and the middle back toward the ceiling (Marjaryasana II).

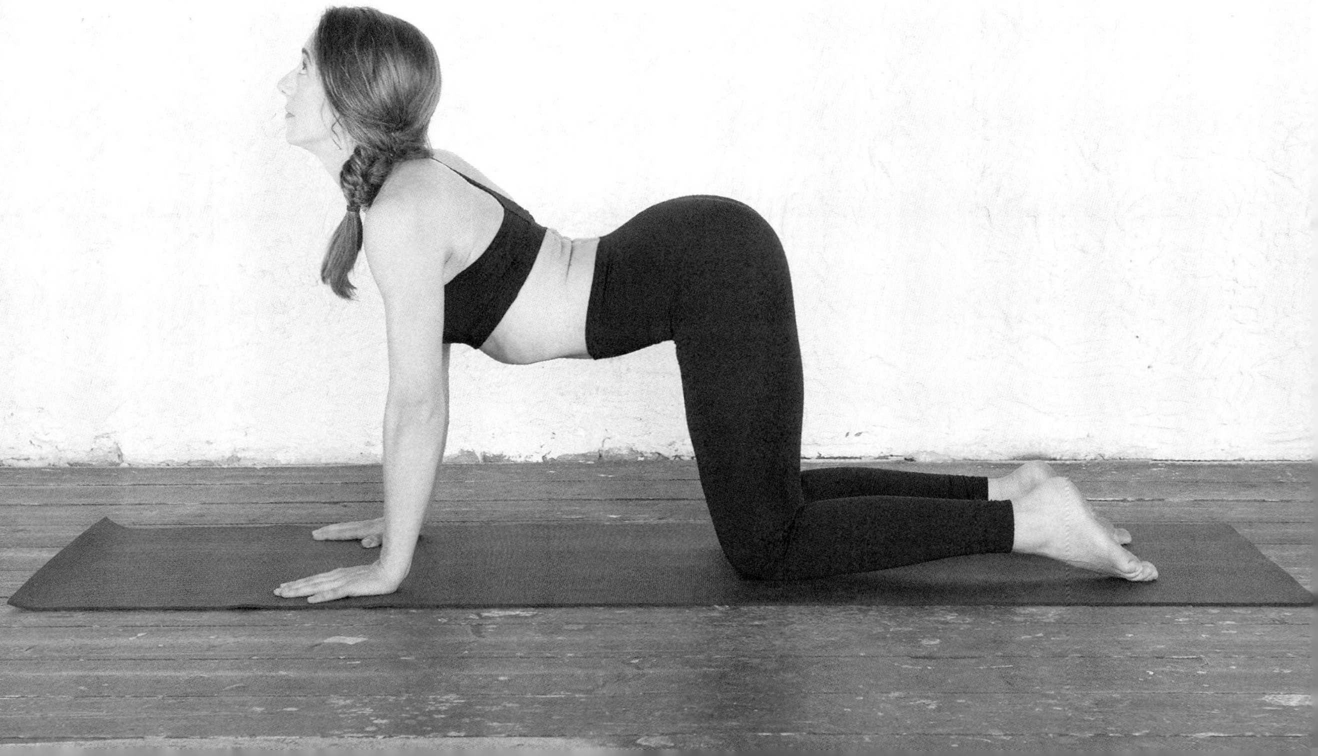

Next pose

Continue with Seated Forward Bend or a variation thereof.

Alignment cues

These poses can be performed either dynamically, moving into Marjaryasana I with every inhalation and into Marjaryasana II with every exhalation, or they can be performed statically, holding each variation around 30 seconds while breathing naturally.

Shoulders are above your wrists, and hips are above your knees.

Toes are pointed, and hands are actively pushing into the floor.

Contraindications & cautions

There are no general contraindications and cautions to this pose. However, respect your limit of movement and do not push further than that, as that can cause strain.

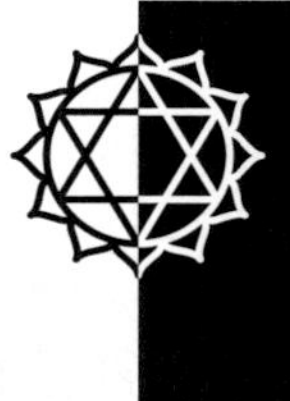

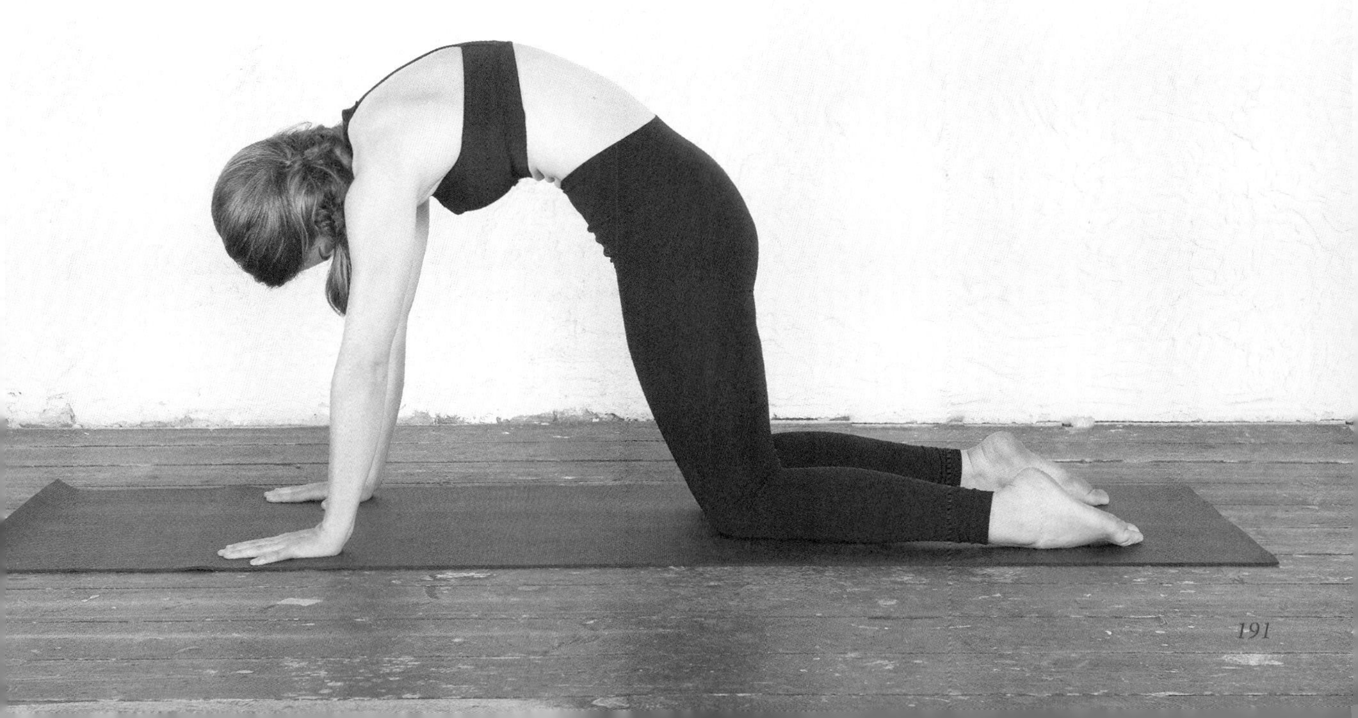

Vyaghrasana I & II
Tiger Pose I & II

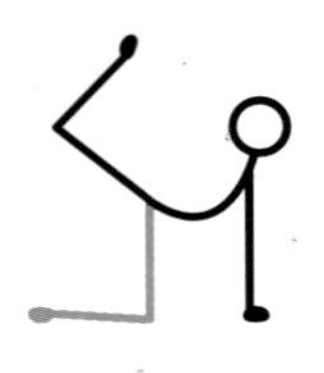

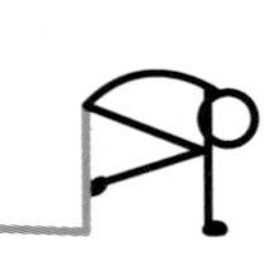

How to come into the pose

Come on to all fours, with your knees right below your hips and your wrists below your shoulders.

As you breathe in, arch your back and look upward and backward.

At the same time, lift your right knee off the floor and reach with the sole of your foot toward the crown of your head (Vyaghrasana I).

As you exhale, bring your right knee to your nose and round your back (Vyaghrasana II).

Come back onto all fours and repeat the same with your left leg.

Next pose

Continue with Seated Forward Bend or a variation thereof.

Alignment cues

These poses can be performed either dynamically—moving into Vyaghrasana I with every inhalation and into Vyaghrasana II with every exhalation—or statically, holding each variation around 30 seconds while breathing naturally.

Shoulders are above your wrists and hips are above your knees.

Elbows are straight, and hands are firmly pushing into the floor.

Your pelvis is kept as square as possible at all times.

Contraindications & cautions

There are no general contraindications and cautions to this pose. However, respect your limit of movement and do not push further than that, because that can cause strain.

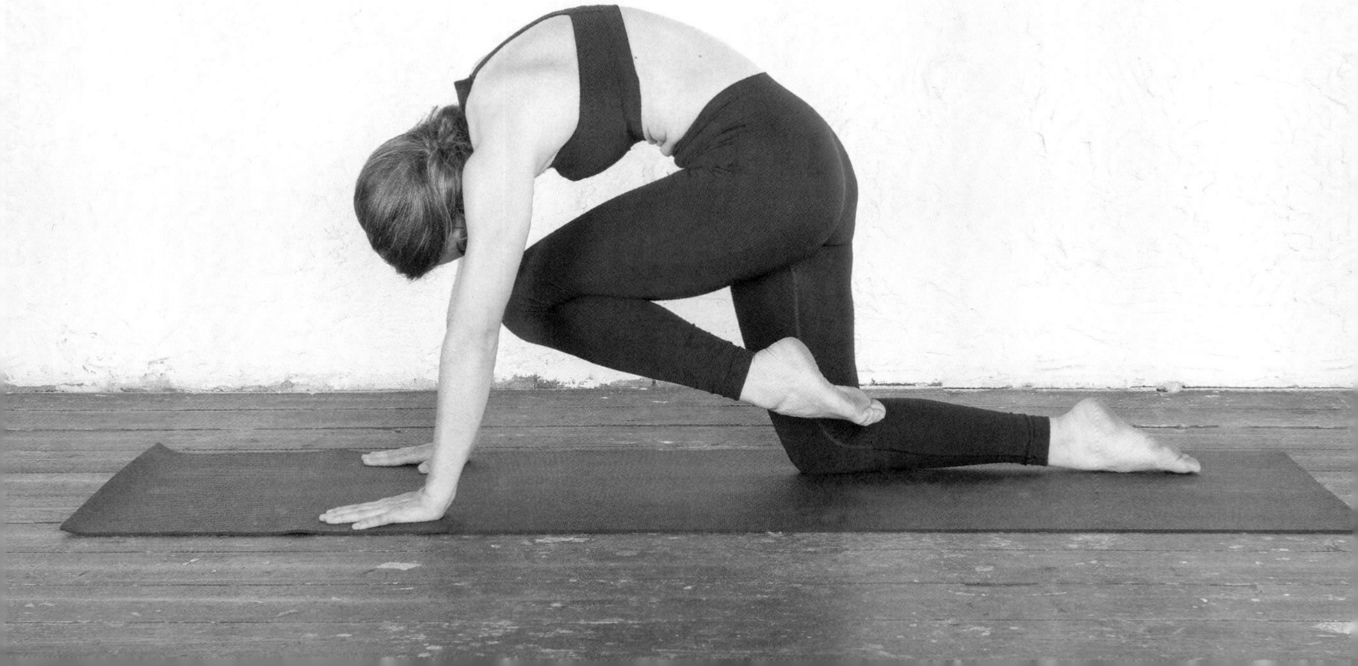

Variations

Eka Hasta Vyaghrasana

One-Handed Tiger Pose

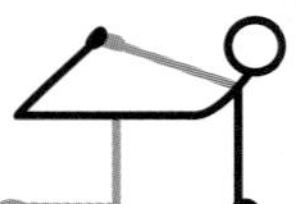

Come on to all fours, with your knees right below your hips and wrists below your shoulders. As you breathe in, arch your back and look up and backward and extend your left arm forward. As you do so, lift your right knee off the floor and reach with the sole of your foot toward the crown of your head. Swipe your left arm sideways and backward and grab hold of the inside of your right ankle. Keeping the elbow straight, create an opposition between your hand and foot, arching your back to the maximum. Look straight ahead and breathe evenly.

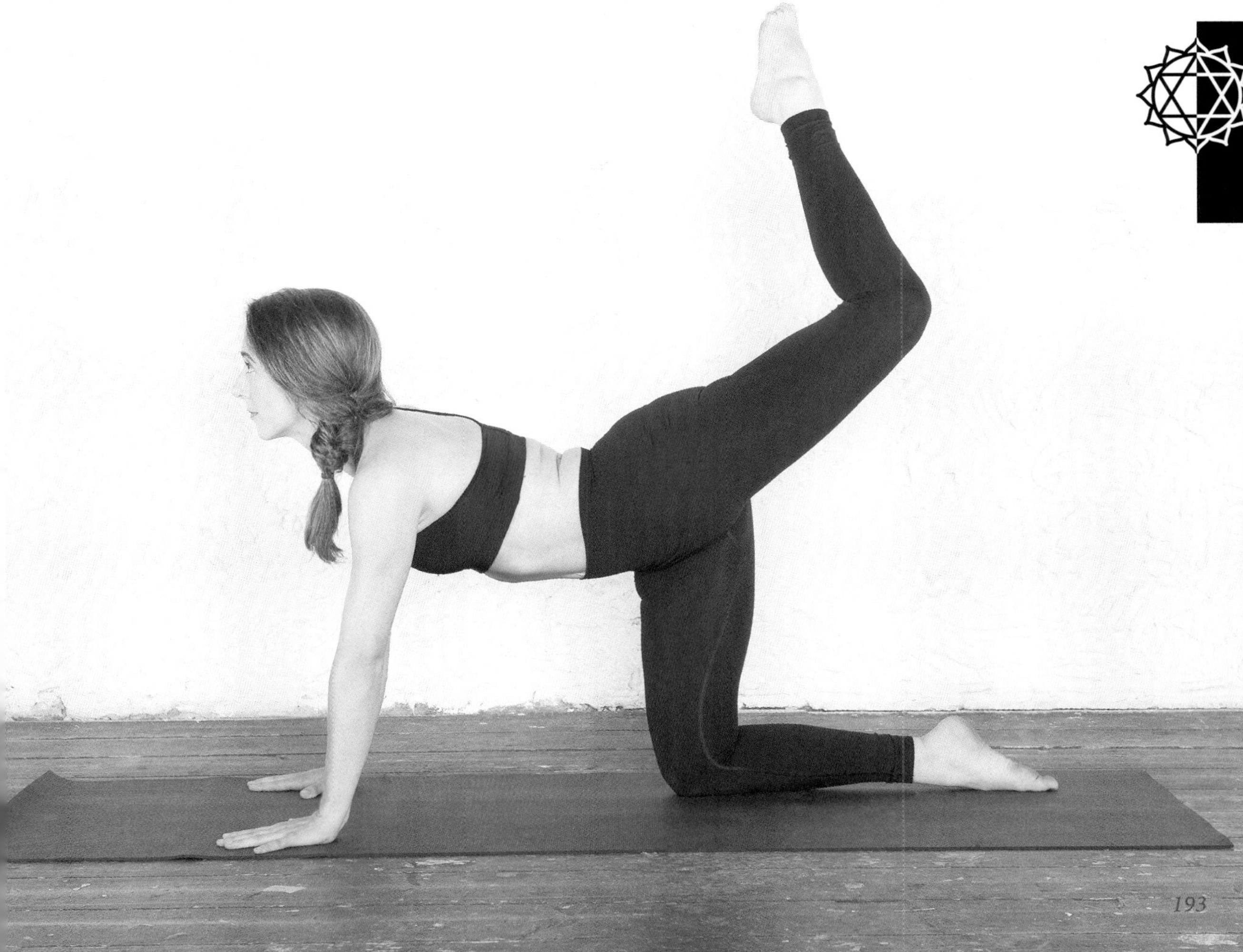

Chapter 15

Variations for the Solar Plexus Chakra

Paschimottanasana (Seated Forward Bend) Variations

Supta Padangusthasana
Reclining Hand-to-Toe Pose

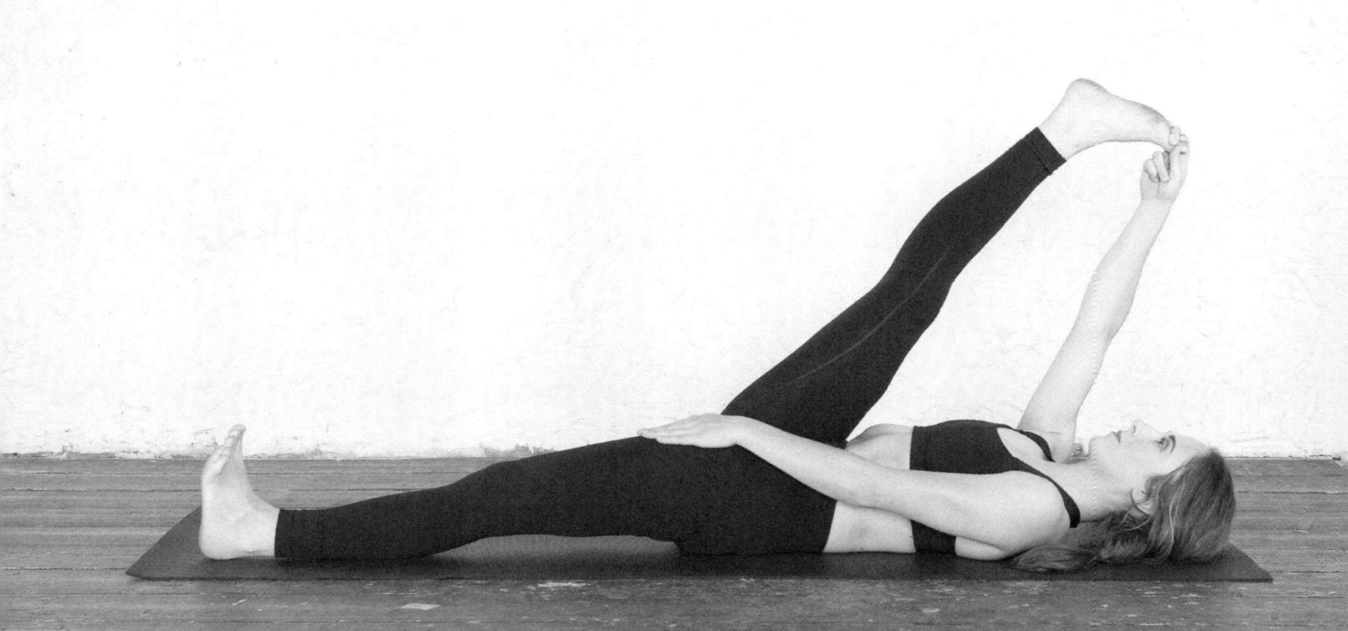

How to come into the pose

Lie supine on the floor, feet together, legs straight.

Bend your right knee and hug your right thigh to your chest.

Hold your right big toe with your right hand and straighten your right leg.

Your left hand is resting on your left thigh.

Breathe evenly and mentally send your breath to your right hamstrings.

After releasing the pose, repeat the same on the other side.

Next pose

Continue with Upward Plank Pose or a variation thereof.

Alignment cues

With the leg on the floor active, push your thigh down toward the mat and push out through the heel.

The back of your head is resting on the floor; shoulders and neck are relaxed.

The lifted leg is straight, and your foot is flexed.

Contraindications & cautions

The same contraindications and cautions apply as in Seated Forward Bend. Also be cautious in this pose if you have hamstring or groin issues.

Modifications & adjustments

If you cannot stretch your leg while holding your big toe, you can wrap a strap around your foot and hold the strap with your right hand. Do not pull forcefully on the strap, because you can injure the hamstrings in this pose.

If you feel tension in your neck and cannot rest your head comfortably on the mat, you can support your head on a low cushion or a folded blanket.

Variations:

Supta Padangusthasana II

Reclining Hand-to-Toe Pose II

From Reclining Hand-to-Toe Pose I (with shoulders and head on the floor), keep holding your big toe or the strap and move your right leg toward your right. Make sure to keep your hips square, with both buttocks and your entire back on the floor. From here you can look straight up toward the ceiling or over your left shoulder.

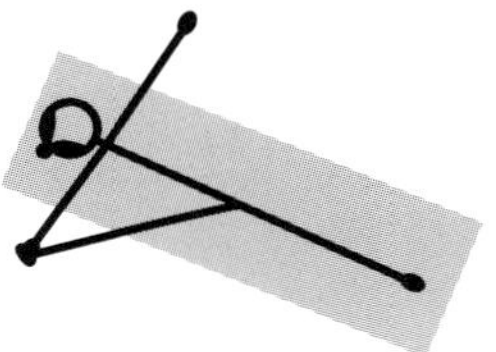

Supta Padangusthasana III

Reclining Hand-to-Toe Pose III

In some traditions, Reclining Hand-to-Toe Pose I is taught with a lifted chest and the nose reaching toward the knee or shin of the lifted leg.

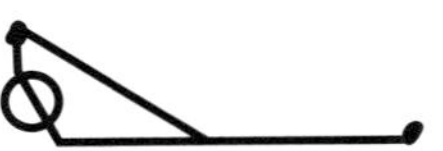

Urdhva Mukha Paschimottanasana I

Upward-Facing Intense-Stretch Pose I

How to come into the pose

Lie on your back with feet together and hands next to you, palms pushing against the floor.

Lift your legs off the floor and catch hold of your calves or ankles.

Gently pull your knees or shins to your nose, keeping your head and shoulders on the floor.

Hold the pose steadily as long as comfortable and breathe evenly.

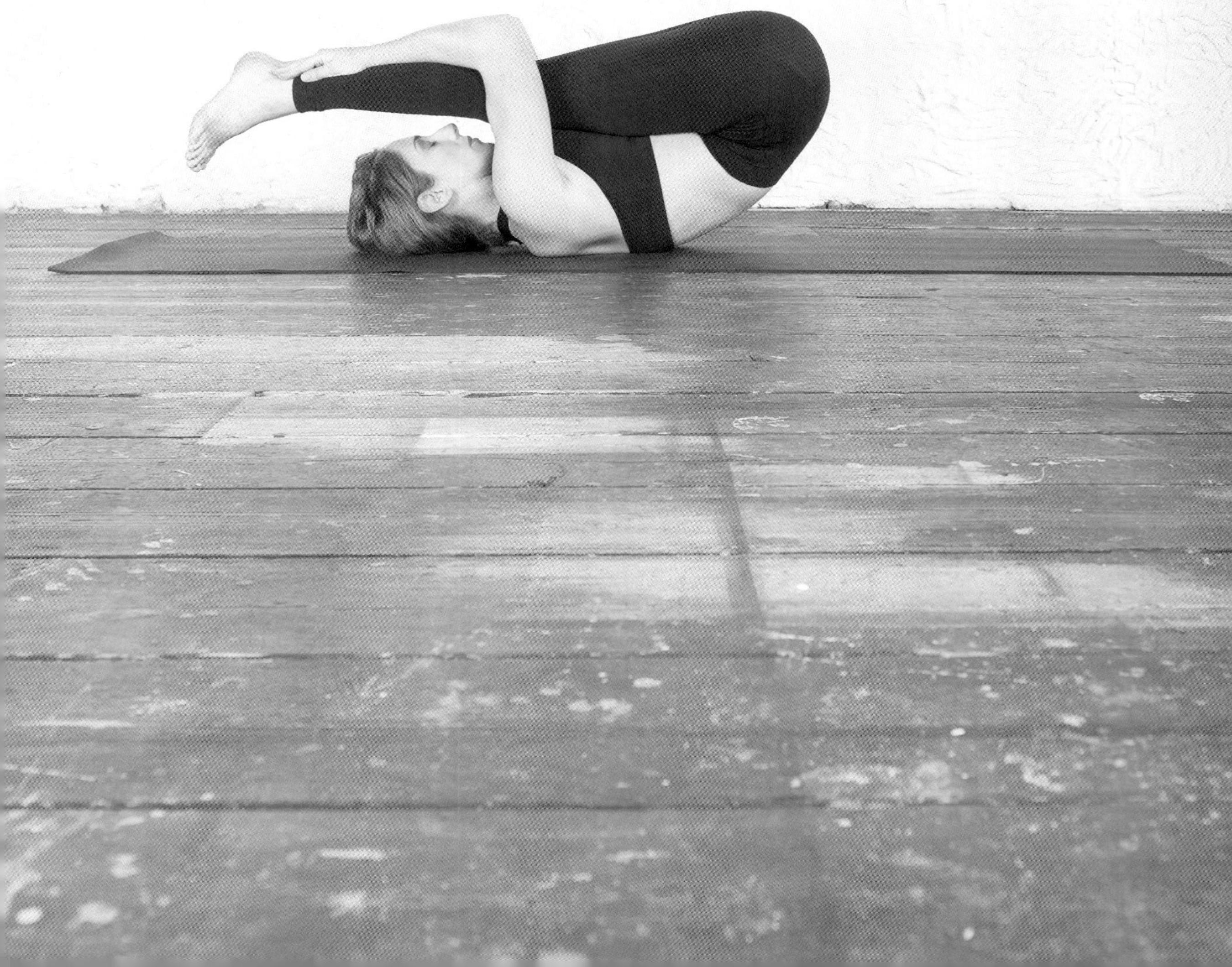

Next pose

Continue with Upward Plank Pose or a variation thereof.

Alignment cues

Head, shoulders, and middle back are relaxed on the floor; your tailbone and lower back can come off the floor.

Legs are straight, and feet are relaxed.

Elbows are tucked in toward your legs; shoulder blades are drawn away from your ears, toward your waist.

Contraindications & cautions

The same contraindications and cautions apply as in Seated Forward Bend.

Modifications & adjustments

If you feel too much strain in your hamstrings or just behind your knees, bend your knees a little.

If you experience tightness in your lower back or hips, you might find the pose more accessible if you open your legs hip-width apart.

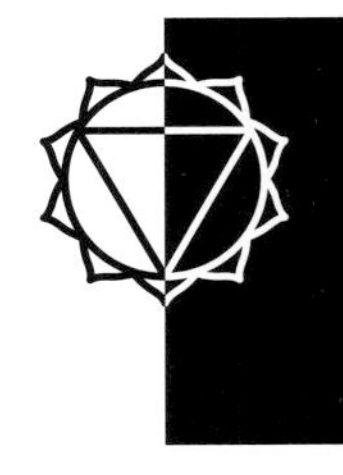

Urdhva Mukha Paschimottanasana II

Upward-Facing Intense-Stretch Pose II

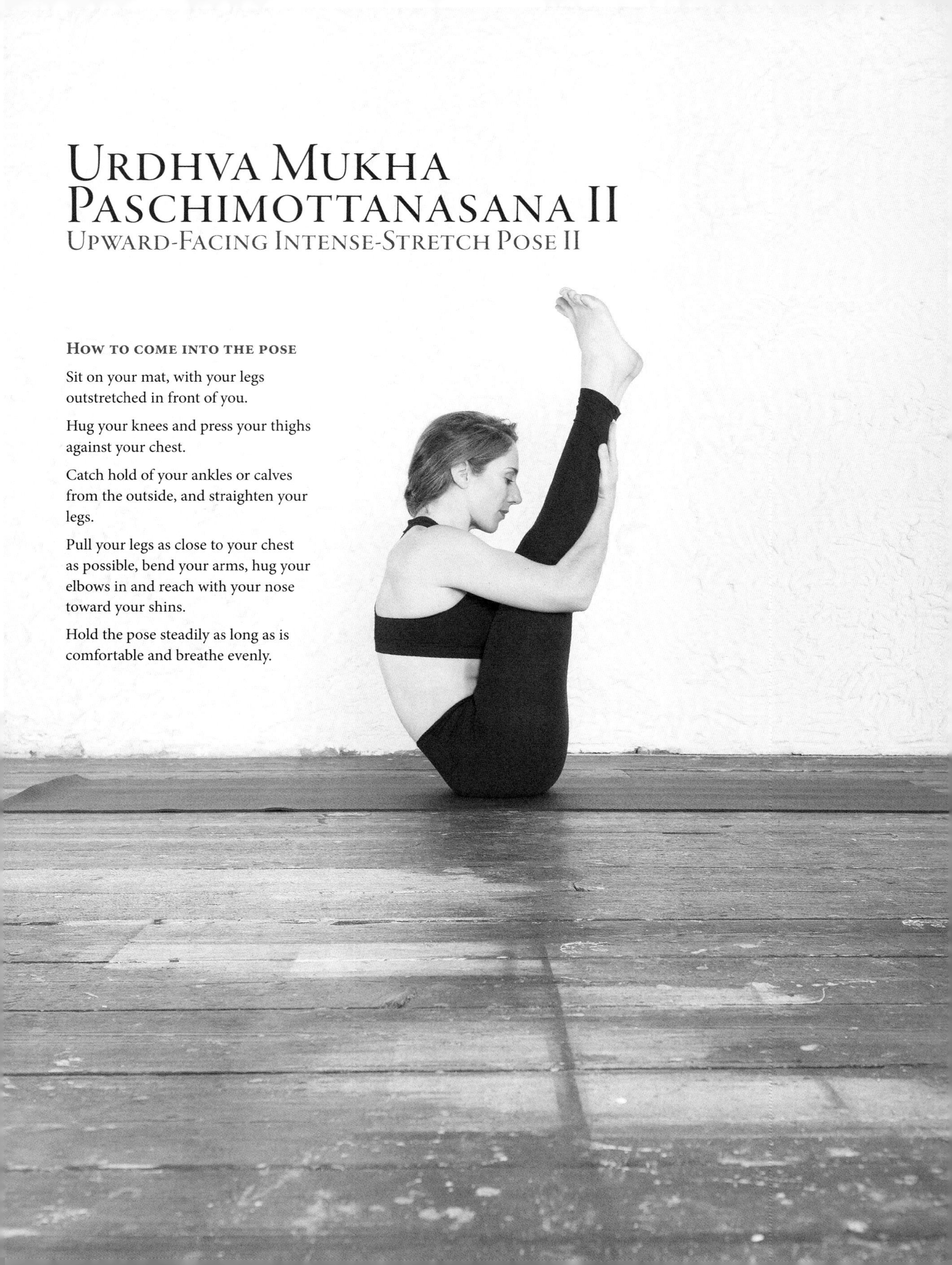

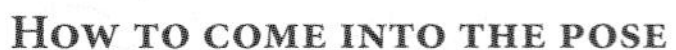

How to come into the pose

Sit on your mat, with your legs outstretched in front of you.

Hug your knees and press your thighs against your chest.

Catch hold of your ankles or calves from the outside, and straighten your legs.

Pull your legs as close to your chest as possible, bend your arms, hug your elbows in and reach with your nose toward your shins.

Hold the pose steadily as long as is comfortable and breathe evenly.

Next pose

Continue with Upward Plank Pose or a variation thereof.

Alignment cues

The back is as straight as possible, chest and thighs are as close together as possible, and shoulder blades are drawn down toward your waist.

Avoid dropping your elbows out by firmly pressing your forearms against the sides of your lower legs.

Contraindications & cautions

The same contraindications and cautions apply as in Seated Forward Bend.

Modifications & adjustments

This pose requires true hamstring flexibility. It is okay to keep your knees slightly bent, if necessary.

If you experience tightness in your lower back or hips, you might find the pose more accessible if you open your legs hip-width apart.

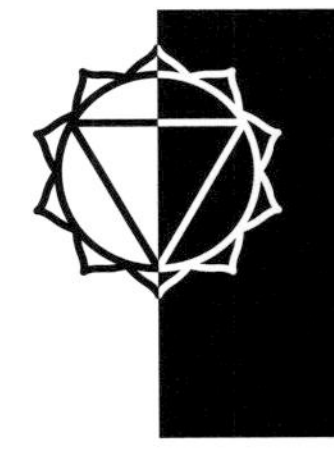

Parivrtta Paschimottanasana
Revolved Seated Forward Bend

How to come into the pose

Sit with your legs straight in front of you, feet together.

Make sure you are sitting high up on your sitting bones.

Breathe in and reach with your hands up to the ceiling.

Breathe out, bend forward, and hold your right big toe with your left hand and your left big toe with your right hand (right arm is crossing above your left arm).

Breathe in and lengthen your spine, gently pulling your toes toward you.

Breathe out and twist your upper body to your right, with the right elbow reaching up toward the ceiling.

Look under your right arm toward the ceiling and reach with your left elbow toward the outside of your right knee.

Hold the pose steadily as long as comfortable and breathe evenly.

To come out of the pose, bring your upper body back to the center, release your hands, and slowly roll upward.

Repeat the same on the other side, with your left arm above your right arm, twisting to your left.

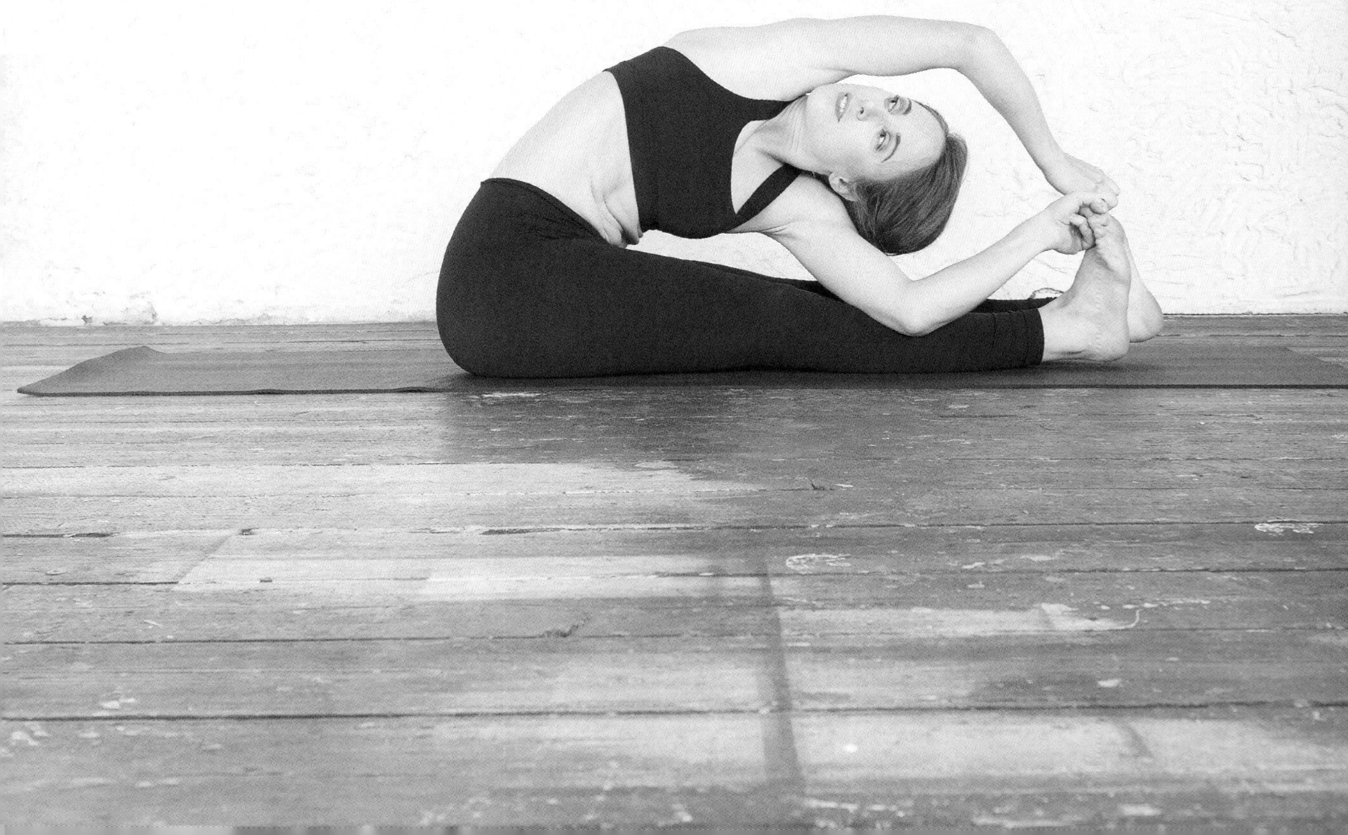

Next pose

Continue with Upward Plank Pose or a variation thereof.

Alignment cues

Legs are straight; feet are together and flexed.

Look underneath the armpit of your upper arm and reach with the elbow of the lower arm to the outside of the opposite knee.

Open your chest as much as possible, trying to bring your shoulders into one vertical line.

Focus on extending and lengthening your spine and creating the rotation from the pelvis.

Contraindications & cautions

The same contraindications and cautions apply as in Seated Forward Bend.

Modifications & adjustments

If tight hamstrings prevent you from reaching your toes while your legs are straight, you can bend your knees and support them with a rolled-up blanket or bolster.

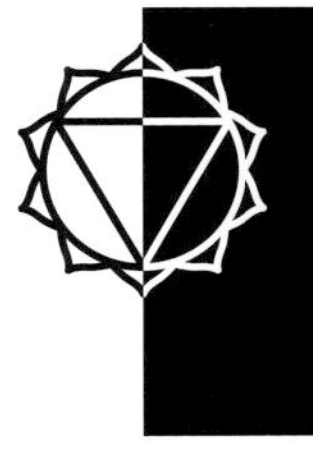

Paschimottanasana A

Seated Forward Bend A

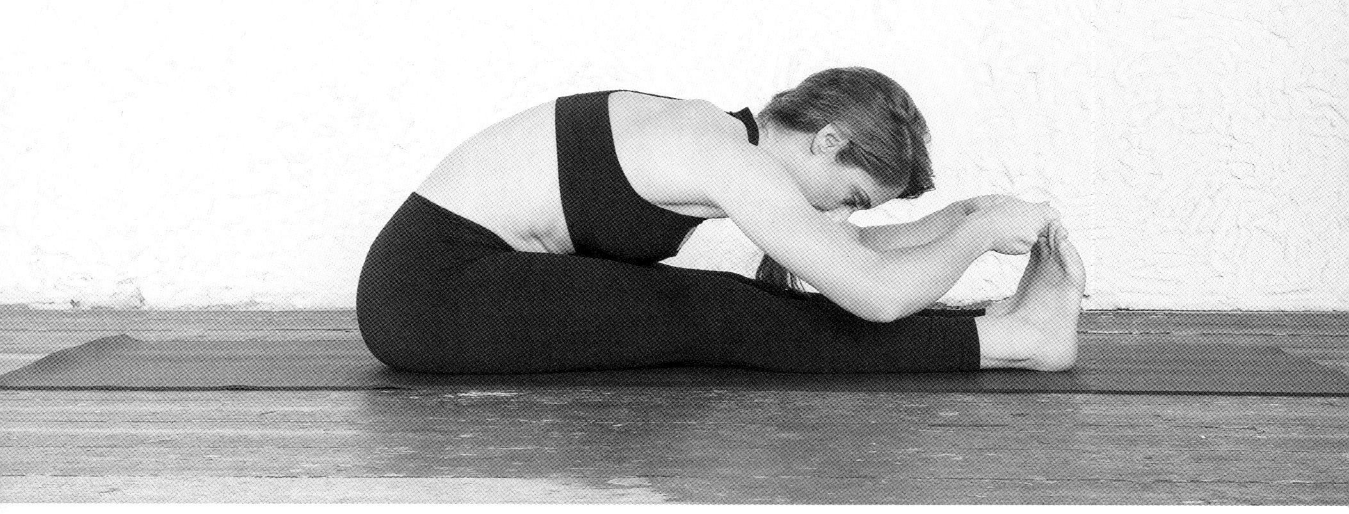

How to come into the pose

Sit on the floor, with your legs straight in front of you, toes pulled toward you, and heels pushing away.

Make sure you are sitting straight up on your sitting bones, with your spine straight. You can remove the flesh from underneath your sitting bones, to help sit up straighter.

Breathe in and stretch your arms up over your head.

Following the direction of your hands, at the same time lengthen your entire spine upward.

Breathe out and bend forward from your hips, keeping your spine as elongated as possible and reaching toward your feet with your hands as you come down. If you can reach your feet, wrap your index fingers around your big toes, with your thumbs resting on the tops of your big toes.

Gently pull on your feet with your arms, folding forward with a straight back and elongated front torso, while keeping your shoulders away from your ears.

Hold the pose steadily as long as comfortable and breathe evenly.

To come out of Seated Forward Bend, breathe in and stretch your hands past your feet and then come up, with a flat back, stretching your arms and spine up as your body comes up.

Breathe out and relax your arms.

Next pose

Continue with Upward Plank Pose or a variation thereof.

Alignment cues

This Seated Forward Bend has a different approach than the one in the Primary Hatha Sequence, where the focus is on bending forward with a slightly rounded back and stretching the back and creating pressure in the abdominal region.

In Paschimottanasana A the focus is to create length in the hamstrings and to keep your spine as straight as possible, initiating the movement from the tilt in your pelvis rather than from your spine.

This is a good variation for people suffering from hernias or SI instability.

Contraindications & cautions

The same contraindications and cautions apply as in Seated Forward Bend.

Modifications & adjustments

If you cannot reach your feet yet, you can use a strap to bridge the gap. Be cautious, though, not to pull yourself forward forcefully, because you could injure your hamstrings!

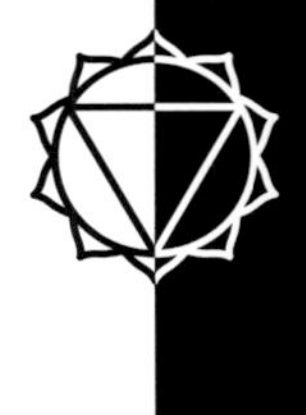

Variations

Paschimottanasana B, C, D

Seated Forward Bend B, C, D

The difference between these variations and Paschimottanasana A is simply the grip. In B, you hold the balls of your feet from the top. In C, you catch hold of the sides of your feet, with the thumb facing toward your head. In D, you bind your hands below the soles of your feet, by catching one wrist with the opposite hand.

Janu Shirshasana
Head-to-Knee Forward Bend

How to come into the pose

Sit with your legs stretched out in front of you.

Bend your right leg and place your right foot against your left inner thigh.

Breathe in, reach your hands up to the ceiling, and lengthen your spine.

Breathe out, bend forward, and catch hold of your left foot.

With every inhalation lengthen the front of your torso and gently reach with your lower belly toward your left thigh.

Hold the pose steadily as long as comfortable and breathe evenly. Repeat the same on the other side.

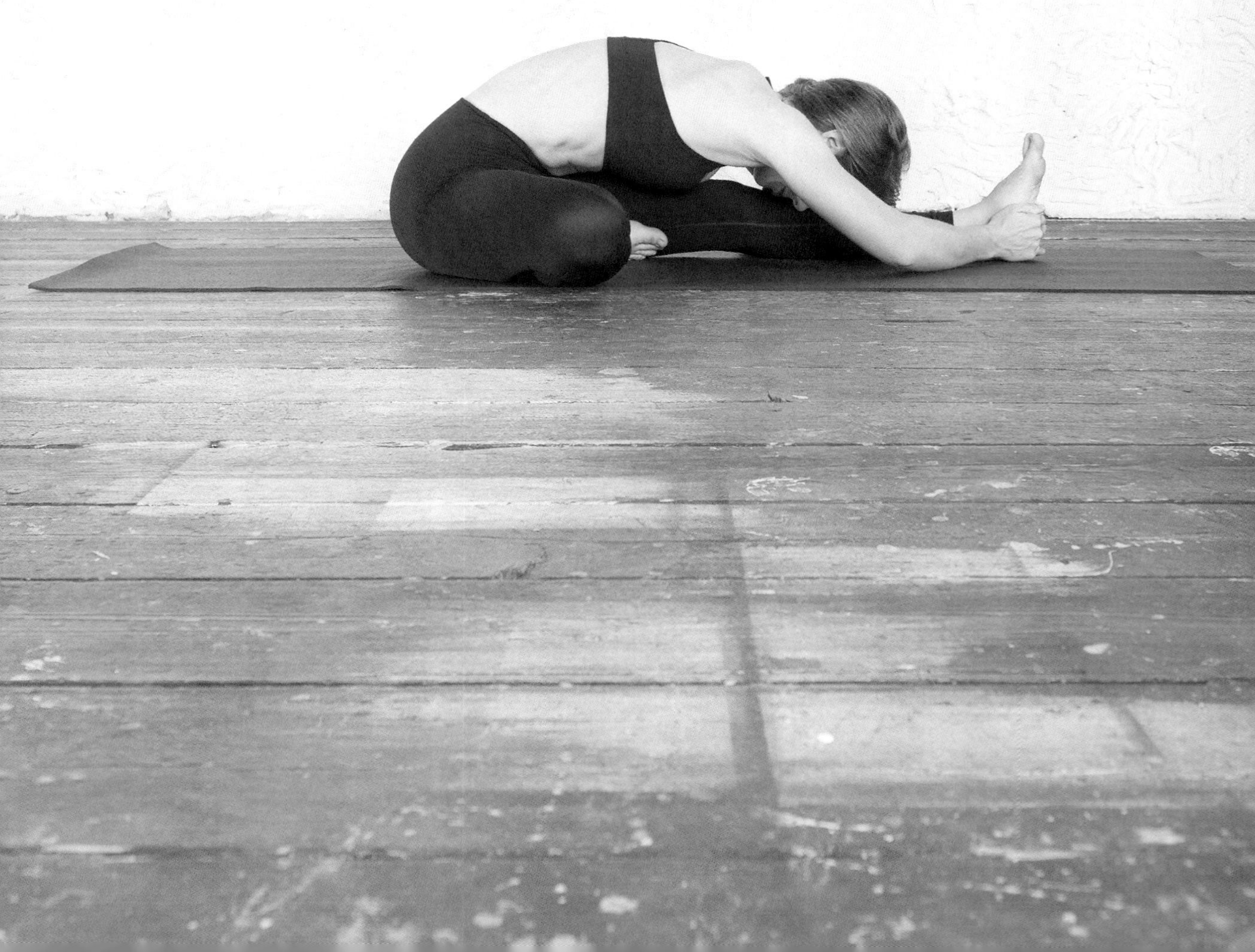

Next pose

Continue with Upward Plank Pose or a variation thereof.

Alignment cues

The foot of your bent leg can come as high as comfortable up along the extended leg. But make sure your pelvis stays straight. If your pelvis is not straight, place your foot a bit lower.

Your spine is elongated; your lower belly is reaching toward the thigh of your extended leg.

Shoulder blades are drawn away from your ears, toward your waist.

If possible rest your chin against your knee or shin, otherwise keep lengthening out through the crown of your head.

Contraindications & cautions

The same contraindications and cautions apply as in Seated Forward Bend.

Modifications & adjustments

If your bent knee comes high off the floor and/or you feel tension in that knee, support it with a bolster.

If tight hamstrings prevent you from holding on to your foot with straight legs, you can slightly bend the knee of your extended leg and support it with a rolled-up blanket or bolster.

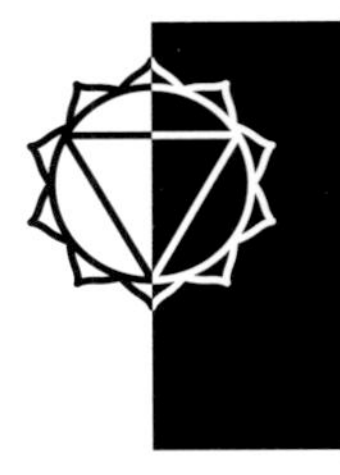

Marichyasana A

Pose Dedicated to Sage Marichi A

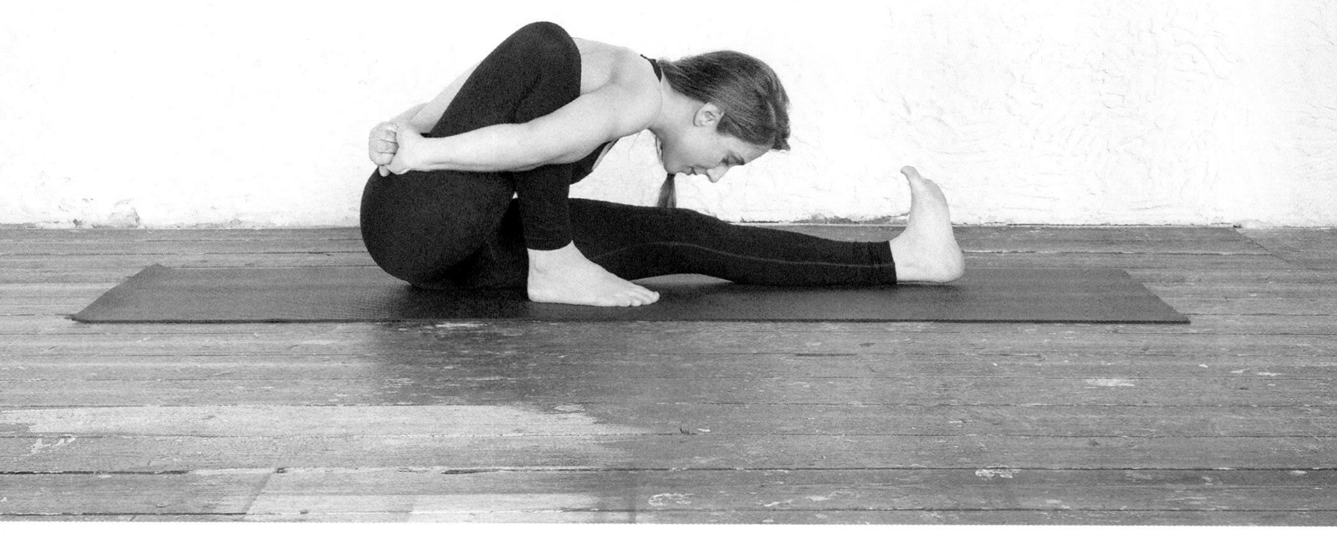

How to come into the pose

Sit with your legs straight in front of you, feet together.

Bend your right knee and place your right foot flat on the floor next to your left inner thigh.

Place your foot up as high as possible toward the buttock, while keeping a distance of at least one foot-width between your right foot and left inner thigh.

Reach your right arm forward and rotate it inward, so the thumb points to the floor and the palm faces out to your right.

As you extend your right arm forward, lengthen your torso forward and aim to bring your right shin into the armpit.

Then breathe out and sweep the forearm around the outside of the leg.

On the next exhalation, sweep the left hand behind your back and clasp your left wrist with your right hand.

Keep a firm grip and breathe in, extending your spine.

Breathe out and reach with your nose toward your left knee.

Breathe evenly, and with every exhalation fold more deeply forward.

Then release and repeat the same on the other side.

Next Pose

Rest in Child's Pose for 30–45 seconds, then continue with Easy Crow Pose or a variation thereof.

Alignment cues

Place the foot of the bent leg as high as possible, making sure you are still sitting firmly on your sitting bones.

Avoid sitting on your tailbone.

The extended leg is active. Focus on pushing out through the heel.

Be sure your shoulders do not scrunch up into your ears; draw your shoulder blades actively down your back.

As you fold forward toward the extended leg, keep the front of your torso as long as possible. Do not collapse in your chest.

Contraindications & cautions

The same contraindications and cautions apply as in Seated Forward Bend.

Modifications & adjustments

If you cannot clasp your hands behind your back, you can use a strap to bridge the gap. To move more deeply into the forward bend in this pose, it is helpful for beginning students to sit up high on a bolster or thickly folded blanket. If bending forward toward your extended knee is still too strenuous, you can also stay upright and work on lengthening your spine by pushing into the floor with your hips and reaching out through the crown of your head.

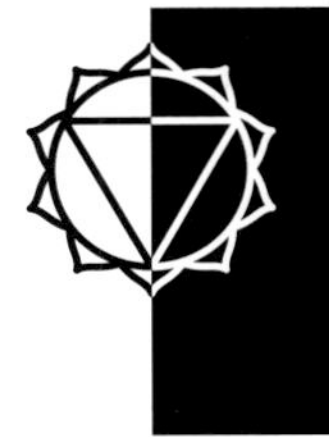

Variations

Marichyasana B

Pose Dedicated to Sage Marichi B

This pose is more challenging, because the previously extended leg (in Sage Marichi's Pose A), is now folded into a Half Lotus position. Attempt this only if you can fold easily and without strain into Half Lotus Pose. Start seated, with your legs in front of you. Then fold your left leg into Half Lotus Pose and follow the instructions as described on the left from the second step onward.

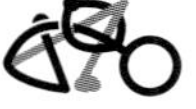

Parighasana
Gate Pose

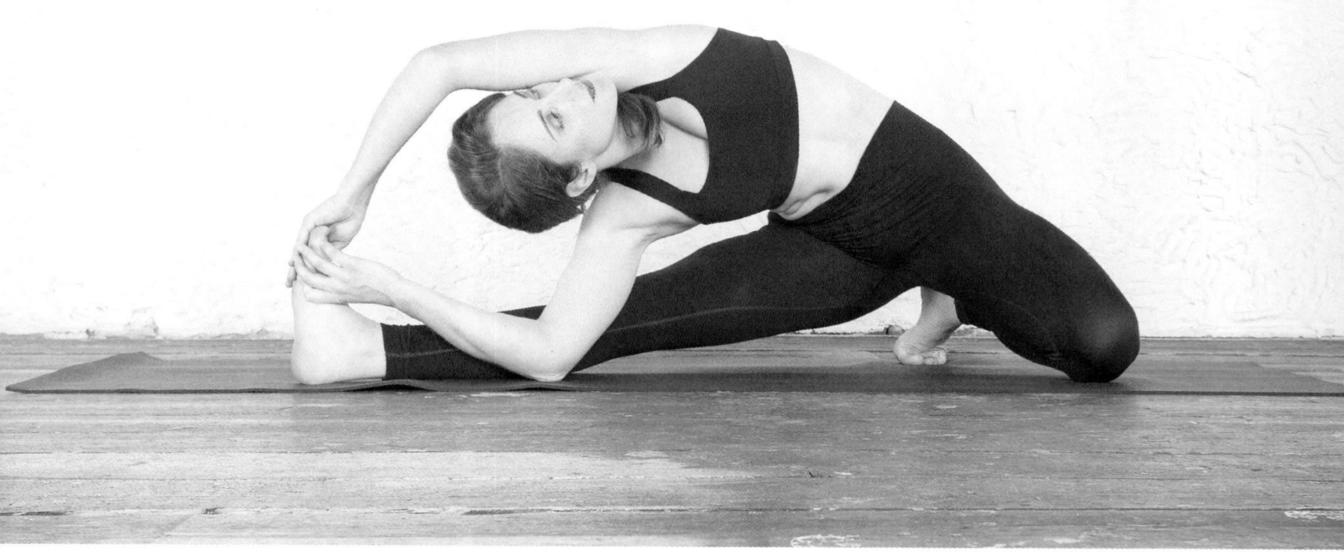

How to come into the pose

Begin by kneeling on the floor, with your hips raised and toes curled under.

Stretch your right leg out to your right and sit down onto your left heel (toes are curled).

Bring your arms out to your sides, with your palms down.

Bend to your right side over your right leg and hold on to the right big toe or your shin or ankle.

Sweep your left arm over your head and to your right, and if possible also catch hold of the right big toe.

Look along your left upper arm toward the ceiling. Hold the pose steadily as long as comfortable and breathe evenly.

To come out of the pose, reach out with your left hand and bring your torso into an upright position again.

Repeat on the other side.

Next pose

Continue with Upward Plank Pose or a variation thereof.

Alignment cues

Keep your shoulder blades down your back and shoulders away from the ears.

The toes of the extended leg are pointing upward.

Keep the sitting bone firmly grounded on the heel.

The focus is on stretching your torso laterally while expanding the chest maximally.

Contraindications & cautions

The same contraindications and cautions apply as in Seated Forward Bend.

Modifications & adjustments

If keeping the toes curled and heel raised is too intense, the foot of the bent leg can also be pointed.

Variations

Sukha Parighasana

Easy Gate Pose

This version of the Gate Pose is less intense for the legs and hips and focuses more on the stretch to the side of the torso. For this, kneel on the mat with your hips raised. Extend your right leg sideways, sole of the foot resting on the ground. Now bring your arms out to your sides, with your palms down, bend to your right side over your right leg, and lay your right hand on your shin, ankle, the floor, or a block. Then sweep your left arm over your head to the left as you roll your shoulders down your back and allow your palm to face the floor.

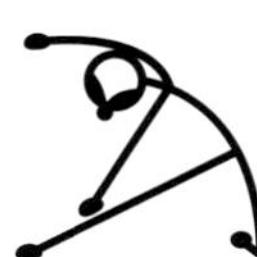

Parighasana II

Gate Pose II

For this version of the Gate Pose, come onto your left knee with your hip resting on the heel. From here extend the right leg sideways. Then sit down on the floor between your legs and start to bend to your right side over your right leg and hold on to the right big toe (or your shin or ankle). Sweep your left arm over your head and to your right, and if possible also catch hold of the right big toe. Look along your left upper arm toward the ceiling.

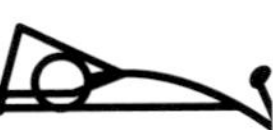

Trianga Mukhaikapada Paschimottanasana
Three Limbs Facing Intense West Stretch Pose

How to come into the pose

Sit on your mat, legs straight in front of you, feet together.

Make sure you sit high up on your sitting bones.

Bend your left leg and place your left heel next to your left hip.

Your left foot is pointed, with the sole of your foot pointing up toward the ceiling.

Breathe in and reach with your hands up toward the ceiling.

Breathe out, bend forward, and catch hold of your right heel or top of your foot.

Lengthen your torso and reach with your nose to your right shin or with your chin toward the ankle.

Hold the pose steadily as long as comfortable and breathe evenly.

Repeat the same on the other side.

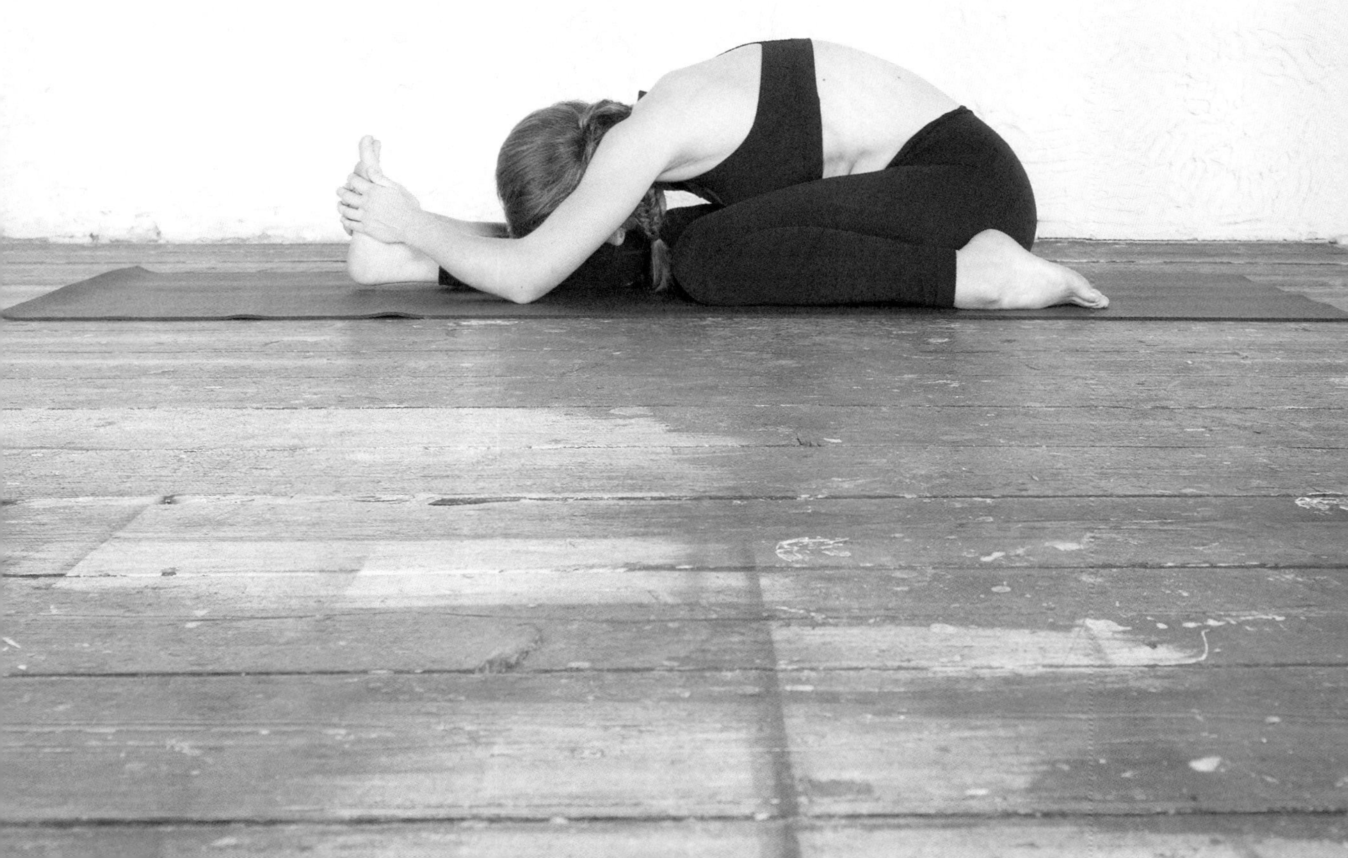

Next pose

Continue with Upward Plank Pose or a variation thereof.

Alignment cues

Sit firmly on both sitting bones while avoiding tipping over to one side.

The foot of your bent leg is pointed, and the sole of your foot is facing up to the ceiling.

The straight leg is active, with your foot flexed and pushing out through the heel.

Try to keep your spine straight, initiate the forward fold from your pelvis, and reach with your chin to the shin or ankle of the extended leg.

Keep the back of your neck elongated and your shoulder blades drawn away from your ears, toward your waist.

Contraindications & cautions

The same contraindications and cautions apply as in Seated Forward Bend. Also be cautious in this pose if you have knee, groin, or hamstring issues.

Modifications & adjustments

There should be no discomfort in your knee joint. If necessary, sit on a folded blanket or block.

If the knee of the straight leg needs to soften due to tightness of the hamstrings, you can support it with a rolled blanket.

If you cannot reach the foot of your straight leg, you can also hold on to the ankle or the shin.

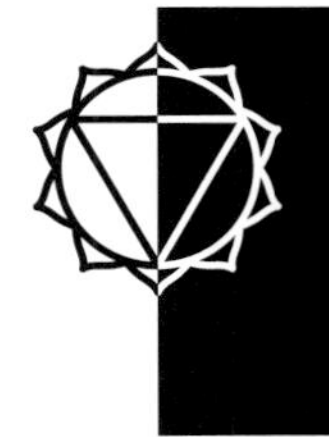

Krounchasana
Heron Pose

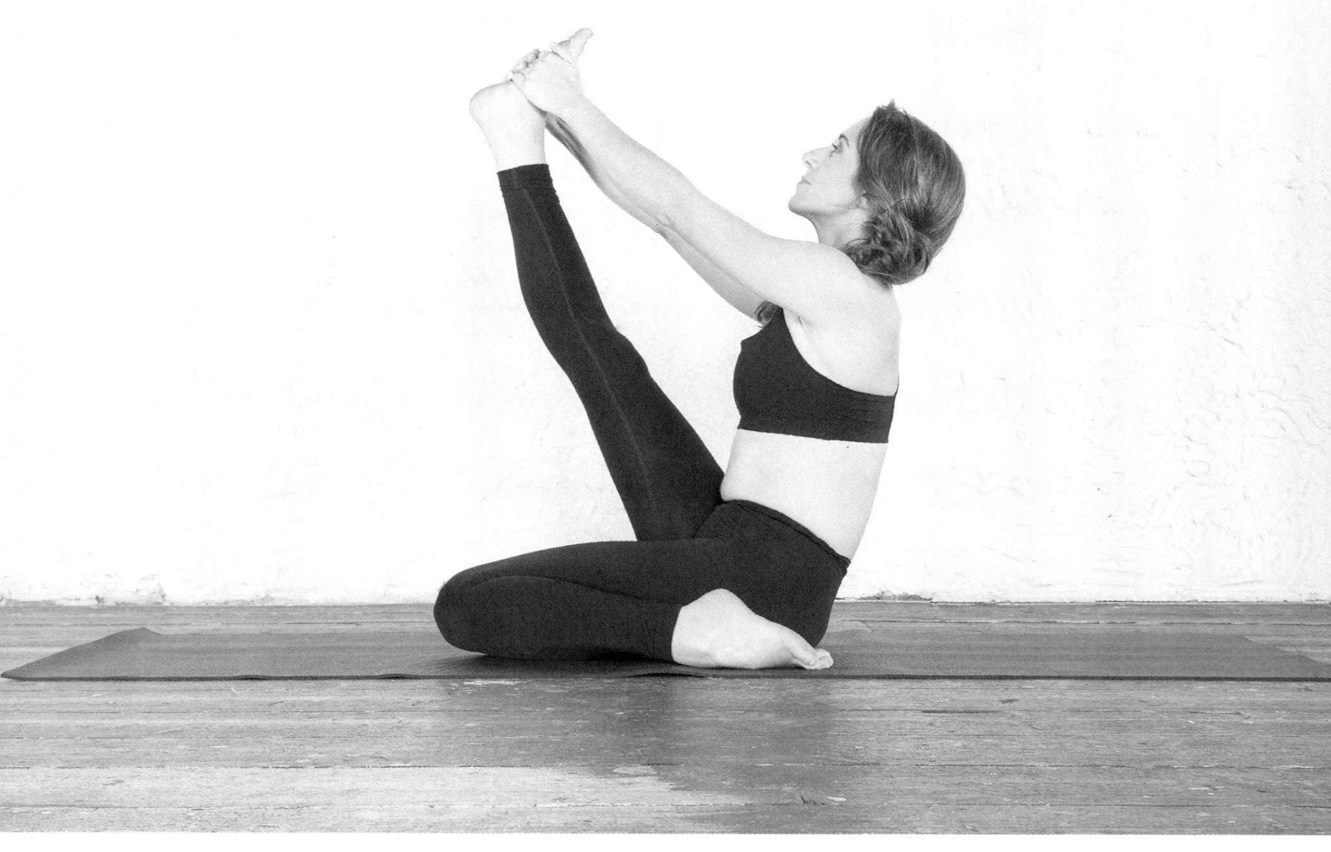

How to come into the pose

Sit on your mat, legs straight in front of you, feet together. Make sure you sit high up on your sitting bones.

Bend your left leg and place your left heel next to your left hip.

Your left foot is pointed, with the sole of your foot pointing up toward the ceiling.

Bend your right leg and catch hold of your right heel with both hands.

Push your right foot into your hands and straighten out your right leg toward the ceiling.

Keep your spine straight, chest open, and shoulders down, and gaze toward your right foot.

Hold the pose steadily as long as comfortable and breathe evenly.

Repeat the same on the other side.

Next pose

Continue with Upward Plank Pose or a variation thereof.

Alignment cues

Sit firmly on both sitting bones.

The foot of your bent leg is pointed, and the sole of your foot is facing up toward the ceiling.

The foot of your straight leg is flexed.

Try to keep your spine straight, initiating the fold from your pelvis and reaching with your chin to the ankle of the extended leg.

Pull your shoulders back and draw your shoulder blades down toward your waist.

Contraindications & cautions

The same contraindications and cautions apply as in Seated Forward Bend. Also be cautious in this pose if you have knee, groin, or hamstring issues.

Modifications & adjustments

There should be no discomfort in your knee joint. If necessary, sit on a folded blanket or block.

If due to tightness in the hamstrings you cannot straighten the extended leg without rolling on your tailbone and rounding your back, you can hold your heel, keeping your knee bent so that the lower leg is parallel to the mat.

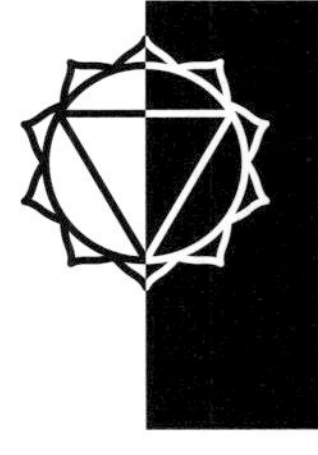

Ardha Baddha Padma Paschimottanasana
Half Bound-Lotus Forward Bend

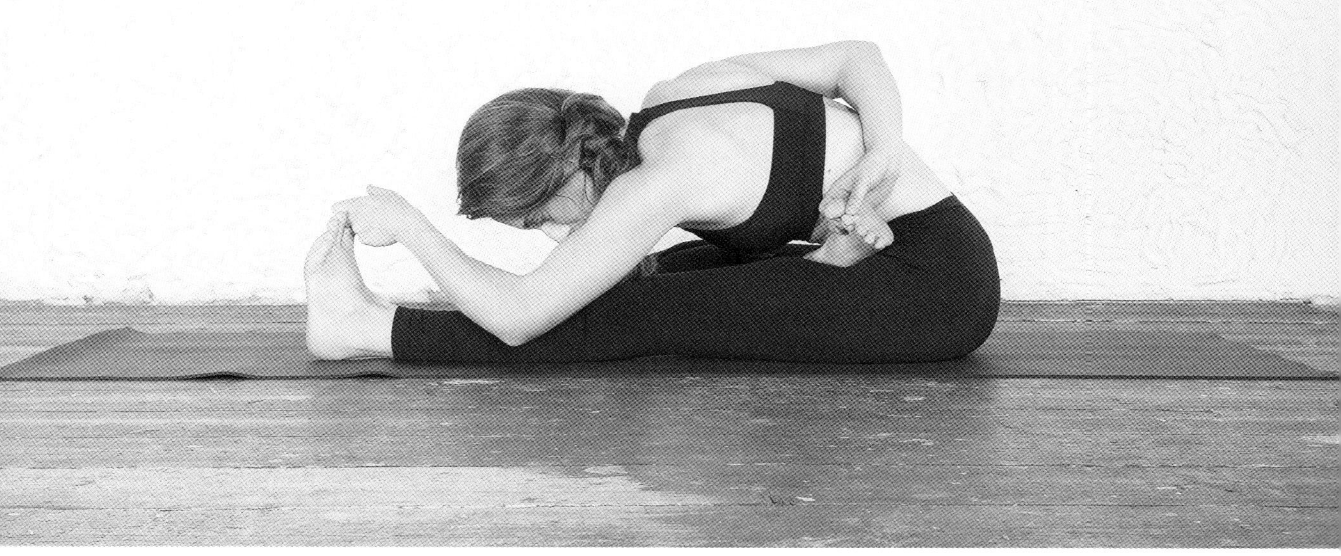

How to come into the pose

Sit on the mat, with your legs straight in front of you.

Place your right leg in Half Lotus Pose.

Bring your right hand behind your back, and hold your right big toe.

Breathe in, reach with your left hand up toward the ceiling, and elongate your spine.

Breathe out, fold forward over your left leg, and hold on to your left big toe.

Keep your spine long and reach out and forward through the crown of your head.

Hold the pose steadily as long as comfortable and breathe evenly.

To come out of the pose, release the grip of your left hand, come up with a straight back, and gently unfold your legs.

Then repeat the same on the other side.

Next pose

Continue with Upward Plank Pose or a variation thereof.

Alignment cues

When bringing your foot into Half Lotus Pose, the rotation should come from your hip joint, not from your knee or ankle.

The ankle that is crossing over in Half Lotus position should be resting in the crease of the opposite hip.

Make sure that your foot is not sickled.

There should be no tension in your knee or ankle.

Try to keep your spine straight, initiate the forward fold from your pelvis, and reach with your chin toward the ankle of the extended leg.

Contraindications & cautions

The same contraindications and cautions apply as in Seated Forward Bend. Also be cautious in this pose if you have tight hips or knee issues.

Modifications & adjustments

Attempt this pose only if you can fold your legs comfortably and without force into a Half Lotus position.

If you can fold into Half Lotus but your knee is higher than the knee of the outstretched leg, place a bolster underneath to prevent your knee from depressing too far down (and therefore causing strain) as you bend forward.

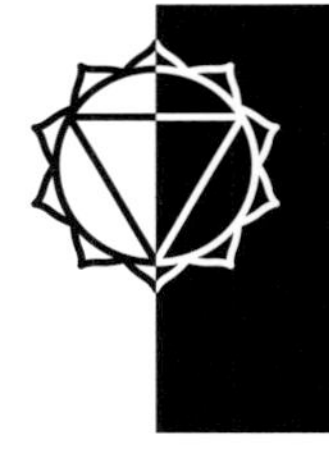

Baddha Konasana
Bound Angle Pose

How to come into the pose

Sit with your legs in front of you.

Bend your knees and bring the soles of your feet together.

Bring your feet as close toward your pelvis as possible, while staying seated on your sitting bones with your spine erect (you should not feel any pain or pressure in the knees).

Hold your feet, breathe in, and lengthen out through the crown of your head.

Breathe out and bend forward with a straight back.

Once bent forward, you can relax your back and, if possible, rest your forehead on your hands or on the floor.

Hold the pose steadily as long as comfortable and breathe evenly.

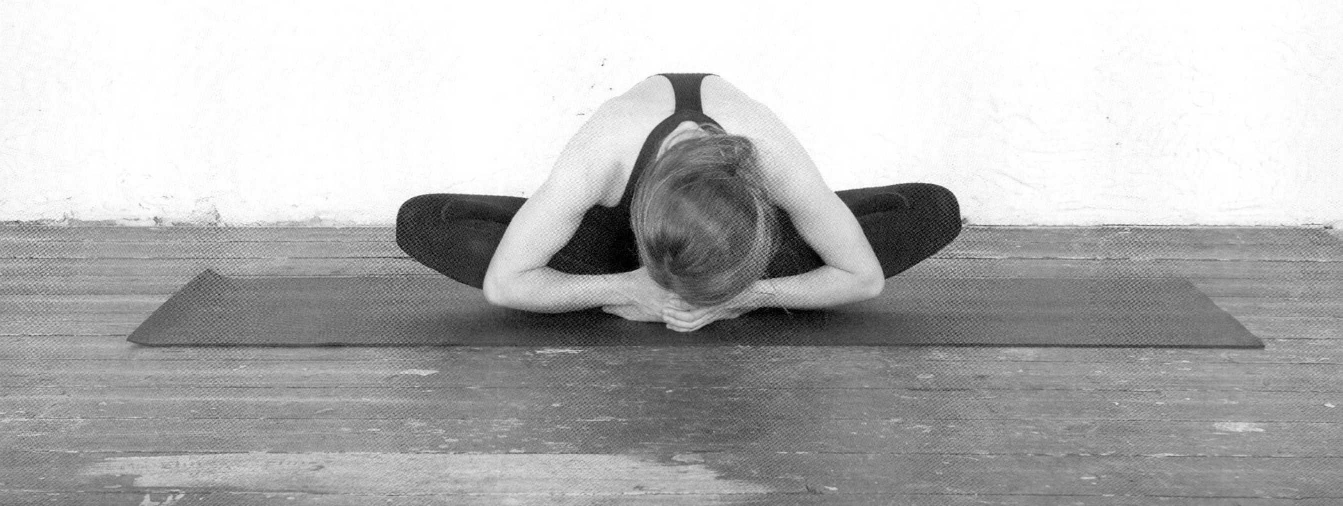

Next pose

Continue with Upward Plank Pose or a variation thereof.

Alignment cues

As you fold forward, focus on releasing the inner thighs, groin, and hip flexors.

Make sure you stay seated on your sitting bones and do not roll back toward your tailbone.

Contraindications & cautions

The same contraindications and cautions apply as in Seated Forward Bend. Also be cautious in this pose if you have knee and groin issues.

Modifications & adjustments

It can be difficult to lower your knees toward the floor. If your knees are too high and your back rounded, be sure to sit on a high support, even as high as 30 centimeters off the floor.

If you feel tension in your knees, place a bolster under each knee, supporting your thighs an inch or so above their maximum stretch. Never force your knees down toward the floor!

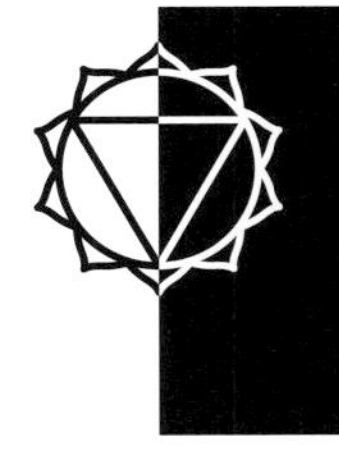

KURMASANA
TORTOISE POSE

HOW TO COME INTO THE POSE

Sit on your mat, with your feet mat-width apart.

Bend your knees and place the soles of your feet on the floor.

Fold forward by tilting your pelvis and slide your arms backward and under your thighs (one at a time), palms facing downward.

Walk your hands back as much as possible.

Start to push out through your heels in order to straighten your legs, and reach with your chin toward the mat.

Hold the pose steadily as long as comfortable and breathe evenly.

To come out of the pose, first bend your legs, and then gently release your arms.

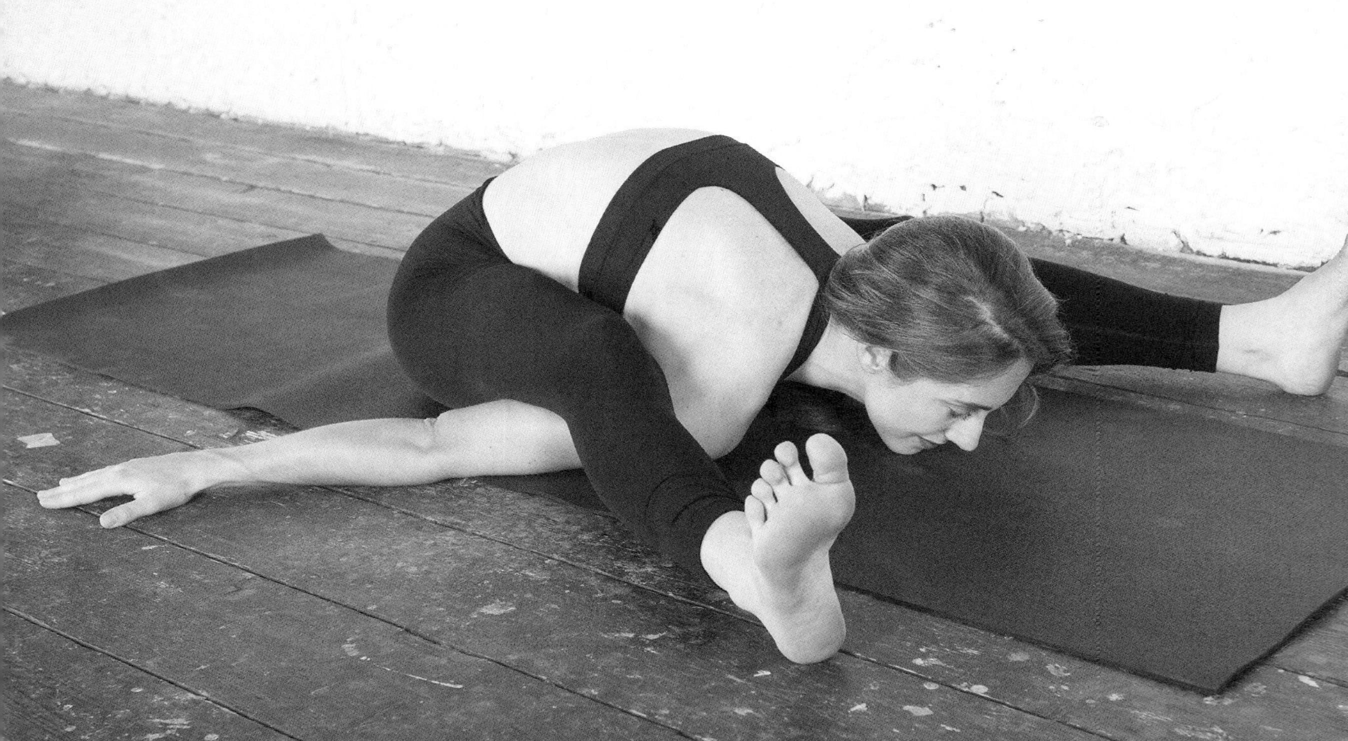

Next pose

Continue with Upward Plank Pose or a variation thereof.

Alignment cues

Your arms are as high under your thighs as possible; palms are facing downward.

Make sure not to press your thighs against your elbows.

Use the straightening action of your legs to bring your chest, shoulders, and chin to the floor.

Even though your back is rounded, try to keep your chest wide and your shoulder blades drawn down and away from your ears.

Contraindications & cautions

The same contraindications and cautions apply as in Seated Forward Bend. Also be cautious in this pose if you have shoulder or groin issues.

Modifications & adjustments

If you feel strain on your neck when reaching with your chin toward the floor, you can also place your forehead on the mat.

If you experience difficulties placing your arms under your legs, you can bend your legs a bit more and initially hold on to the outside of the ankles. Initiate the tilt from your pelvis, keeping your back flat. Once your shoulders are at knee level or lower you can bring your arms underneath your thighs. Initially you might find it easier to reach your hands more sideways, with the palms facing upward.

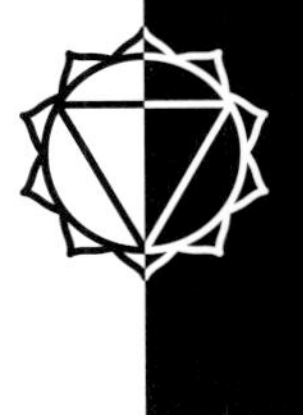

Variations

Supta Kurmasana

Sleeping-Tortoise Pose

From Tortoise Pose, bend your knees and walk your feet a little back toward your hips. Turn your palms up toward the ceiling and clasp your hands behind your lower back. Draw your feet toward each other and if possible cross your right ankle over your left, keeping your left heel on the floor. If that is not accessible, you can also place the soles of the feet as close together as possible, and if necessary you can release the bind of your hands and keep them flat on the floor. The full pose, in fact, entails placing your feet over your head.

Mandukasana
Frog Pose

How to come into the pose

Sit on your knees, with your hips resting on your heels.

Clench both fists and place them on your thighs as close as possible to your abdomen.

Breathe in, open your chest, breathe out, and bend forward, placing your forehead on the floor.

Hold the pose steadily as long as comfortable and breathe evenly.

To come out of the pose, slowly roll up and relax your hands.

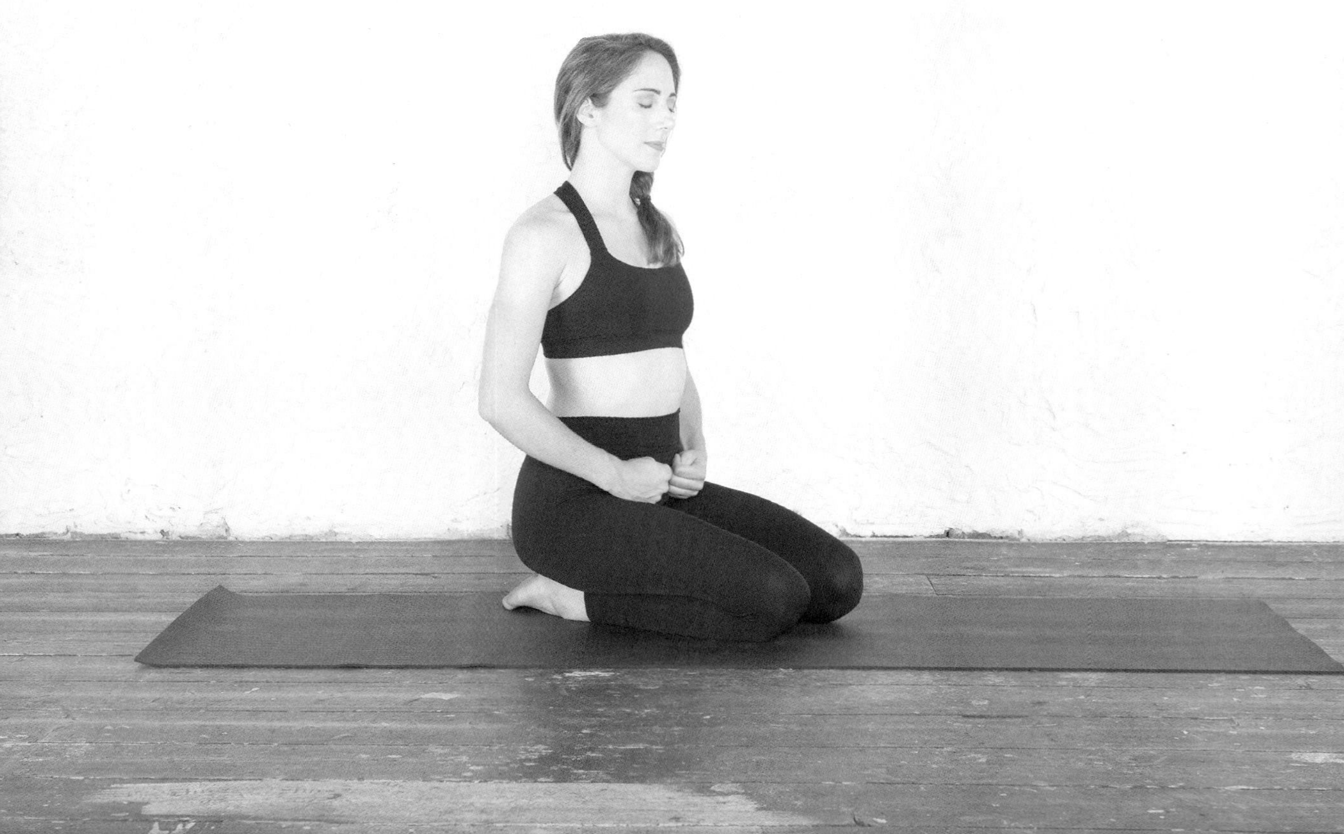

Next pose

Continue with Upward Plank Pose or a variation thereof.

Alignment cues

Forehead is resting on the floor, and hips are resting on your heels.

The thumbs, even though they are folded into the fists, should be pointing upward. Do not allow your fists to roll forward as you fold forward.

Contraindications & cautions

The same contraindications and cautions apply as in Seated Forward Bend. Also be cautious if you have knee issues.

Modifications & adjustments

If you cannot sit comfortably on your heels, due to knee problems, you can support your hips on a cushion or block with your knees hip-width apart.

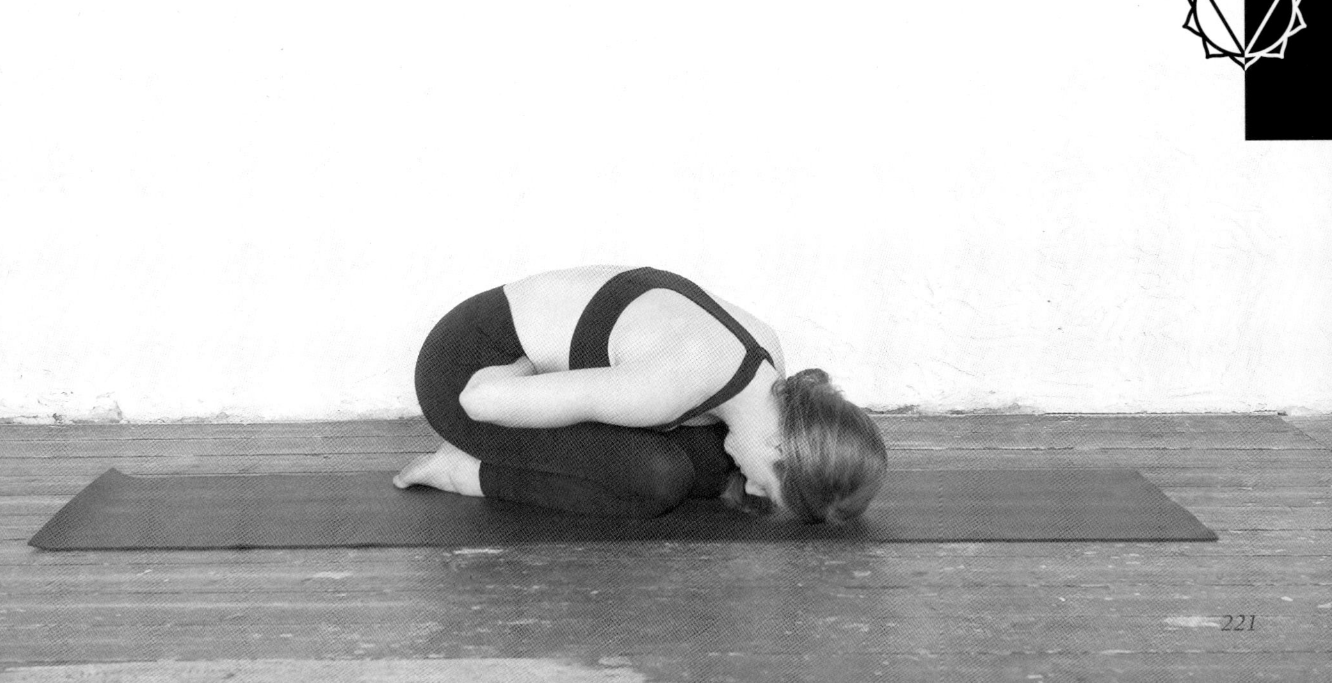

Adho Mukha Shvanasana
Downward-Facing Dog Pose

How to come into the pose

Come on to your hands and knees.

Set your knees directly below your hips and your hands slightly forward from your shoulders.

Spread your palms, index fingers parallel or slightly turned out, and tuck your toes under.

Spread your fingers wide apart, with your palms shoulder-width apart.

Press out through your fingers and the edges of your hands.

Using straight (but not locked) arms, press your hips up and back, reaching the chest toward your thighs.

Lift up through your tailbone to keep your spine straight and long.

Place your feet hip-width apart, with your toes facing forward.

Press your heels toward the floor, feeling a stretch in the backs of your legs.

Draw your shoulder blades down toward your waist, letting your head and neck hang freely from your shoulders.

Hold the pose steadily as long as comfortable and breathe evenly.

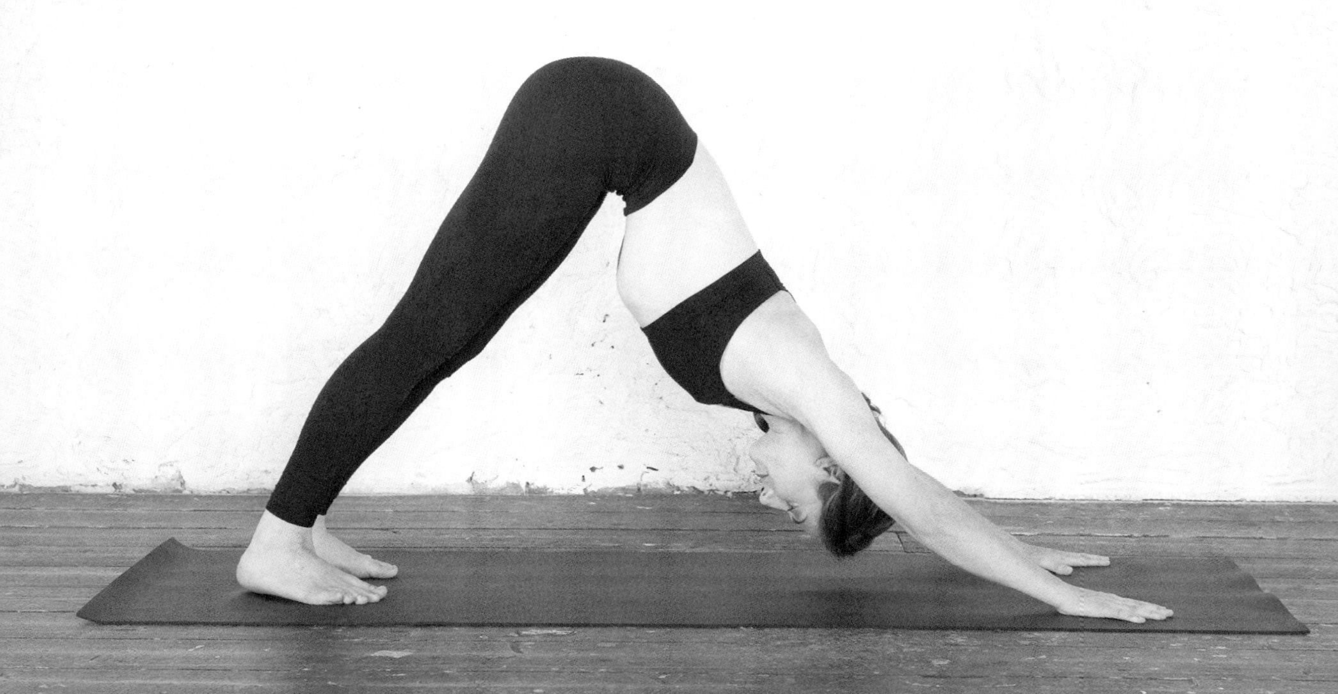

Next pose

Rest in Child's Pose for 30–45 seconds, then continue with either Upward Plank Pose or a variation thereof or with Cobra Pose or a variation thereof.

Alignment cues

Firm the outer arms and press the root of the palm, the knuckles, and the fingertips actively into the floor.

Firm your shoulder blades against your back, then spread them and draw them toward the tailbone.

Your legs are straight, or you can have a small bend at your knees to keep the back flat.

Heels are reaching toward the floor, but do not have to touch the floor.

Create an opposition between the crown of your head and your tailbone, lengthening your spine.

Contraindications & cautions

The same contraindications and cautions apply as in Seated Forward Bend. Also be cautious in this pose if you have shoulder or wrist issues.

Modifications & adjustments

If you have stiff hamstrings, you can slightly bend your knees and push your chest toward your thighs.

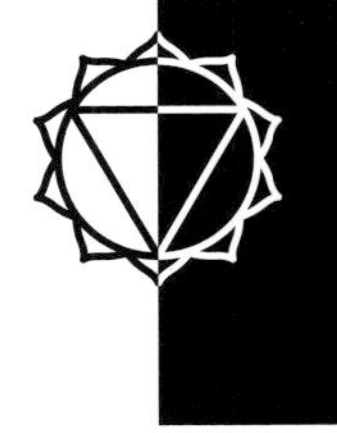

Variations

Eka Pada Adho Mukha Shvanasana

One-Legged Downward-Facing Dog

Come into Downward-Facing Dog and then proceed to raise your right leg back and upward, pressing through the heel. Aim to keep your hips as square as possible. Reach with your chest toward your left leg and release your head toward the floor. Release with an exhalation and repeat on your left for the same length of time.

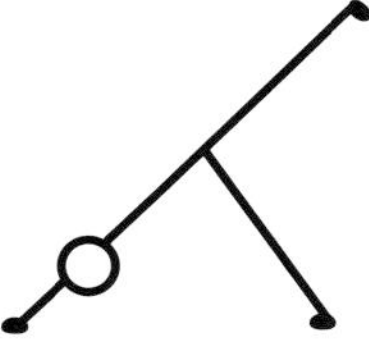

Akarna Dhanurasana
Archer's Pose

How to come into the pose

Sit on the floor, with your legs straight in front of you, feet together.

Breathe in, reaching your hands up toward the ceiling.

Breathe out, bend forward, and hold your big toes with your first two fingers and thumb of each hand.

Bend your right knee, holding the big toe with your right hand, and place your right heel on the floor a few inches away from your inner left knee.

Pause here, press the back of your left leg into the floor, roll forward onto your right sitting bone, and press it down into the floor.

Breathe in, bend your right arm, and bring your right foot as close to your right ear as possible. Right elbow is pointing diagonally back and up. Hold as long as comfortable and breathe evenly, then release and repeat on the other side.

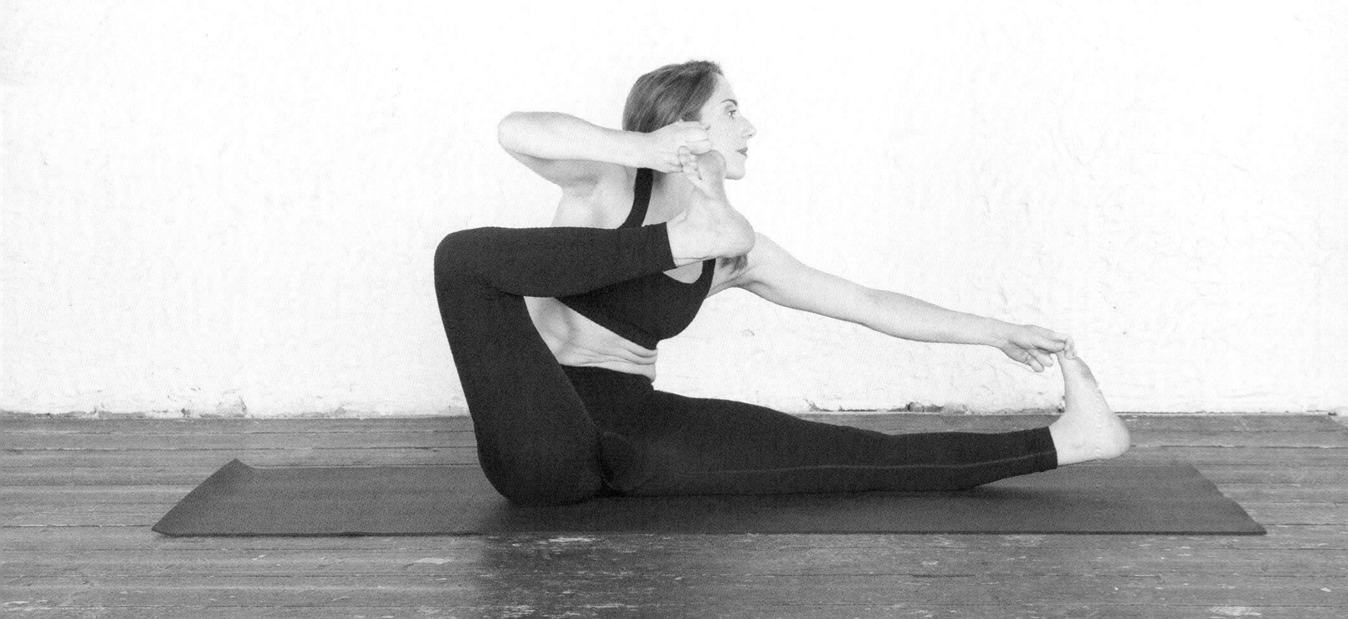

Next pose

Continue with Upward Plank Pose or a variation thereof.

Alignment cues

Keep your spine as straight as possible and avoid rounding your lower back.

To release the hip on the side of your bent leg, allow the sole of your foot to turn toward your face.

Draw your shoulder blades down and toward your waist and keep your neck and throat relaxed.

Contraindications & cautions

The same contraindications and cautions apply as in Seated Forward Bend. Also be cautious in this pose if you have groin or hamstring issues.

Modifications & adjustments

If it is uncomfortable to hold your big toes you can also hold the balls of your feet from the outside.

If your hamstrings are tight, hold on to the shin of the extended leg instead. If your lower back rounds or feels strained, sit up on a folded blanket.

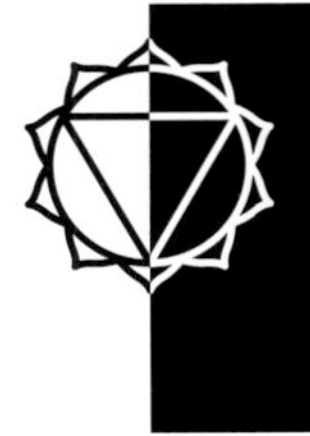

Variations

Parivrtta Akarna Dhanurasana

Revolved Archer's Pose

Start as described, but hold on to the opposite big toe. First hold on to your left foot with your right hand and then hold your right big toe with your left hand. Keep the arm holding the toe of the straight leg on top of the other arm. Now pull your left foot toward your right chest, so that your left shin comes parallel to the chest. Look forward over your right foot.

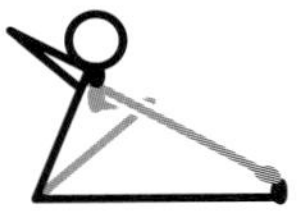

Ubhaya Padangusthasana

Big-Toe Pose

How to come into the pose

Sit with your legs straight in front of you and feet together.

Bend your knees and clasp your your big toes with two fingers of each hand.

Keeping your lower back lifted, draw your knees toward your chest.

Push your feet into your hands and straighten your legs diagonally up toward the ceiling until your arms are fully extended.

Keep your lower back lifted, pulling your shoulders back, open your chest, and look diagonally upward.

Hold the pose steadily as long as comfortable and breathe evenly.

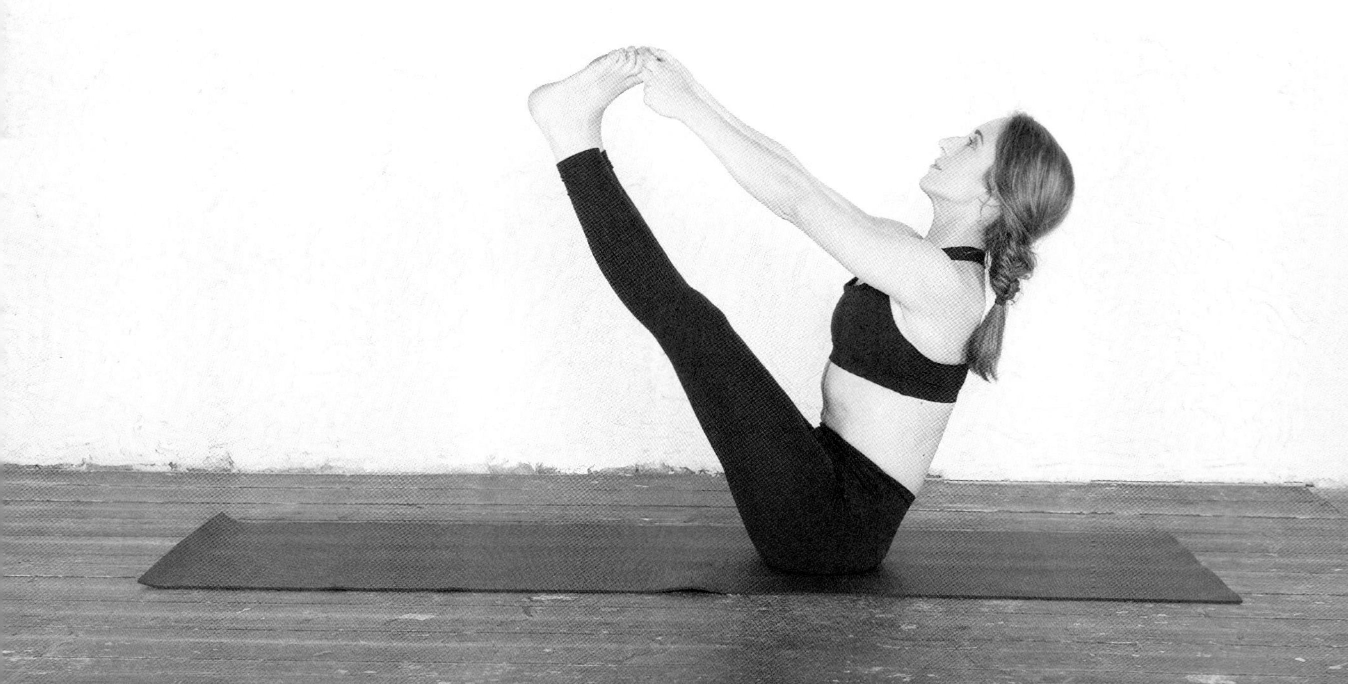

Next pose

Continue with another seated forward-bending posture or move on to Upward Plank Pose or a variation thereof.

Alignment cues

Arms and legs are straight, feet pushing into your hands and hands drawing back.

Sit up as high as possible on the sitting bones and avoid rolling back toward the tailbone.

Spine is straight, chest open, and shoulder blades drawn down away from your ears.

Look diagonally up, without dropping your head backward.

Contraindications & cautions

The same contraindications and cautions apply as in Seated Forward Bend. Also be cautious in this pose if you have knee, groin, or hamstring issues.

Modifications & adjustments

If you cannot straighten your legs while holding your feet, you can either keep your knees shoulder-width apart and slightly bent or you can use a strap around your feet and then straighten your legs.

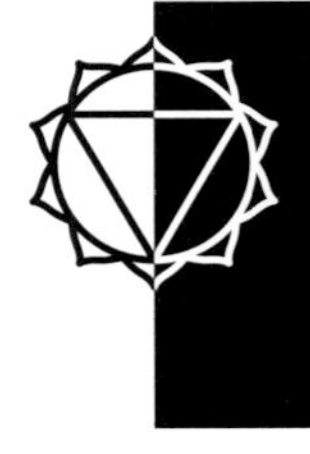

Upavistha Konasana
Wide-Angle Seated Forward Bend

How to come into the pose

Sit with your legs straight in front of you.

Lean your torso backward slightly on your hands and lift and open your legs to an angle of about 90 degrees.

Press your hands against the floor and slide your buttocks forward, widening your legs another 10 to 20 degrees.

Press out through the heels of your feet while keeping your knees pointed straight upward.

Create a hinging motion from your pelvis, and walk your hands forward in between your legs.

If flexibility allows, catch hold of your big toes or the outside of your feet and place your chest and chin on the floor.

Hold the pose steadily as long as comfortable and breathe evenly.

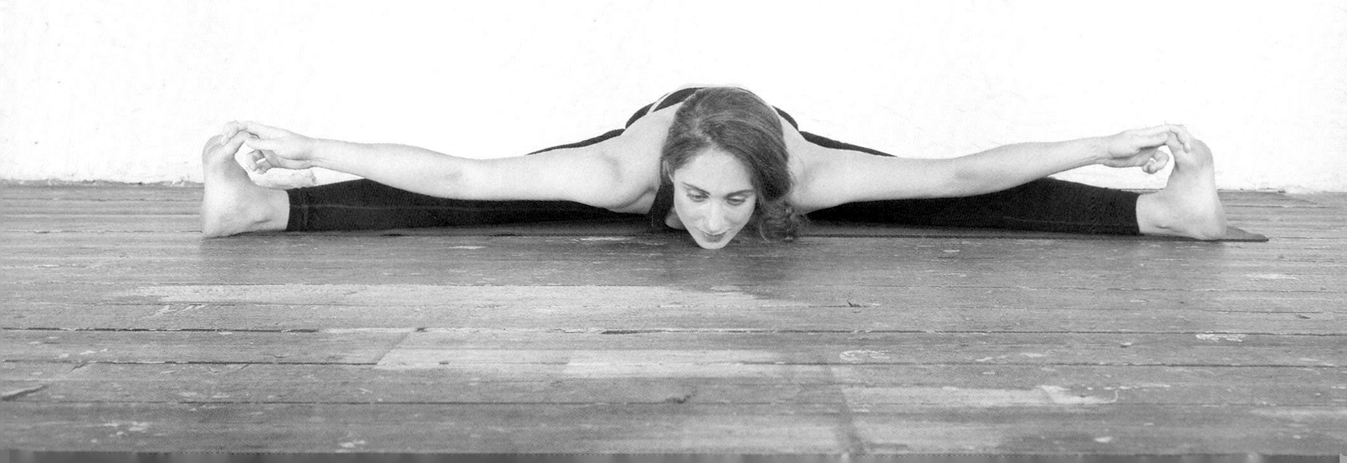

Next pose

Continue with Upward Plank Pose or a variation thereof.

Alignment cues

Sit high up on your sitting bones, with a natural lumbar curve.

Avoid rounding your lower back and rolling toward your tailbone.

Keep your thighs firmly floored, knees pointing straight up toward the ceiling, and feet flexed.

Create the forward fold from your pelvis and aim to keep the length in the front of your torso.

Hands are clasping your big toes or the outside of your feet.

Contraindications & cautions

The same contraindications and cautions apply as in Seated Forward Bend. Also be cautious in this pose if you have groin or hamstring issues.

Modifications & adjustments

If you cannot sit comfortably on your sitting bones, raise your buttocks on a folded blanket.

If tight hamstrings force you to round your lower back, keep your knees bent and the soles of your feet on the floor. Draw your feet in as far as necessary, until you can sit high up on your sitting bones.

The completed pose involves holding the feet or toes. But respect your limits and stay within the range of slight discomfort. You should not experience pain in your hamstring, groin, or inner thighs. If your legs are straight, but it is too intense to fold down entirely, you can keep either the palms or the forearms on the floor between your legs. Then keep reaching out through the crown of your head and down toward the floor from your belly button.

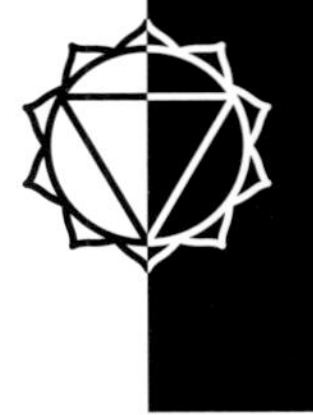

Variations

Upavistha Konasana B

Wide-Angle Seated Forward Bend B

From Wide-Angle Seated Forward Bend, bend your knees slightly and rock back to your sitting bones, lifting your feet off the floor and diagonally up toward the ceiling. Keep a tight grip around your big toes or outside of your feet and simultaneously press your feet away, creating a stabilizing, opposing action. Engage your core, lift up from your lower back, open your chest, and look diagonally up.

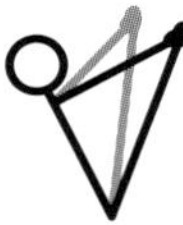

Adho Mukha Gomukhasana

Downward-Facing Cow Face Pose (aka Shoelace Pose)

How to come into the pose

Sit on your heels, with your knees together.

Shift your weight to your left, and sit on your left hip.

Cross your right leg over your left leg, placing your right heel next to your left hip.

Your right knee is on top of your left knee.

Breathe in, push both your sitting bones into the floor, and elongate your spine.

Breathe out and fold your torso forward across your right leg.

Rest your hands on the floor and your forehead on your knee or the floor in front of you.

Breathe evenly and allow your body to further relax into the pose with every exhalation.

Then release, unwind your legs, and repeat on the other side.

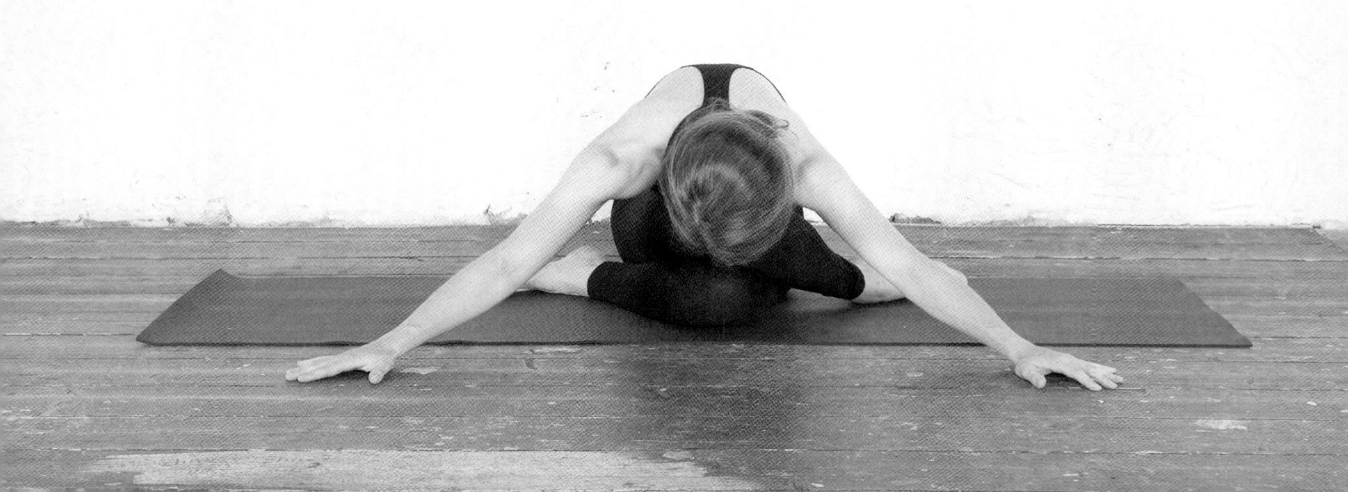

Next pose

Continue with Upward Plank Pose or a variation thereof.

Alignment cues

Sitting bones should be on the floor, while avoiding sitting on the opposite heel.

Contraindications & cautions

The same contraindications and cautions apply as in Seated Forward Bend. Also be cautious in this pose if you have knee issues.

Modifications & adjustments

If this pose is challenging due to tightness in the hips or knees, you can support either both or one hip with a folded blanket or a block. Keeping the lower leg stretched out in front makes this pose much more accessible.

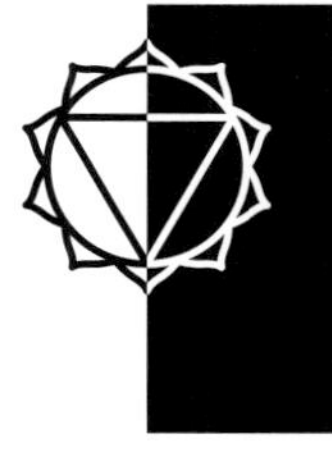

Agnistambhasana
Fire Log Pose

How to come into the pose

Sit on your mat, with your legs straight in front of you, spine straight, and arms by your sides.

Bend your right knee and hug it to your chest.

Then bring your right ankle to rest just above your left knee cap.

Bend your left knee and slide your left shin beneath your right shin.

Aim to bring your left ankle directly underneath your right knee.

If it is accessible for you, slide your right ankle a little more to your left until the ankle rests on your left knee.

Your right foot will hover over the floor, to the side of your left knee.

Work toward bringing your shins parallel to the top edge of your mat, keeping your right shin stacked directly above your left shin.

Both shins should be at a 90-degree angle to each thigh.

Flex your feet and press through your heels.

With your fingertips resting on the floor at either side of your body, press your sitting bones into the floor and lengthen your spine, then fold your hands in Prayer position and breathe evenly.

Hold the pose steadily as long as comfortable, then release and repeat on the other side.

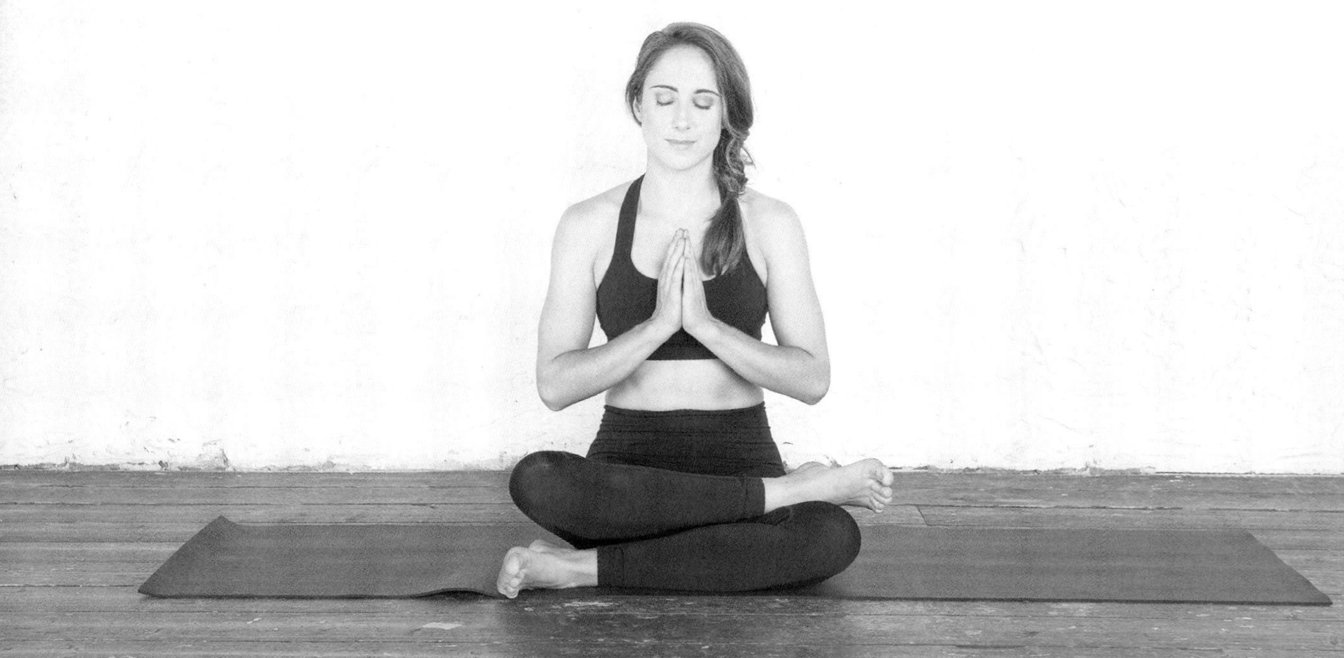

Next pose

Continue with Upward Plank Pose or a variation thereof.

Alignment cues

Keep your sitting bones on the floor.

Keep your feet actively flexed and aim to rest the top ankle over the lower knee. Do not allow your foot to sickle.

If your top knee is not resting on the bottom knee, do not force it down. Instead support it with a block or bolster and focus on releasing the tension in your hip flexors.

Contraindications & cautions

The same contraindications and cautions apply as in Seated Forward Bend. Also be cautious in this pose if you have knee issues.

Modifications & adjustments

If this pose is challenging due to tightness in the buttocks or knees, you can support either both or one side with a folded blanket or block.

To deepen the pose, gently walk your hands forward along the floor and fold your torso over your crossed legs. Make sure to create a hinging motion in your pelvis as you fold forward.

Once you have reached your maximum range, you can allow your back to round and your head to rest on your hands, legs or on the floor.

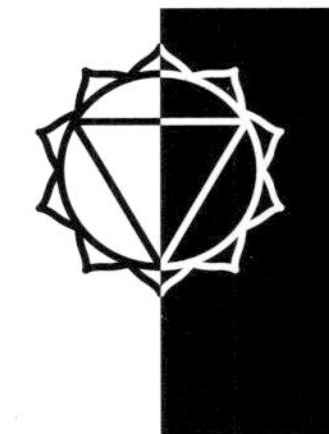

Paripurna Navasana
Boat Pose

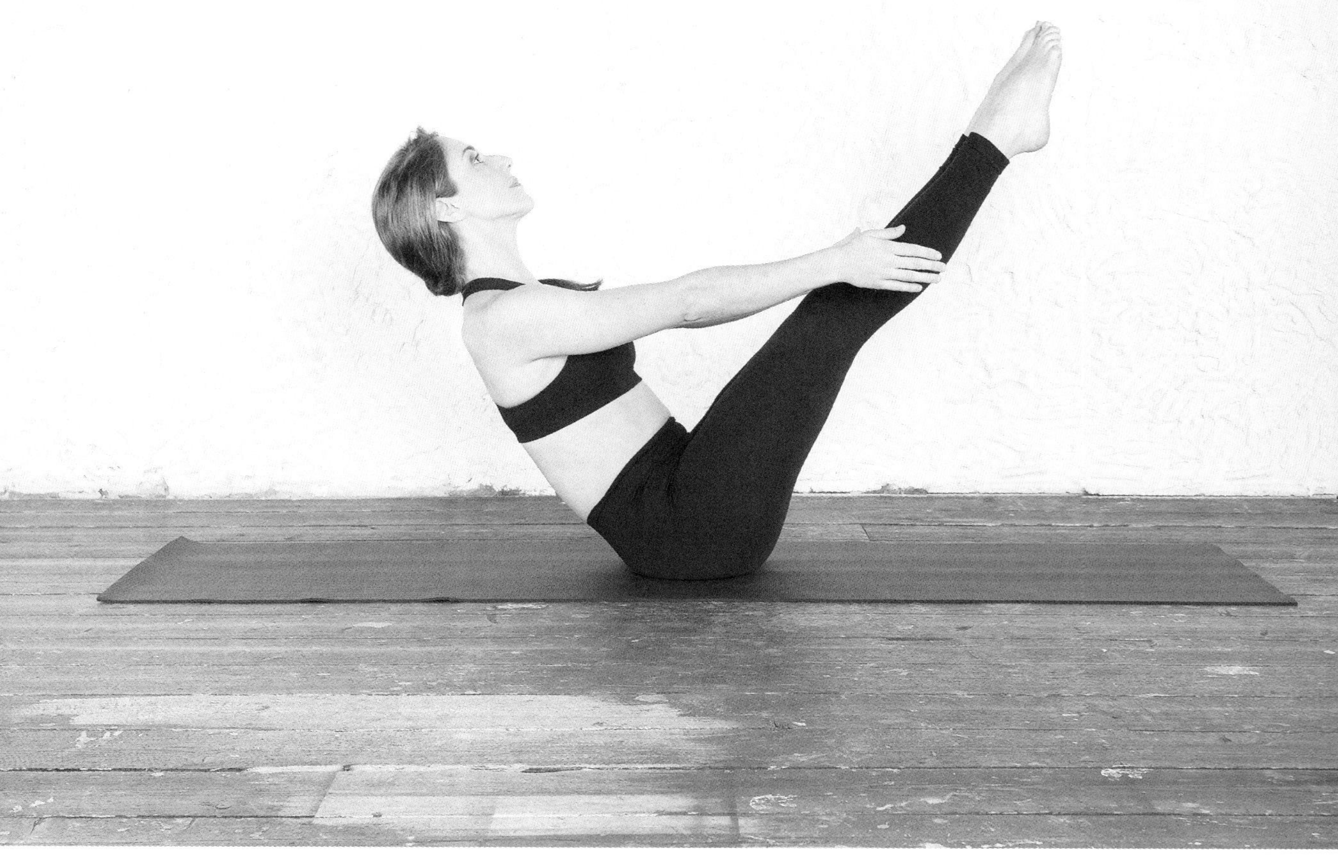

How to come into the pose

Sit with your feet together, knees bent, and feet resting on the floor.

Lean back slightly and place your hands behind you on the mat.

Lift your feet off the floor, and straighten your legs until they form an approximately 50-degree angle with the floor.

Lift your hands off the floor and extend them forward, at shoulder level, with your palms facing each other.

Look straight forward or slightly upward and hold the pose steadily as long as comfortable, breathing evenly.

Next pose

Continue with Upward Plank Pose or a variation thereof.

Alignment cues

There should be an approximately 90-degree angle between your torso and your legs.

Your hands are reaching forward along your knees, with palms parallel to each other and the floor.

Legs are straight, inner thighs are engaged, and feet gently pointed.

Your spine is straight, chest open, and your shoulder blades are drawn down and away from your ears.

Contraindications & cautions

The same contraindications and cautions apply as in Seated Forward Bend.

Modifications & adjustments

If this pose is challenging due to less strength or flexibility, you can start off with bent knees, shins parallel to the floor.

For extra support you can also hold on to the backs of your knees.

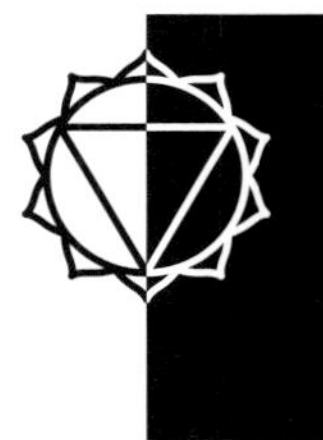

Variations

Ardha Navasana
Half Boat Pose

Lie on your back and extend both legs up toward the ceiling. Point your feet, and flex your toes back toward you. Keep the inner thighs engaged, and with control lower your legs down to about 30 degrees from the floor (or as low as you can while still keeping your lower back relatively flat against the floor). Extend your arms forward, parallel to the floor, with palms facing inwards. Curl your head and shoulder blades off the floor and gaze toward your lower belly. Draw your belly in, and round your back.

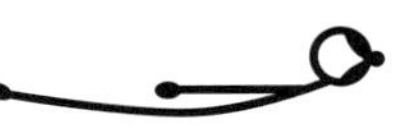

Ardha Purvottanasana

Reverse Table Pose

How to come into the pose

Sit on your mat, with your legs straight in front of you.

Bend your knees and place the soles of your feet on the mat.

Place your hands next to your hips, with your palms flat on the floor.

Fingers can be pointing toward or away from your toes.

Lift your pelvis from the floor, bringing your upper body and thighs parallel to the floor, making sure that your hands are below your shoulders and your feet below your knees.

Look diagonally up or straight up toward the ceiling.

Hold the pose steadily as long as comfortable and breathe evenly.

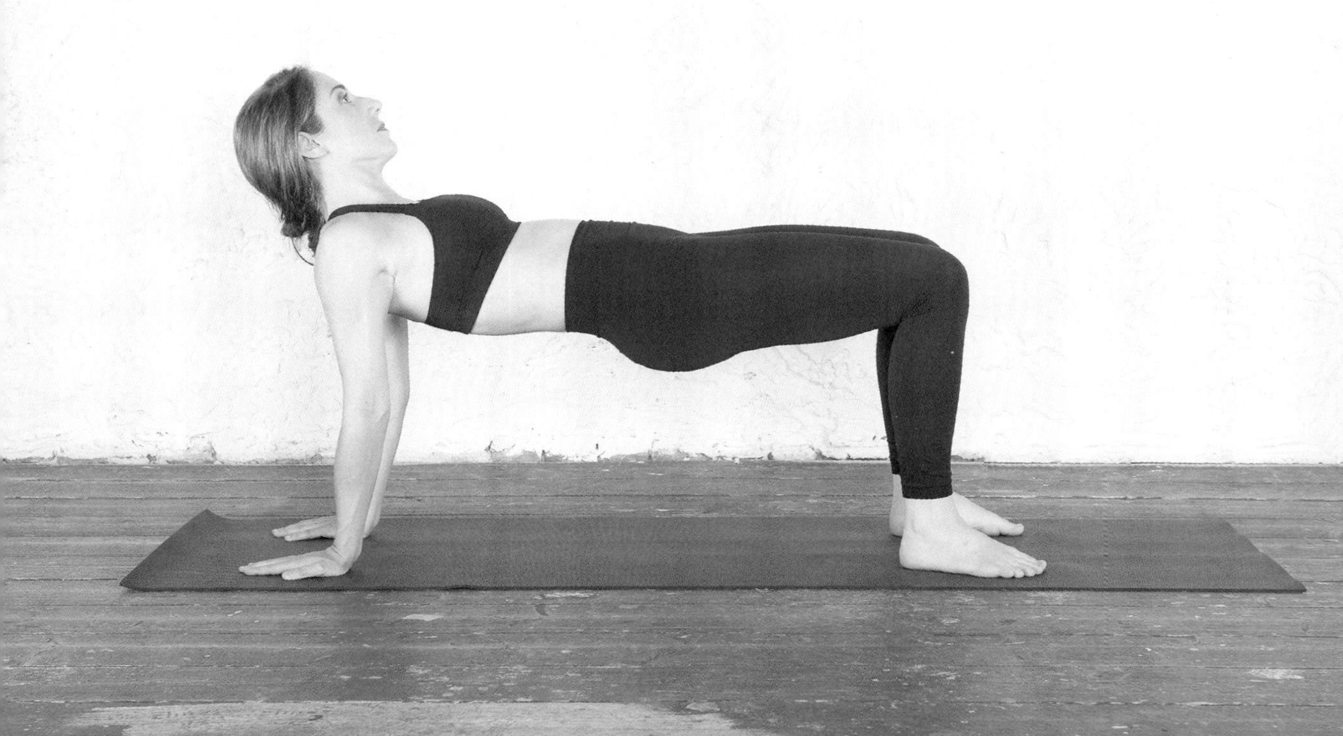

Next pose

Continue with Cobra Pose or a variation thereof.

Alignment cues

Keep the back of your neck elongated and shoulders away from your ears.

Make sure your knees and ankles are in one perpendicular line.

Contraindications & cautions

The same contraindications and cautions apply as in Upward Plank Pose.

Modifications & adjustments

If you feel tension or pain in your neck in this pose, you can look at your navel.

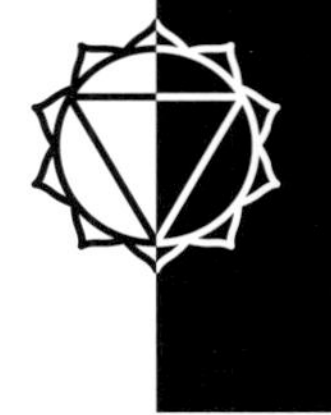

Variations

Eka Pada Ardha Purvottanasana

One-Legged Reverse Table Pose

To make the pose more challenging, you can lift up one leg at a time toward the ceiling. Aim to keep your hips in the same position as in the basic version. Flex your foot and push out through your heel.

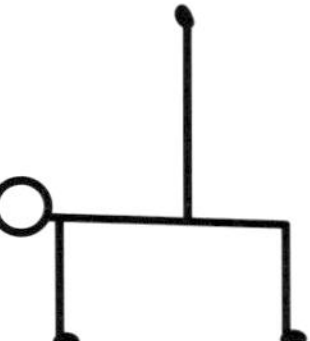

Supta Virasana
Reclining Hero Pose

How to come into the pose

Kneel on the floor, with your thighs perpendicular to the floor, and touch your inner knees together.

Slide your feet apart, slightly wider than your hips, with the tops of your feet flat on the floor.

Sit down, with your buttocks in between your heels.

If your buttocks are resting easily on the floor and you do not experience any strain in your knees, lean back on your hands and walk them backward away from you.

Gently ease yourself down until you can lie down.

Bring your arms above your head and hold on to your opposite elbows.

Hold the pose steadily as long as comfortable and breathe evenly.

To come out of the pose, gently push yourself up on your elbows until you are seated.

From here, press your hands against the floor and lift your buttocks slightly upward and release one leg at a time.

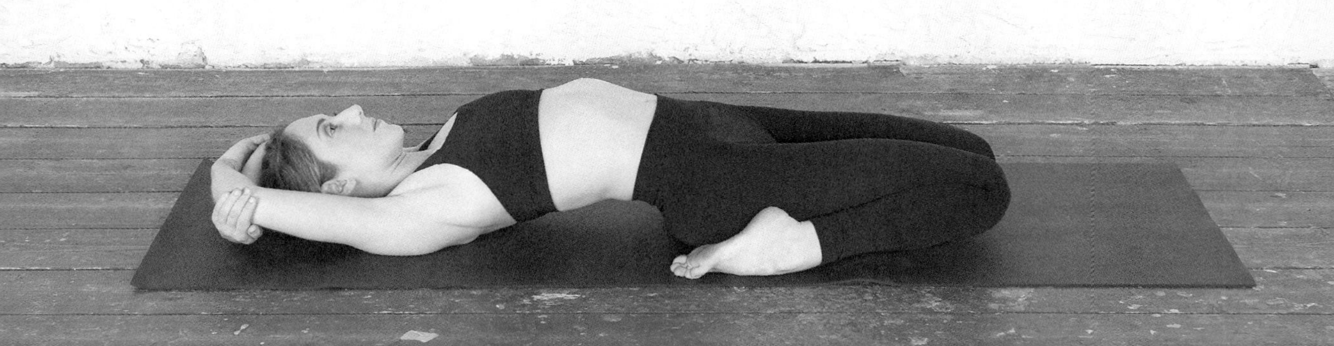

Next pose

Continue with Cobra Pose or a variation thereof.

Alignment cues

Ease into the pose very slowly and consciously.

At no time should you feel strain in your knees.

Sit firmly on the floor, in between your heels.

When you are in the reclined position, your lower back can arch and rise slightly off the floor.

Contraindications & cautions

The same contraindications and cautions apply as in Upward Plank Pose. Also be cautious in this pose if you have tight knees and hip flexors and/or knee issues.

Modifications & adjustments

If you cannot sit down in between your heels comfortably, place a block or cushion between your feet and make sure both sitting bones are resting on it equally.

If you feel tension in your knees when keeping them together, you can open your knees a little apart.

If lying down all the way is too much, you can build up gradually, by leaning on your hands or forearms and staying there. You can also use a bolster or cushion to rest your upper body on.

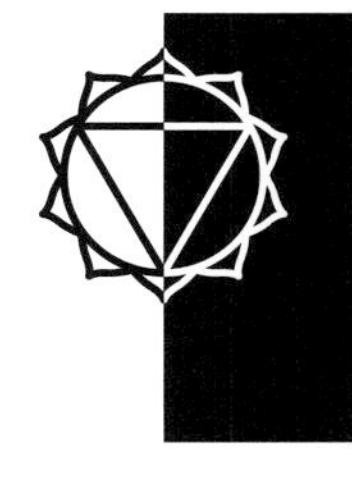

Bhujangasana (Cobra Pose) Variations

VISTRIT BHUJANGASANA
EXTENDED COBRA POSE

HOW TO COME INTO THE POSE

Lie down on your stomach with your forehead on the floor and your hands next to your chest.

Legs are hip-width or shoulder-width apart.

Breathe in, pushing your hands against the floor, and reach forward and up with your torso.

Lift your entire torso as far off the floor as possible, while keeping the front of your pelvis firmly on the floor.

Bring your entire spine into a backward arch by firmly pressing your hands against the floor.

Look diagonally up or even up and back, keeping your neck elongated.

Hold the pose steadily as long as comfortable and breathe evenly.

To release the pose, lead with your sternum forward and out and gently lower your upper body downward.

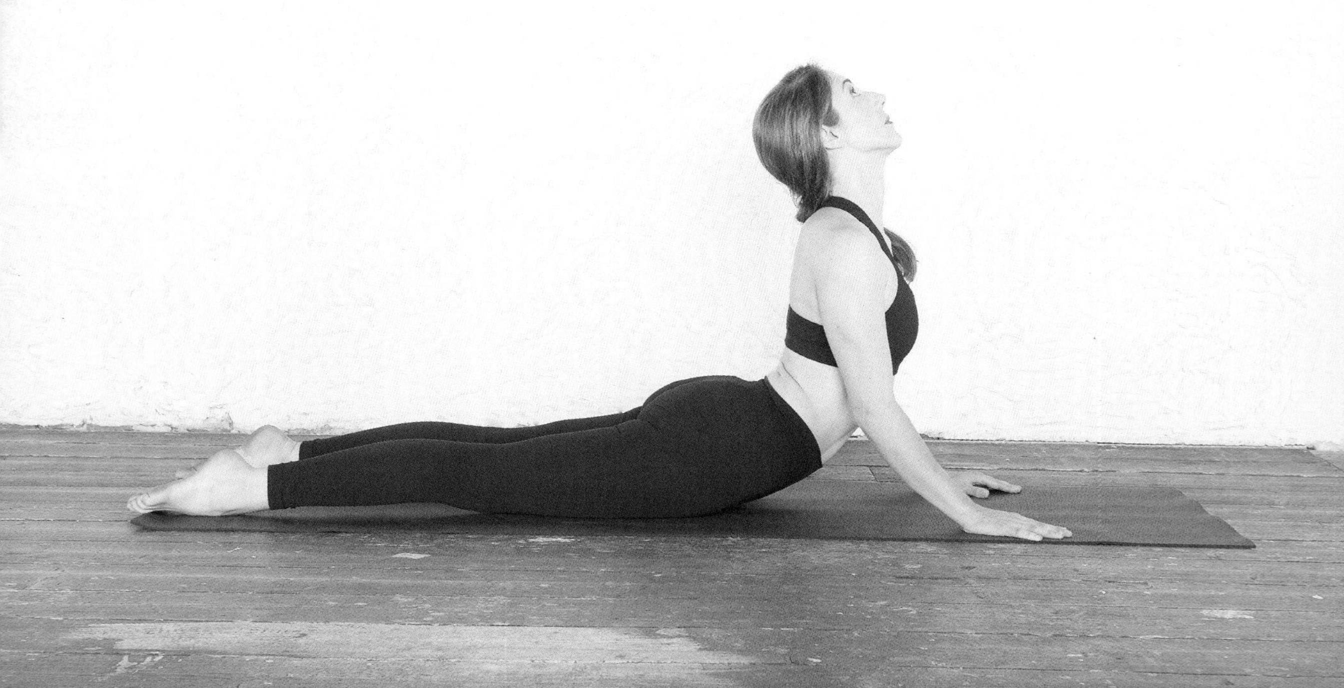

Next pose

Rest in Crocodile Pose for 30–45 seconds, then continue with Locust Pose or a variation thereof.

Alignment cues

Your arms are not locked but slightly bent, with your elbows hugging the side of your torso.

Your pubic bone and thighs stay firmly on the floor.

Shoulders blades are drawn down toward your waist.

Your neck is an extension of your spine. Do not drop your head back.

Depending on your flexibility you are either looking forward, diagonally upward, or up and backward.

Contraindications & cautions

The same contraindications and cautions apply as in Cobra Pose. Also be cautious in this pose if you have wrist issues.

Modifications & adjustments

Depending on the flexibility of your spine, you need to keep your arms bent. The more your arms are bent, the heavier it feels. If it becomes too heavy, you can walk your hands forward so that your elbows straighten out more. But make sure not to allow your shoulders to lift up to your ears.

If you suffer from lower-back issues, backbends often are allowed and even advised. However, make sure to not push yourself to your full movement capacity, but rather stay at around 70 percent of your flexibility. For extra support and stability, keep your core active, by pulling your belly button in toward your spine.

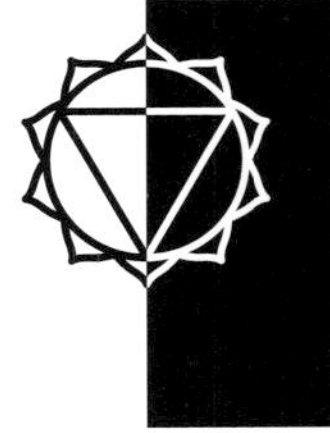

Variations

Raj Bhujangasana

King Cobra Pose

Start as in Extended Cobra Pose. This time, though, keep your legs wider apart than your shoulders, bend your knees, and bring your big toes together. Rest your forehead on the floor and set up your hands next to your rib cage (slightly lower than in Extended Cobra Pose). Now breathe in, pushing your hands into the floor, reach with your head toward your feet, and pull your feet in toward your head. Even as you look backward toward your feet, keep your neck elongated. Your pelvis and even your upper thighs might lift off the floor, but make sure not to lift them up actively but rather try to release them toward the floor to accomplish the deep arch.

URDHVA MUKHA SHVANASANA
UPWARD-FACING DOG POSE

HOW TO COME INTO THE POSE

Come onto all fours, with your knees below your hips and your wrists below your shoulders, toes curled.

From here drop your hips forward toward the floor.

Press your palms firmly into the floor, drop your shoulders down and back, and press your chest forward as you reach the crown of your head up toward the ceiling.

Breathe in and lift your thighs and legs off the floor by pressing the balls of your feet and toes down against the floor and pushing out through your heels.

Engage your core and legs.

To deepen the pose, you can look up and backward, without dropping your head.

Hold the pose steadily as long as comfortable and breathe evenly.

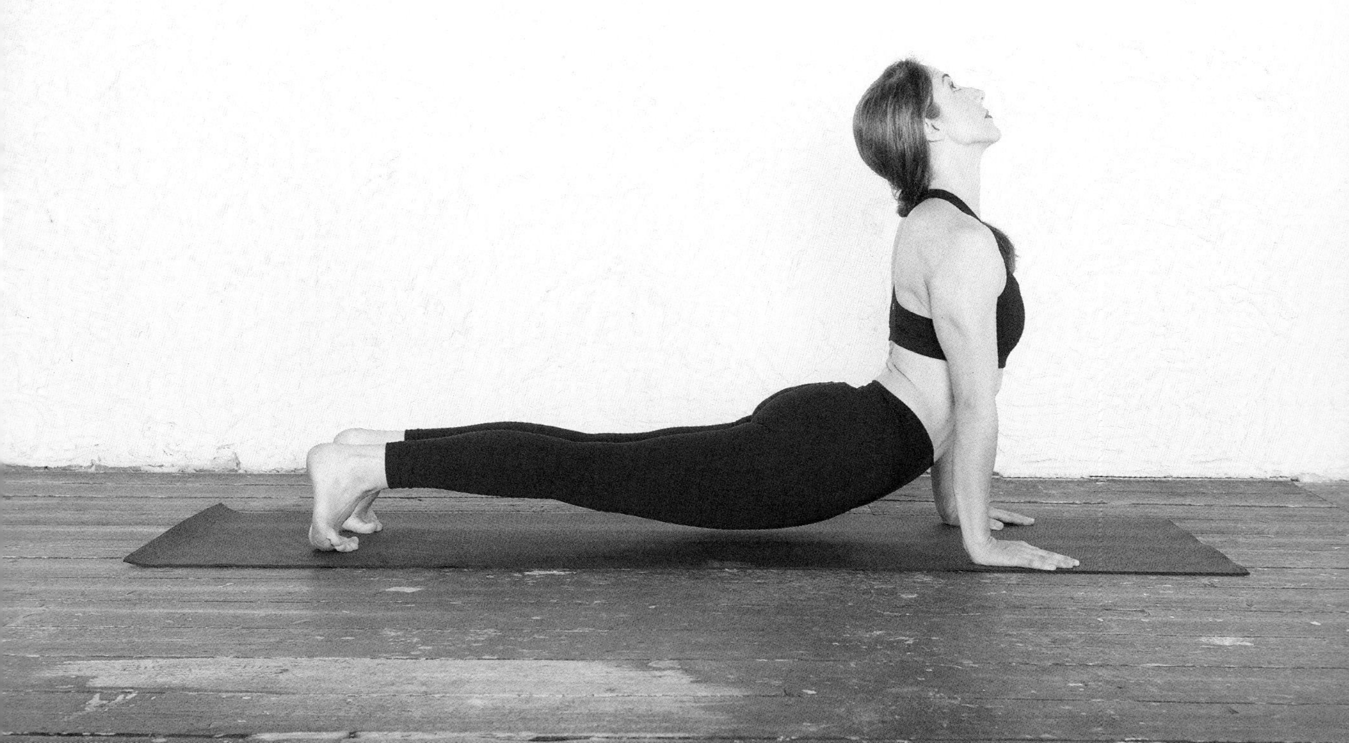

Next pose

Rest in Crocodile Pose for 30–45 seconds, then continue with Locust Pose or a variation thereof.

Alignment cues

The only connection points with the floor are your hands and balls of your feet. Your legs, pelvis, and torso are all lifted.

Keep your entire body (especially legs and core) engaged, pressing out through your heels in order to lessen the strain on your knees, elbows, and lower back.

Arms are straight, with your shoulders down and away from your ears.

Make sure that your shoulders are right above your wrists or slightly behind them. Do not allow your shoulders to drop in front of your wrists, because that can cause strain and eventually injury to your wrist joints.

Keep your neck as an extension of your spine. If flexibility allows, look up and backward.

Contraindications & cautions

The same contraindications and cautions apply as in Cobra Pose. Also be cautious in this pose if you have wrist or shoulder issues.

Modifications & adjustments

This is quite a tiring pose and requires strength and control in order to keep the joints and back safe. A good alternative to this pose, if it is too intense, is Extended Cobra Pose, in which you also work on your lower-back flexibility and chest opening.

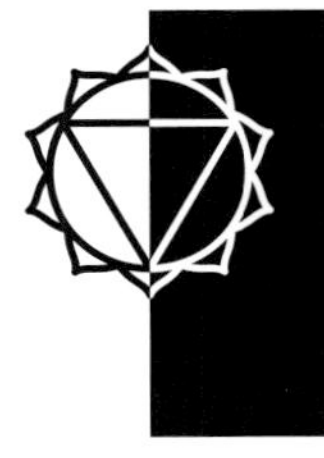

Shalabhasana (Locust Pose) Variations

Ardha Shalabhasana

Half Locust Pose

How to come into the pose

From Crocodile Pose, roll to your right side and clasp your hands tightly in a kind of volleyball position, then push your hands below your pelvis.

Roll back on your stomach and keep your shoulders as close together as possible.

Look forward and place your chin flat on the floor.

Breathe in, push your upper arms against the floor, and lift your right leg up as high as possible, while keeping your pelvis squared.

Hold the pose steadily as long as comfortable and breathe evenly, then release and repeat the same with your left leg.

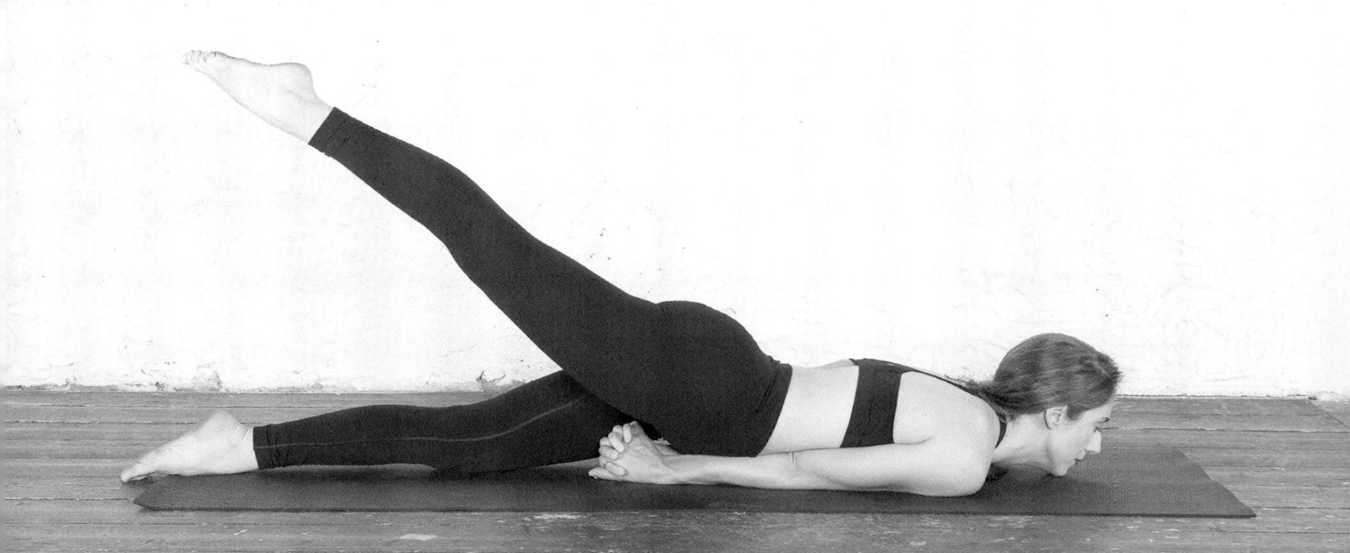

Next pose

Rest in Crocodile Pose for 30–45 seconds, then continue with Bow Pose or a variation thereof.

Alignment cues

Arms are completely straight; shoulders are rolled forward and inward so that your elbows and wrists are touching their opposite counterparts.

Your hands are pushed as low as possible below your pelvis.

Avoid tilting your pelvis as you lift your leg up.

Your legs are straight, and your feet are pointed.

This pose can also be performed dynamically, alternately lifting the legs with an inhalation and releasing them down to the floor with the exhalation. In this case, it can be repeated for 3–5 rounds (right and left alternating is one round).

Contraindications & cautions

The same contraindications and cautions apply as in Locust Pose.

Modifications & adjustments

If you feel pain in your arms or elbows you can place a rolled blanket under your elbows. If you feel tension in your neck or cannot place your chin flat on the floor, you can place a blanket underneath your chest. You can modify your hand position by making two fists next to each other or hands flat next to each other, with palms facing downward. If you suffer from tension or pain in your neck, you can place your forehead (instead of your chin) on the floor.

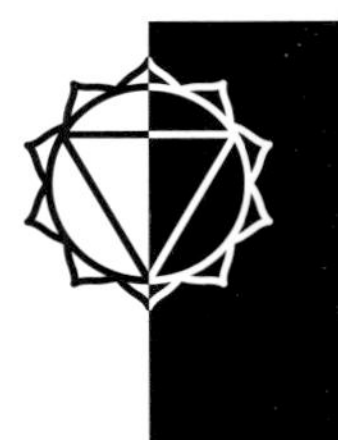

Variations

Salamba Ardha Shalabhasana

Supported Half Locust Pose

Come into the starting position as described in Half Locust Pose. Then breathe in, push your upper arms against the floor, and lift your right leg up as high as possible, while keeping your pelvis squared. Support the right leg with the sole of your left foot, letting the thigh, knee, or shin gently rest on the left foot. Breathe evenly and hold the pose steadily, then repeat on the other side.

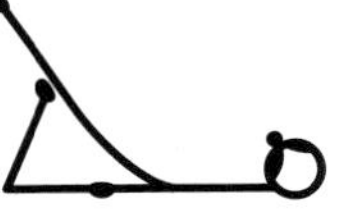

Vistrit Shalabhasana
Extended Locust Pose

How to come into the pose

From Crocodile Pose, roll to your right side and clasp your hands tightly in a kind of volleyball position, then push your hands below your pelvis.

Roll back on your stomach and keep your shoulders as close together as possible.

Look forward and place your chin flat on the floor.

Breathe in, curl your toes, and, pushing your feet into the floor, lift your pelvis upward.

Walk your feet close toward your chest, hips reaching up toward the ceiling.

Lift one leg high up, aiming to bring your hips above your shoulders.

Push off with your foot on the floor and take a gentle hop.

As you hop, allow your back to arch more and reach with your feet toward your head.

Firmly push your arms into the floor, keep lifting your pelvis upward, and find your balance.

Hold the pose steadily as long as comfortable and breathe evenly.

To release the pose, firmly press your arms into the floor and roll your torso back down.

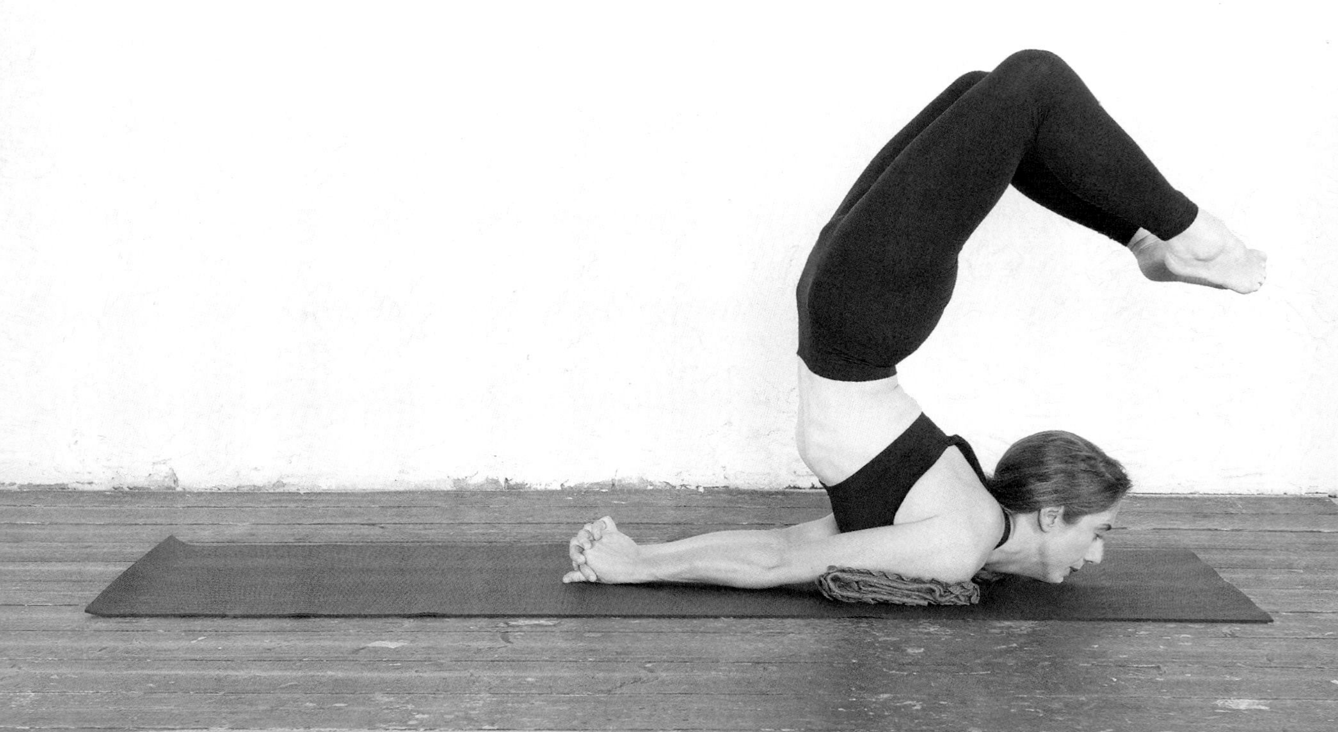

Next pose

Rest in Crocodile Pose for 30–45 seconds, then continue with Bow Pose or a variation thereof.

Alignment cues

Arms are completely straight; shoulders are rolled forward and inward, so that elbows and wrists are touching their opposite counterparts.

Hands are pushed as low as possible below your pelvis.

Do not collapse in your lower back.

Especially if you have a very flexible back, make sure to keep your core, back, and buttocks engaged to protect your back.

Contraindications & cautions

The same contraindications and cautions apply as in Locust Pose. Also be cautious in this pose if you have lower-back issues or hypertension.

Modifications & adjustments

If you feel pain in your arms or elbows you can place a rolled blanket under your elbows. If you feel tension in your neck or cannot place your chin flat on the floor you can place a blanket underneath your chest. You can modify your hand position as follows: clench both fists next to each other or hands flat next to each other, with palms facing downward.

Variations

Vistrit Shalabhasana II

Extended Locust Pose II (Straight Legs)

Follow the instructions as described of Extended Locust Pose, but instead of bending your knees and reaching with your feet to your head, keep your legs straight with feet reaching toward the ceiling.

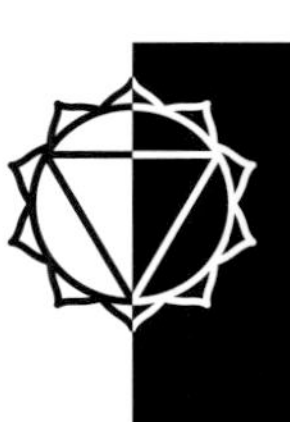

Accomplished Vistrit Shalabhasana

(Coming Up Without Hopping)

To increase the level of difficulty, you can aim to come into the pose without hopping. Come into the starting position with your hands below your pelvis and your feet hip- or shoulder-width apart. From there, lift your legs up, allowing your knees to bend, and project them over your head. This variation requires not only a considerable amount of flexibility but also immense core awareness and control. You can practice this initially by hopping into the pose and then coming down in a very slow and controlled manner.

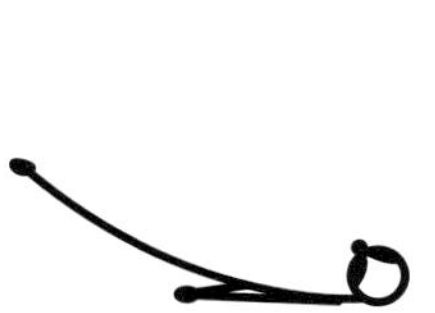
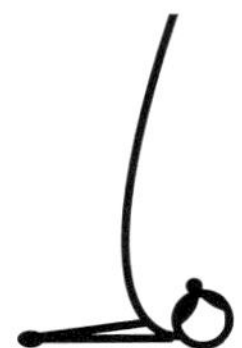
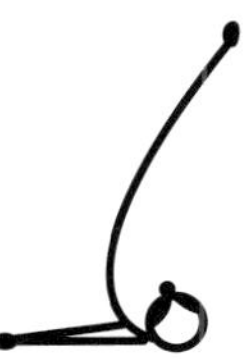
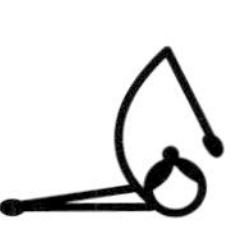

Ganda Bherundasana
Formidable-Face Pose (aka Chin Stand)

How to come into the pose

Start in Downward-Facing Dog Pose, with your hands shoulder-width apart.

Then walk your feet a little closer toward your hands.

Keep your hips raised toward the ceiling and shift your shoulders forward past your wrists.

Engage your arms, pressing your elbows in toward your torso and lower your chin toward the floor.

With control, lift your left leg upward, engaging your buttocks and leg muscles.

Then, push off the ball of your right foot to lightly kick this second leg up toward the ceiling.

Activate your core muscles and firmly press your legs together, pointing your feet and reaching with your toes up toward the ceiling or drop your feet toward your head.

Hold the pose steadily as long as comfortable and breathe evenly.

To release the pose, firmly press your hands into the floor and release one leg at a time back to the floor.

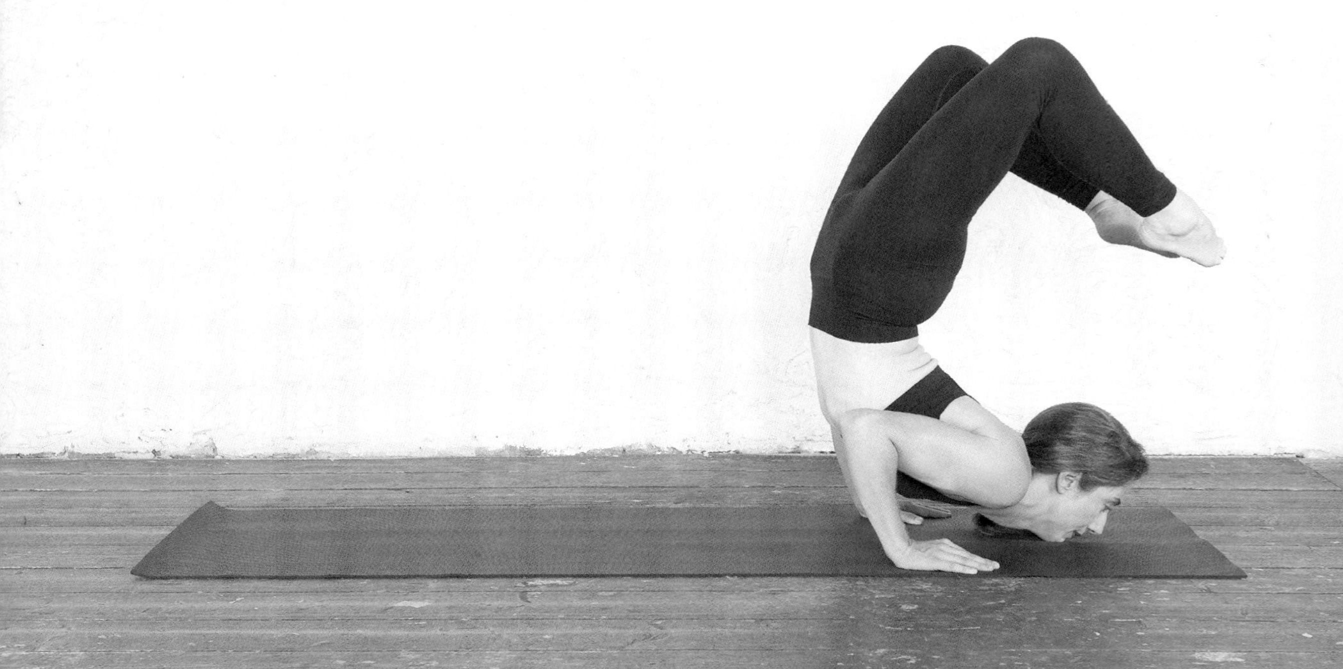

Next pose

Rest in Crocodile Pose for 30–45 seconds, then continue with Bow Pose or a variation thereof.

Alignment cues

Press your elbows firmly against your torso.

Keep your shoulders drawn away from your ears and maintain length in your neck.

Place little to no weight on the chin and do not thrust your head back or allow your shoulders to collapse.

Direct the energy of the pose up the length of your spine toward your feet rather than down into your chin and the floor.

Contraindications & cautions

The same contraindications and cautions apply as in Locust Pose. Also be cautious in this pose if you have lower-back issues or hypertension.

Modifications & adjustments

For a supported variation, place a block under each shoulder as you kick up into the pose. The blocks help support your body weight and reduce the risk of injury and strain in your neck and shoulders. Starting in Downward-Facing Dog Pose, place a block directly in front of the fingertips of each hand. As you shift forward, place your shoulders on the blocks, then lift one leg up and kick the second one up with control.

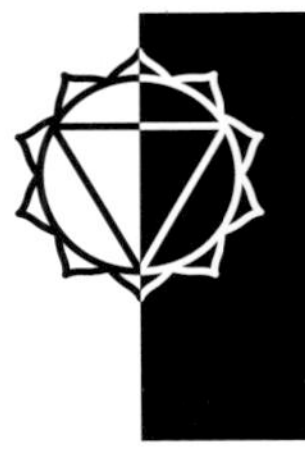

Dhanurasana (Bow Pose) Variations

Eka Pada Dhanurasana

One-Legged Bow Pose

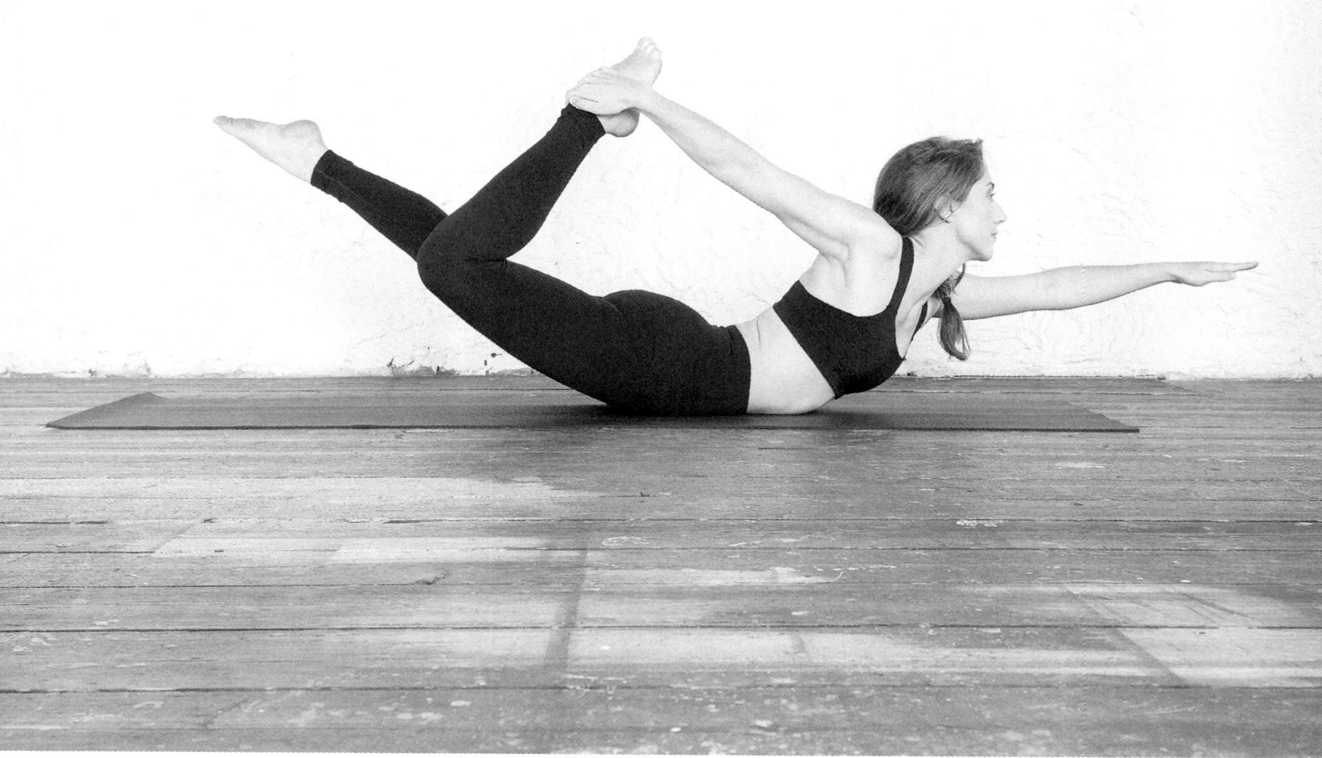

How to come into the pose

Lie down on your abdomen, with your forehead on the floor, knees shoulder-width apart.

Bend your right knee and clasp your right ankle from the outside with your right hand.

Extend your left arm forward, palm facing downward.

Breathe in, pushing your right foot into your hand, and lift your chest and knee.

At the same time, reach out and upward with your left hand and foot and lift them off the floor.

Push your belly button down toward the floor, looking diagonally upward and taking small and easy breaths.

Hold the pose steadily as long as comfortable.

Release the pose and repeat on the other side.

Next pose

Rest in Crocodile Pose for 30–45 seconds, then continue with Half Spinal Twist or a variation thereof.

Alignment cues

Elbows are straight.

Use the opposing force of your foot kicking against the hand to lift yourself higher upward.

Aim to keep your weight on your abdomen and bring your chest and knees in one parallel line to the floor.

Lift the straight leg and arm just as high up as the bound opposite side.

Maintain your neck as an extension of your spine.

If flexibility allows, look diagonally upward, otherwise gaze forward.

Contraindications & cautions

The same contraindications and cautions apply as in Bow Pose. Also be cautious in this pose if you have lower-back issues or hypertension.

Modifications & adjustments

This pose is ideal for anyone who finds it too challenging to bind both hands to the ankles, as in Dhanurasana. If it is still challenging to catch the one ankle, you can use a strap to bridge the gap.

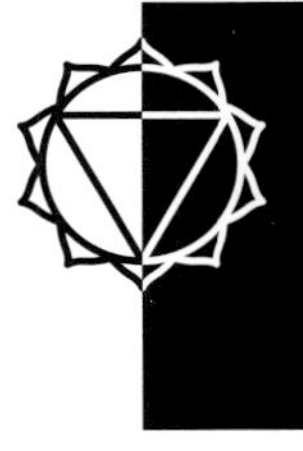

Viparita Navasana
Reverse Boat Pose

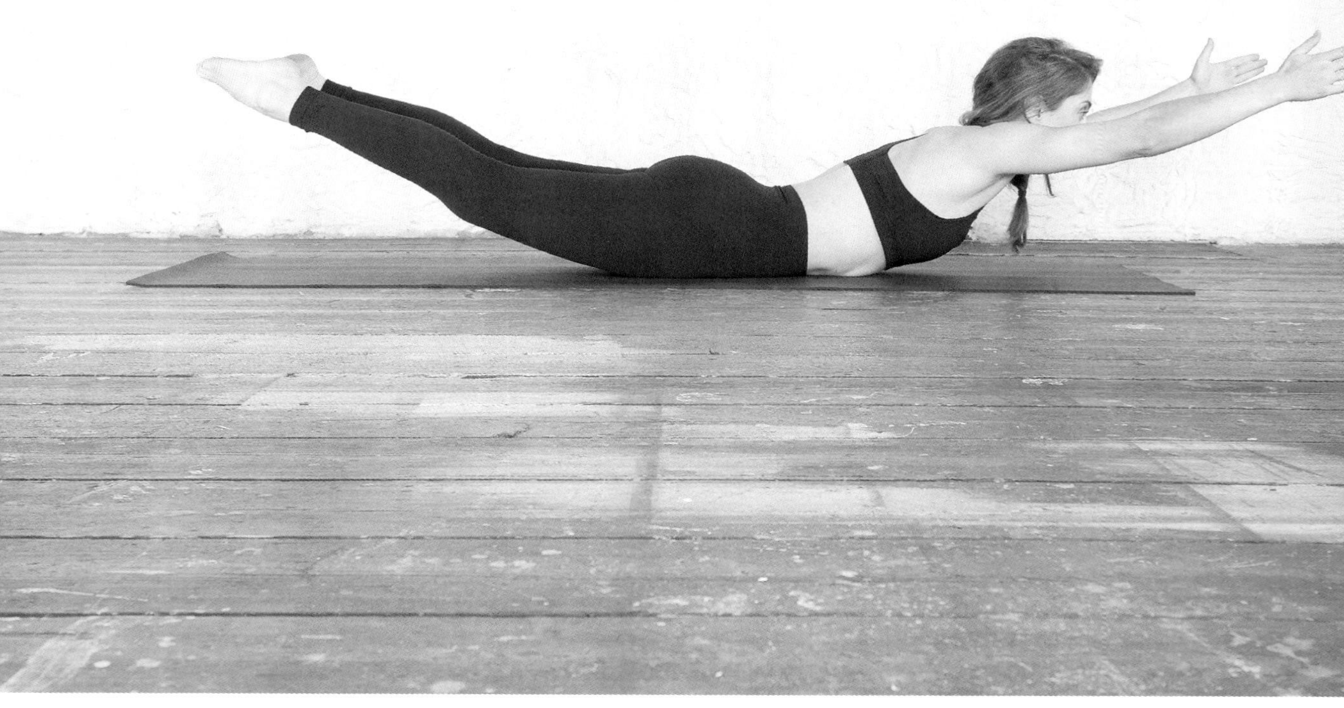

How to come into the pose

Lie on your stomach, with your forehead on the floor, your arms reaching forward above your head, and your feet together.

Breathe in, lifting your arms, chest, and legs off the floor as high as possible.

Feet are pointed, fingertips reaching out as far as possible.

Look forward or diagonally upward.

Hold the pose steadily as long as comfortable and breathe evenly.

Next pose

Rest in Crocodile Pose for 30–45 seconds, then continue with Half Spinal Twist or a variation thereof.

Alignment cues

Palms can be either facing downward or facing toward each other.

Rather than making an effort to raise your hands and legs more, focus on stretching your arms and legs away from your torso.

Keep the neck elongated.

Contraindications & cautions

The same contraindications and cautions apply as in Bow Pose. Because the knees are straight, this is an ideal Bow Pose variation for anyone suffering from knee issues.

Modifications & Adjustments

If you find this pose heavy on your shoulders or feel tension in your neck, you can also keep your arms next to your body, with your fingers pointing toward your feet.

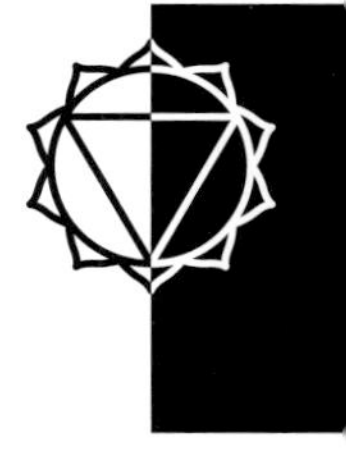

Eka Pada Rajakapotasana
One-Legged King Pigeon Pose

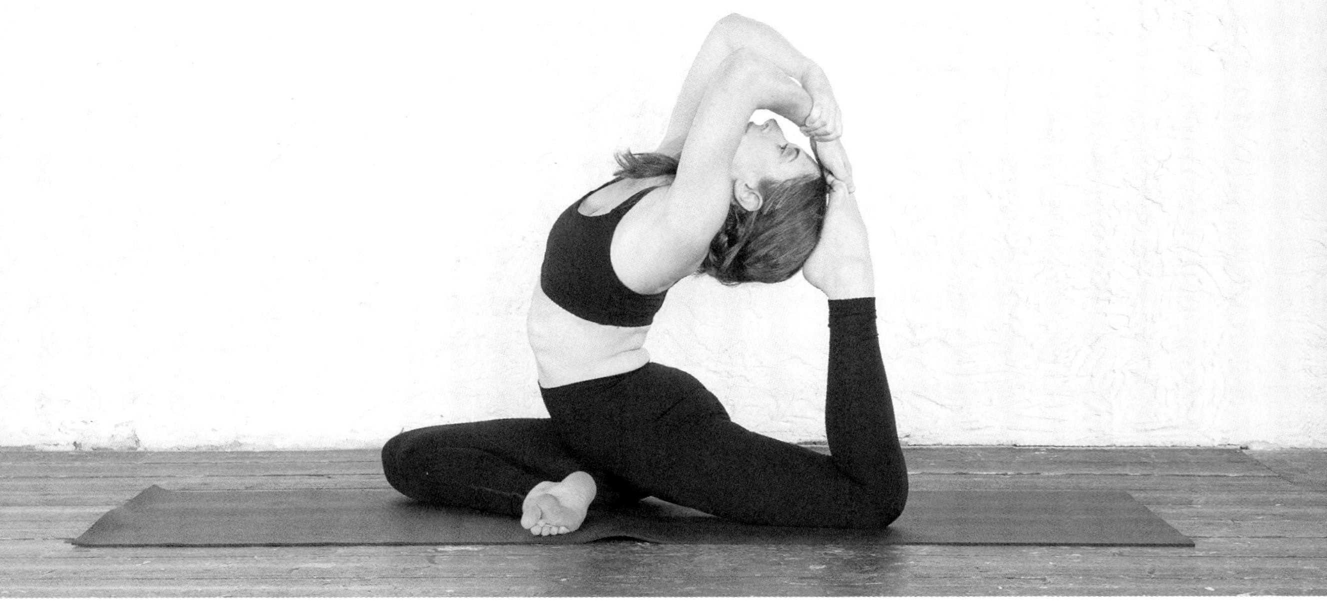

How to come into the pose

Begin on all fours, with your knees directly below your hips, and your hands slightly ahead of your shoulders.

From there, slide your right knee forward to the outside of your right wrist; at the same time bring your right foot to the front of your left knee, resting the outside of your right knee on the floor.

Slowly slide your left leg backward, straightening your knee and lowering the front of your thigh to the floor. Lower the outside of your right buttock to the floor.

Position your right heel just in front of your left hip and push your fingertips firmly to the floor. Roll your left hip joint toward your right heel, squaring your pelvis as much as possible.

Then, with your hands pushing against the floor, bend the back knee and bring your foot as close to the top of your head as possible.

Breathe in, reach with your right arm toward the ceiling, and then breathe out, bending the elbow, and, reaching back, grasp the inside of your left foot.

After a few breaths, reach back with your left hand and grasp the outside of your foot.

Draw the sole of your foot as close as possible toward the crown of your head.

Hug both elbows into your midline and look up.

Keep your lower belly and leg active in order to stay in balance. Hold the pose steadily as long as comfortable and breathe evenly.

To come out of the pose, place your hands back on the floor and step back to Downward-Facing Dog Pose, before moving on to the other side.

Next pose

Rest in Child's Pose for 30–45 seconds, then continue with Half Spinal Twist or a variation thereof.

Alignment cues

The front knee can be slightly angled outwards, outside the line of the hip.

Make sure to create the rotation from your hip joint; do not twist your knee joint in an effort to bring your front shin more forward and parallel to the mat.

Your back leg should extend straight out of your hip and should be rotated slightly inwards, so its midline presses against the floor.

Proceed to the full version, as described above, only if you are able to square your hips and maintain an upright position of your pelvis and spine without the support of your hands against the floor or knee.

If that is not possible, work toward the pose with the variations described below.

Contraindications & cautions

The same contraindications and cautions apply as in Bow Pose. Also be cautious in this pose if you have lower-back issues (especially SI-joint issues), tight hips, or knee, groin, or hamstring issues.

Modifications & adjustments

This pose requires a considerable range of rotation in the hip joints, psoas, and chest. It is often difficult to bring the buttock of the front leg all the way down to the floor. You can place a rolled or folded blanket underneath the hip for support. Before attempting the full expression of this pose, practice the variations as described below.

Variations

Supta Eka Pada Kapotasana

Sleeping One-Legged Pigeon Pose

Follow the first four steps described to the left, then gently walk your hands forward until your chest rests on your front knee and your forehead on the floor.

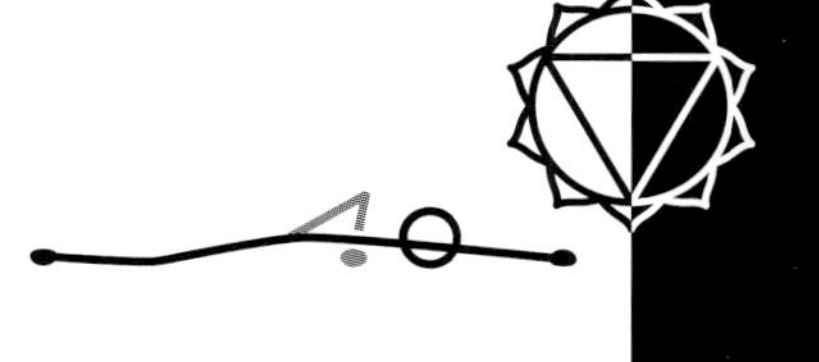

Sukha Eka Pada Kapotasana I

Easy One-Legged Pigeon Pose I

Follow the first five steps as described to the left, then hold on to the inside of your left ankle with your right hand. Create opposition by kicking your left foot away, and if you are stable, extend your left hand diagonally upward. Gaze at a point slightly above eye level.

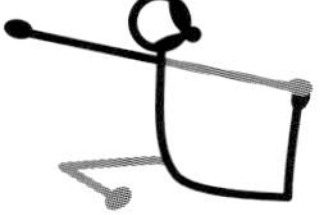

Sukha Eka Pada Kapotasana II

Easy One-Legged Pigeon Pose II

Follow the first five steps as described to the left, then wrap your left elbow around your left ankle. Now clasp your hands together and bring them behind your head as you gaze forward and slightly upward.

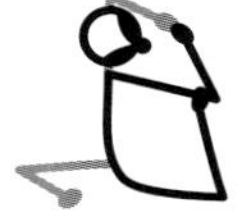

Hanumanasana
Monkey Pose

How to come into the pose

Start in low lunge, with your right foot in front, your right knee over your right ankle.

Place both hands on the floor along your right foot.

Your left knee is resting on the floor, toes pointed.

To come into the split-legs phase, lift the ball of the front foot upward and start sliding your right heel forward as far as your hamstrings permit.

Keep pushing the back knee backward so your left thigh is getting closer to the floor.

Keep your hips square toward the front of the mat, and when you reach the floor, straighten your spine and lift your hands up toward the ceiling in Prayer position (in line with your forehead).

Lift your chest and chin slightly and look at the eye-shaped space between your palms.

To release the pose, carefully lean to the side of your front leg, sit on your outer hip, and bring your legs together.

Then repeat on your left.

Hold the pose steadily as long as comfortable and breathe evenly.

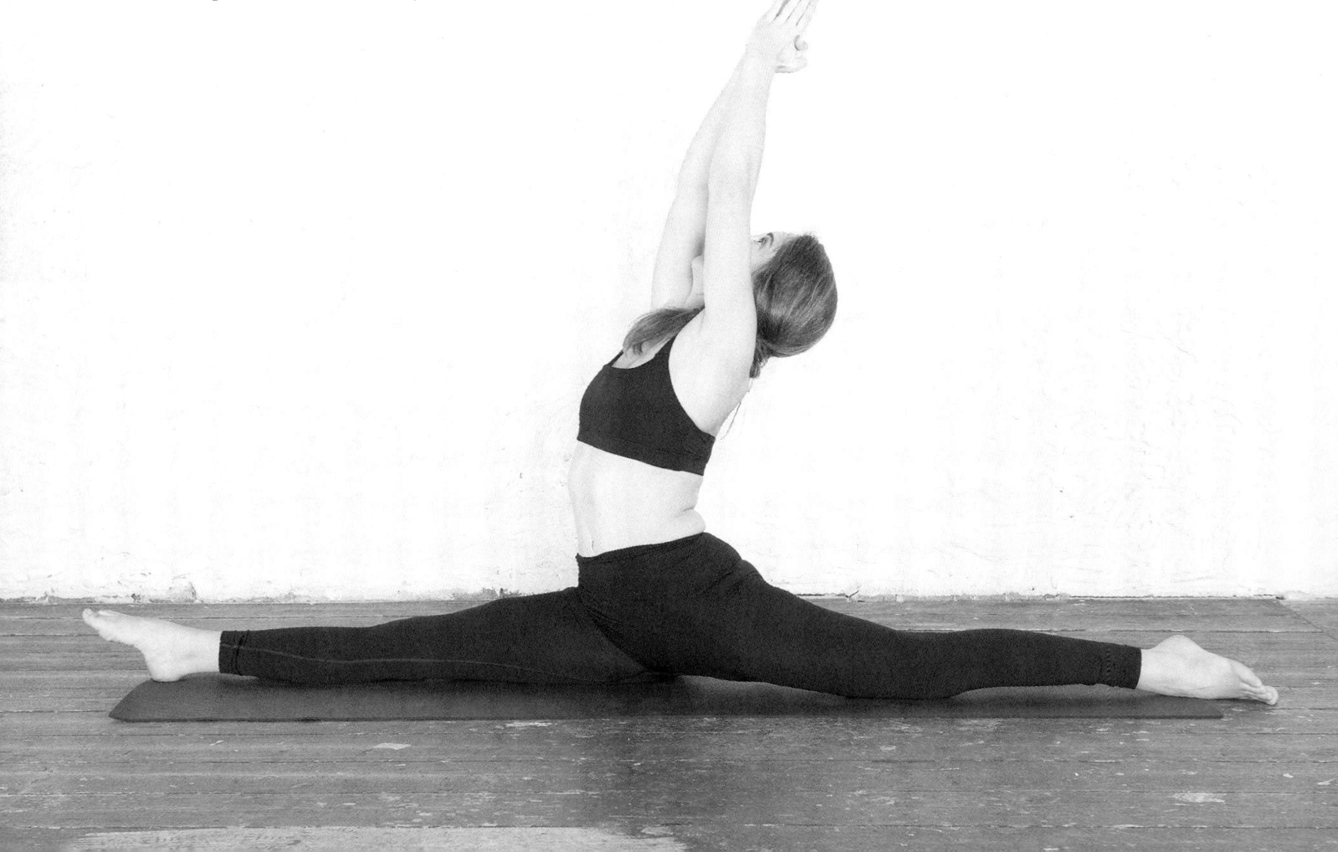

Next pose

Rest in Child's Pose for 30–45 seconds, then continue with Half Spinal Twist or a variation thereof.

Alignment cues

Make sure your hips are square and your back leg remains straight from the hip and is not pointing sideways.

Focus on leveling your pelvis instead of reaching to the floor.

Even as you are looking up, keep your neck as an extension of your spine. Do not drop your head backward.

Contraindications & cautions

The same contraindications and cautions apply as in Bow Pose. Also be cautious in this pose if you have groin or hamstring issues.

Modifications & adjustments

This pose requires truly flexible hamstrings. Never force yourself into this pose, but proceed with caution. In this pose, the hamstring muscles are intensely exposed and can easily become injured. Until you can easily release your pelvis to the floor, keep a firm foundation with your hands. You can also use a bolster and block underneath the top of your front thigh, so that you do not have to rely solely on your hands. To build up toward the full expression of the pose, you can start by practicing Easy Monkey Pose, as described below.

Variations

Sukha Hanumanasana

Easy Monkey Pose

Start in a low lunge, with your hands along the front foot on the floor. The knee of your back leg is on the floor, foot pointed. Now push the back leg as far away as possible, while still maintaining the front-knee-above-ankle alignment. Lift your chest, push your pelvis forward toward your front leg, and reach with your hands above your head, palms together. Reach upward and backward with your hands, allowing your spine and especially chest to arch even more, and look up toward the eye-shaped space between your palms.

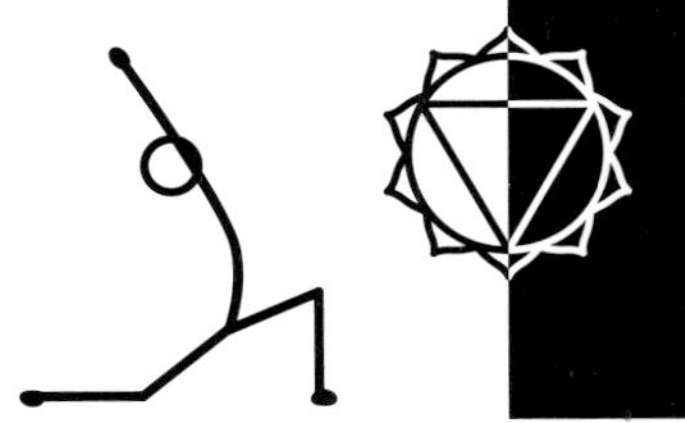

Eka Pada Raja Hanumanasana

One-Legged King Monkey Pose

Come into Hanumanasana, as described on the left. Once you are comfortable in the pose, with your hips square, start to bend your back knee and reach back with your left hand with your palm up and elbow bent. Grab on to your left big toe and, maintaining the rotation of your palm, rotate your elbow outward, upward, and inwards. As you do so, draw your arm to your face. Brace yourself with your right hand against the floor. When stable, reach it upward, bend the elbow, and walk down your right forearm to find your foot. Hold on to your left foot with both hands, pulling your foot toward your head. Hug both elbows into your midline and look up. Keep your lower belly and legs active in order to stay in balance.

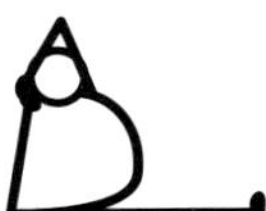

Ardha Matsyendrasana (Half Spinal Twist) Variations

Parivrtta Janu Shirshasana

Revolved Head-to-Knee Pose

How to come into the pose

Sit with your legs stretched out in front of you.

Bend your right leg and place your right foot against your left inner thigh.

Place your right hand behind your spine and cross your left hand over your right knee, palm facing upward.

Breathe in, and lengthen your spine.

Breathe out, look over your right shoulder, and twist to your right.

Breathe in, reach out with your right hand, and lift your hand up to the ceiling. Breathe out, bend sideways over your left leg, and catch hold of the outside edge of your left foot with your right hand.

Press your left arm against your right knee (elbow straight) and use the opposition between your two hands to help twist your upper torso further.

Turn your head to look at the ceiling.

Hold the pose steadily as long as comfortable and breathe evenly.

To come out, first untwist your torso, and, without coming upright, sweep it to your right midway between your legs.

Then inhale and roll up to an upright position. Repeat on the other side.

Continue with Upward Plank Pose or a variation thereof.

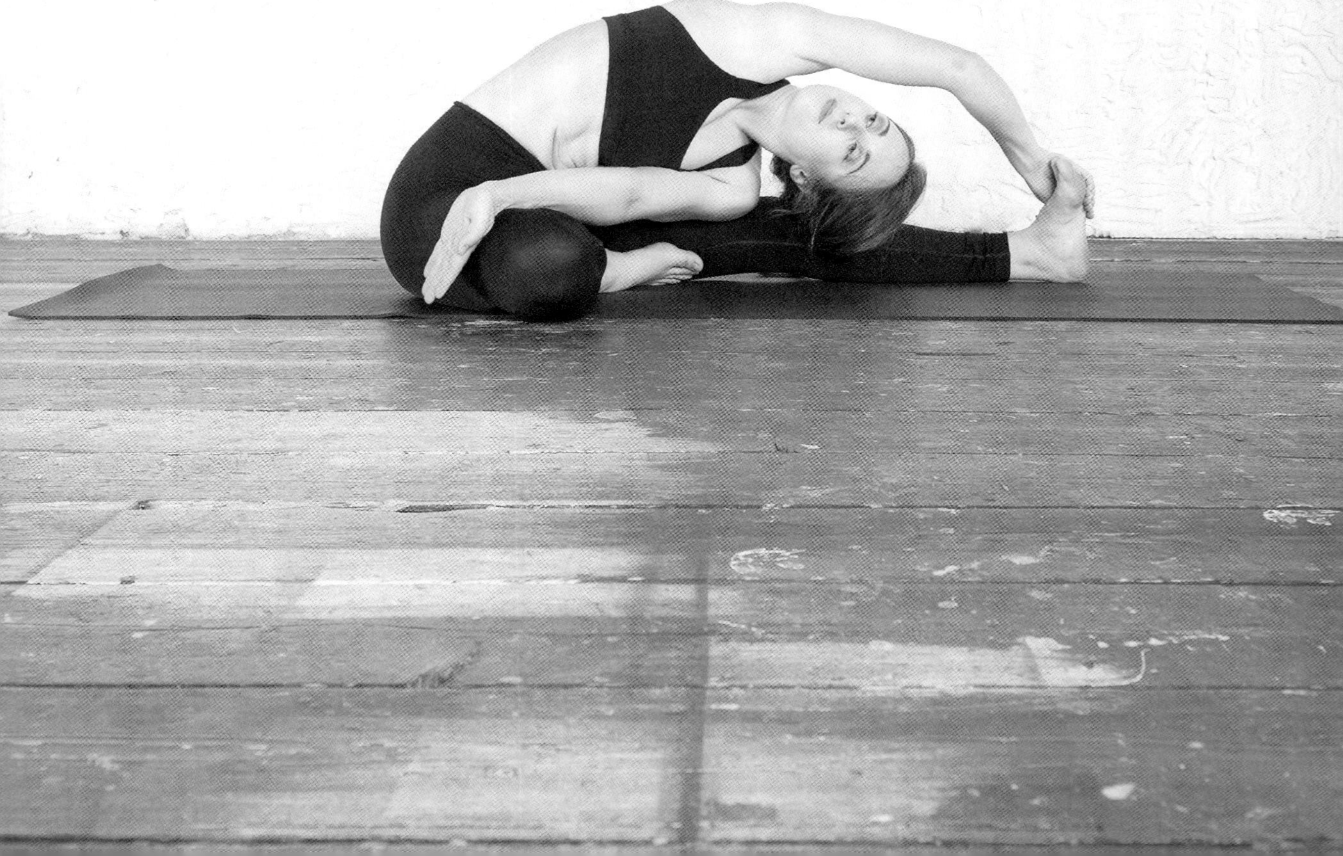

Alignment cues

The foot of your bent leg can come as high as comfortable up along the extended leg. But make sure your pelvis stays straight. If your pelvis is not straight, place your foot a bit lower.

The aim is to twist your upper body, stacking your shoulders vertically above each other, while keeping your pelvis square.

Both sitting bones are rooted firmly into the floor, and the hand crossing your knee helps to secure your hips in a square position.

The focus is on twisting your spine and expanding the chest maximally.

Contraindications & cautions

The same contraindications and cautions apply as in Half Spinal Twist.

Modifications & adjustments

If your bent knee comes high off the floor or you feel tension in that knee, support it with a bolster.

If tight hamstrings prevent you from holding on to your foot with a straight leg, you can lightly bend your knee and support it with a rolled-up blanket.

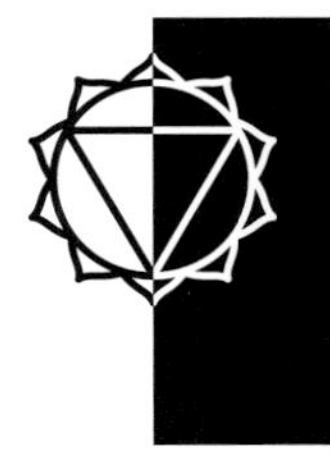

Marichyasana C
Pose Dedicated to Sage Marichi C

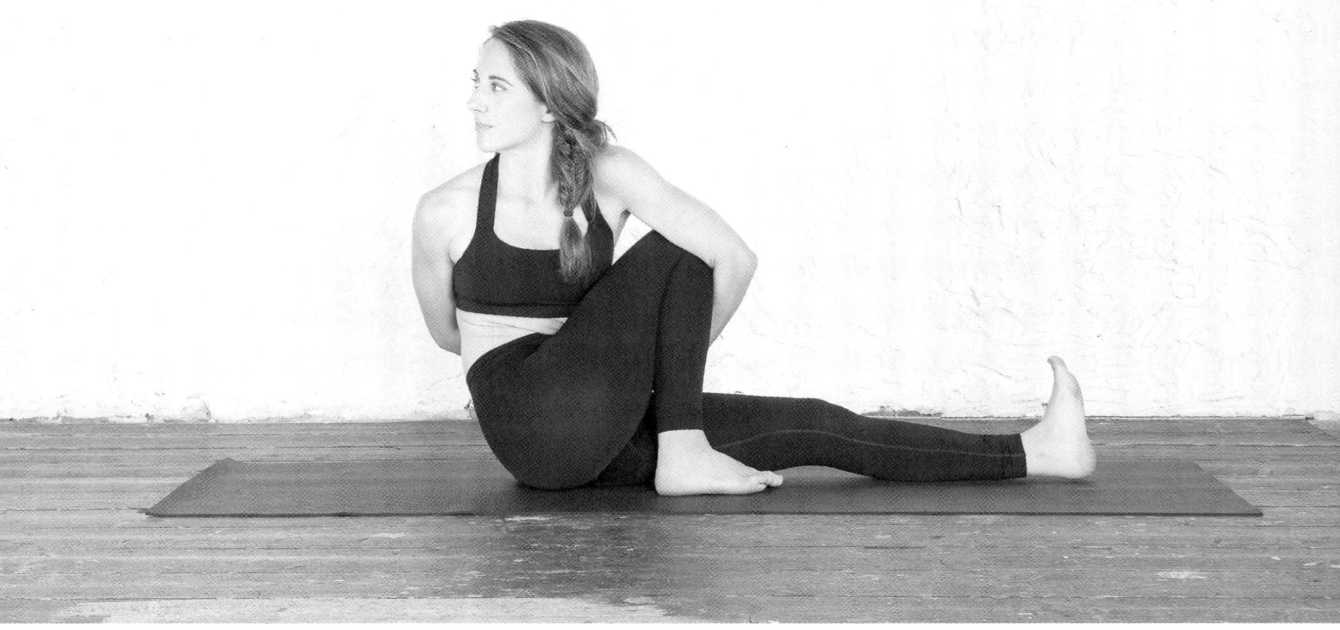

How to come into the pose

Sit with your legs straight in front of you, feet together.

Bend your right knee and place your right foot flat on the floor next to your left inner thigh.

Place your foot up as high as possible toward the buttock while keeping a distance of 1 foot-width between your right foot and left inner thigh.

Hug your right knee tightly to your chest and then shift your chest sideways toward your right.

Reach your left arm forward at the outside of your right knee and rotate it inward, so the thumb points to the floor and the palm faces out to your left.

As you reach your left arm forward, twist your torso to your right and aim to bring the outside of your right shin into your left armpit.

Then breathe out and sweep your left forearm around the outside of your right leg.

Your left hand will press against the outside of your left thigh or buttock.

On the next exhalation, sweep the right hand behind your back and clasp your hands or wrist.

Breathe in, lengthen your spine, and gaze over your right shoulder.

Breathe evenly, and gently move and relax further into the twist with every exhalation.

To release, gaze to the front and release the grip, then repeat the same on the other side.

Next pose

Rest in Child's Pose for 30–45 seconds, then continue with Easy Crow Pose or a variation thereof.

Alignment cues

Place the foot of the bent leg as high as possible, making sure you are still sitting firmly on your sitting bones.

Avoid sitting on your tailbone.

The extended leg is active. Focus on pushing out through your heel.

Be sure your shoulders do not scrunch up into your ears; draw your shoulder blades actively down your back.

Once your hands are firmly bound or braced against the floor, try pressing both hips into the floor and creating length in your spine.

Contraindications & cautions

The same contraindications and cautions apply as in Half Spinal Twist. Also be cautious in this pose if you have groin or hamstring issues.

Modifications & adjustments

If you cannot bind your hands behind your back, you can use a strap to bridge the gap (if it is a small gap). Otherwise, you can keep your right hand on the floor behind you and press your left elbow against the outer right knee and look over your right shoulder.

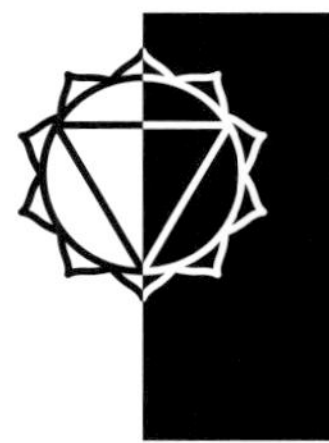

Variations

Marichyasana D

Pose Dedicated to Sage Marichi D

This pose is even more challenging, because the previously extended leg (in Sage Marichi's Pose C), is now folded into a Half Lotus position. Attempt this only if you can fold easily and without strain into Half Lotus Pose. Start seated, with your legs in front of you. Fold your left leg into Half Lotus Pose and then follow the instructions from the second step onwards, as described on the left.

Bharadvajasana
Pose Dedicated to Bharadvaja

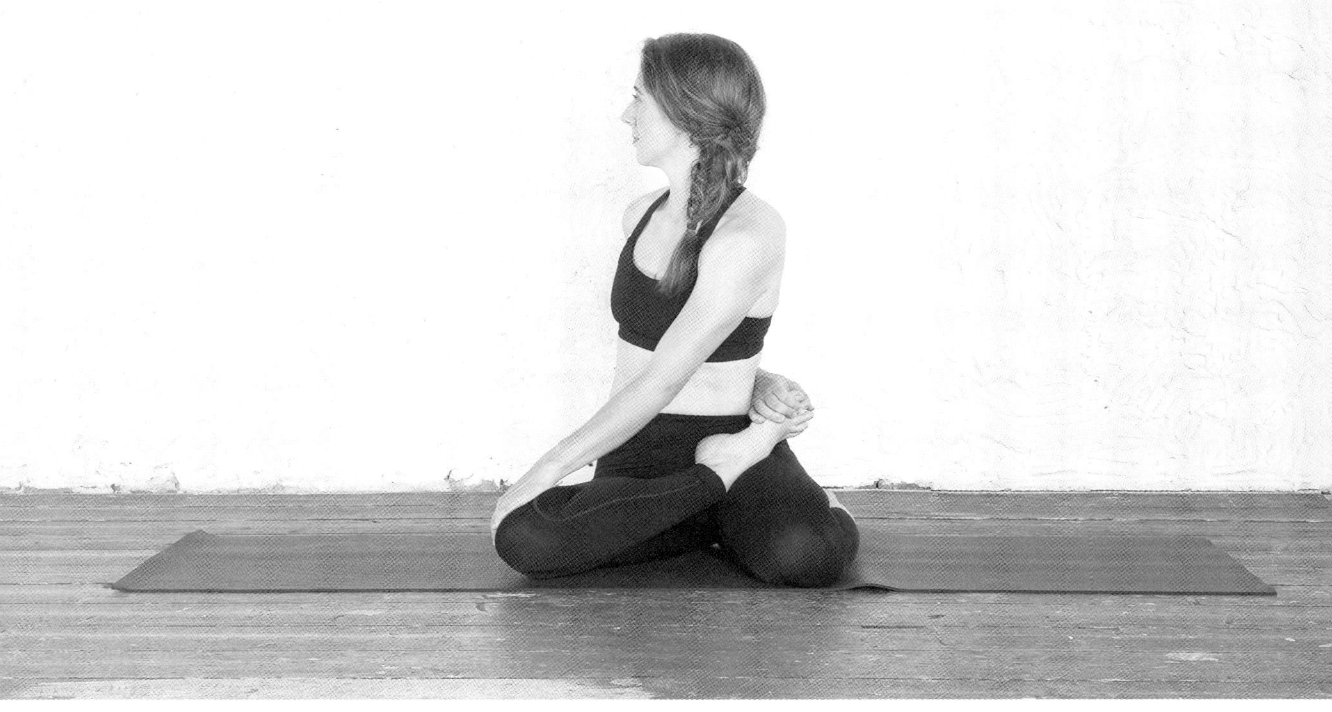

How to come into the pose

Begin seated on the floor, with your legs extended in front of you, arms resting at your sides.

Now fold your left leg into Hero Pose.

From here fold your right leg into Half Lotus position.

On an inhalation, lengthen your spine as long as you can and reach your right hand around your back to hold on to your lotus foot.

Exhaling, twist your upper torso to your right and place your left hand on top of your right knee or (for a deeper twist) below your right knee on the floor, with your fingertips pointing toward your left knee.

On each inhalation, lengthen your spine, and on each exhalation, twist more deeply.

Turn your head to gaze over your right shoulder.

Hold the pose steadily as long as comfortable and breathe evenly.

To release, breathe out and unwind your torso and legs.

Repeat the twist for the same length of time on the opposite side.

Next pose

Rest in Child's Pose for 30–45 seconds, then continue with Easy Crow Pose or a variation thereof.

Alignment cues

Both sitting bones are firmly pressed into the floor.

Both knees should be resting on or close to the floor.

If they are lifting up, you are most probably placing too much strain on them and should rather do the modified version, as described to the right.

If your left hip is lifting off the floor, place a folded, firm blanket beneath your right sitting bone to regain balance.

Draw your shoulder blades down your back and in toward your back ribs.

Avoid leaning forward or backward, but aim to twist around your spine from your tailbone to the crown of your head.

Contraindications & cautions

The same contraindications and cautions apply as in Half Spinal Twist. Also be cautious in this pose if you have tight hips or knee issues.

Modifications & adjustments

If you cannot fold into Half Lotus or Half Hero Pose easily and safely, from Diamond Pose simply shift your weight to your right buttock. Bend your knees and bring your legs to your left. Rest your legs on the floor, and place your left inner ankle in the arch of your right foot. Breathe in and lengthen your spine as long as you can. Breathe out, and twist your upper torso to your right. Place your right hand on the floor behind your body, and rest your left hand on your outer right thigh. Turn your left palm upward. Look over your right shoulder. On each inhalation, lengthen your spine, and on each exhalation, twist more deeply.

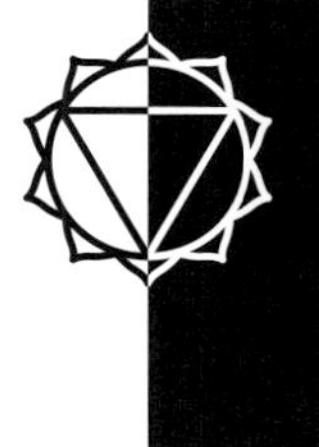

Jathara Parivartanasana
Abdominal Twist

How to come into the pose

Lie on your back, with your legs together and your arms at a 90-degree angle from your body, palms facing upward.

Lift your left knee to your chest and drop it to your right, until your left foot is resting on the floor.

Place your right hand on your left knee, look over your left shoulder, and with every breath focus on releasing your left knee toward the floor while pressing your left shoulder blade toward the floor.

Hold the pose steadily as long as comfortable and breathe evenly.

To come out of the pose, slide your left foot over the floor to join your right and allow your body to roll back into a supine position.

Then repeat on the other side.

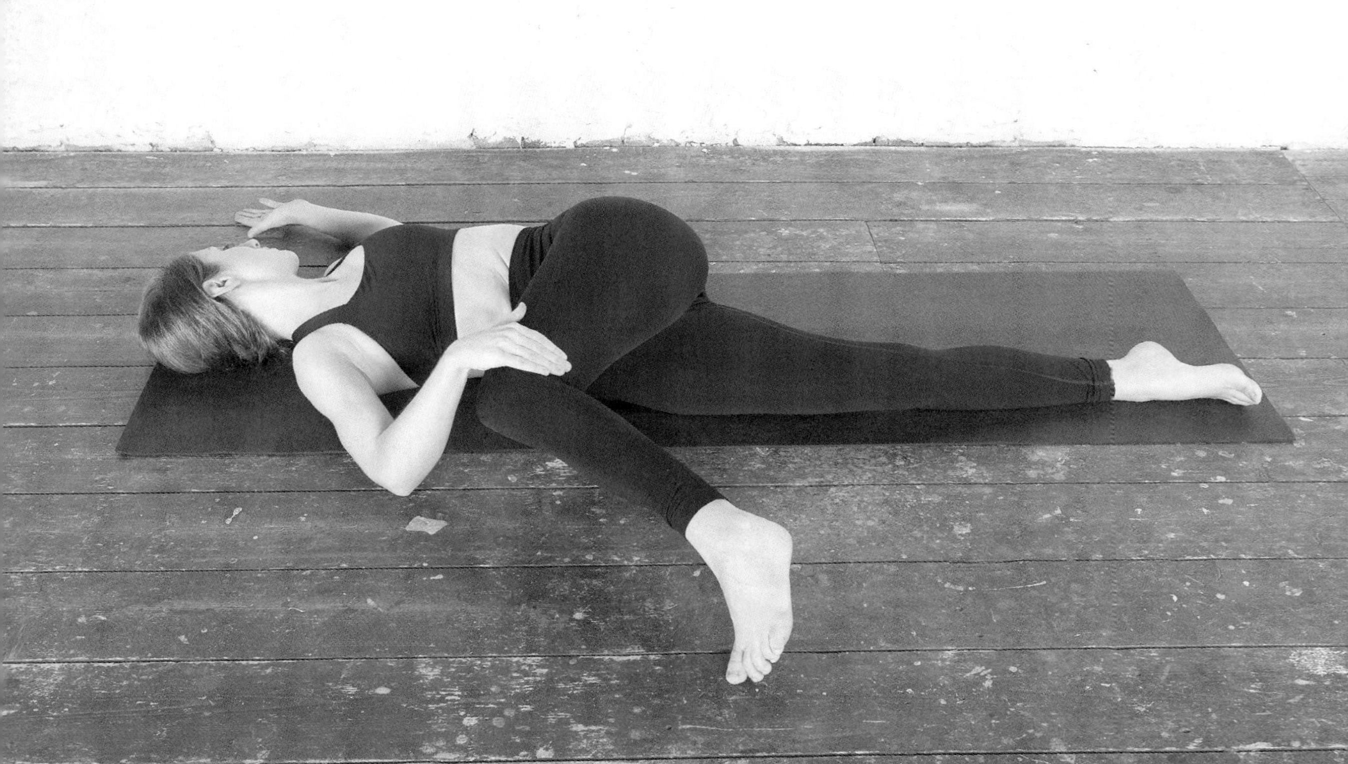

Next pose

Continue to Easy Crow Pose or a variation thereof.

Alignment cues

The entire spine is off the floor. Only the one side of the hip and the opposite shoulder blade should be firmly pressing into the floor to create opposition.

The knee of your upper leg should be at approximately hip level. Do not keep it too low, because then the stretch comes mainly to the buttocks rather than the back.

Make sure that the upper foot is resting on the floor, and keep the lower leg active and straight to create opposition.

Contraindications & cautions

This is quite a restorative and gentle pose in general. It is a good alternative for those for whom seated twists are not recommended.

Modifications & adjustments

To decrease the intensity of the twist, you can place a bolster or rolled-up blanket either under the shoulder that should remain on the floor or under the lower leg or knee.

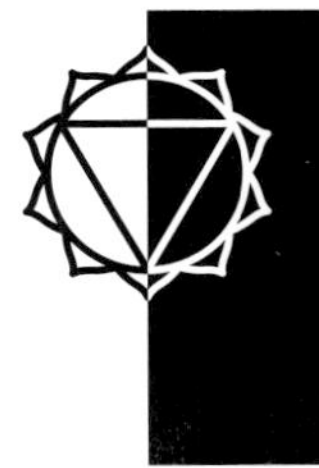

Variations

Jathara Parivartanasana II

Abdominal Twist II

Begin with the same starting position as described on the left, but with your knees lifted up toward your chest. Now gently lower both legs toward your left and let them rest on the floor. Look over your right shoulder and press your right shoulder blade toward the floor.

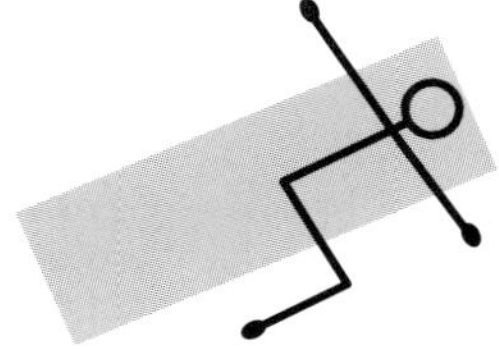

Chapter 16

Variations for the Sacral Chakra

Sukha Kakasana (Easy Crow Pose) Variations

Kakasana
Classical Crow Pose

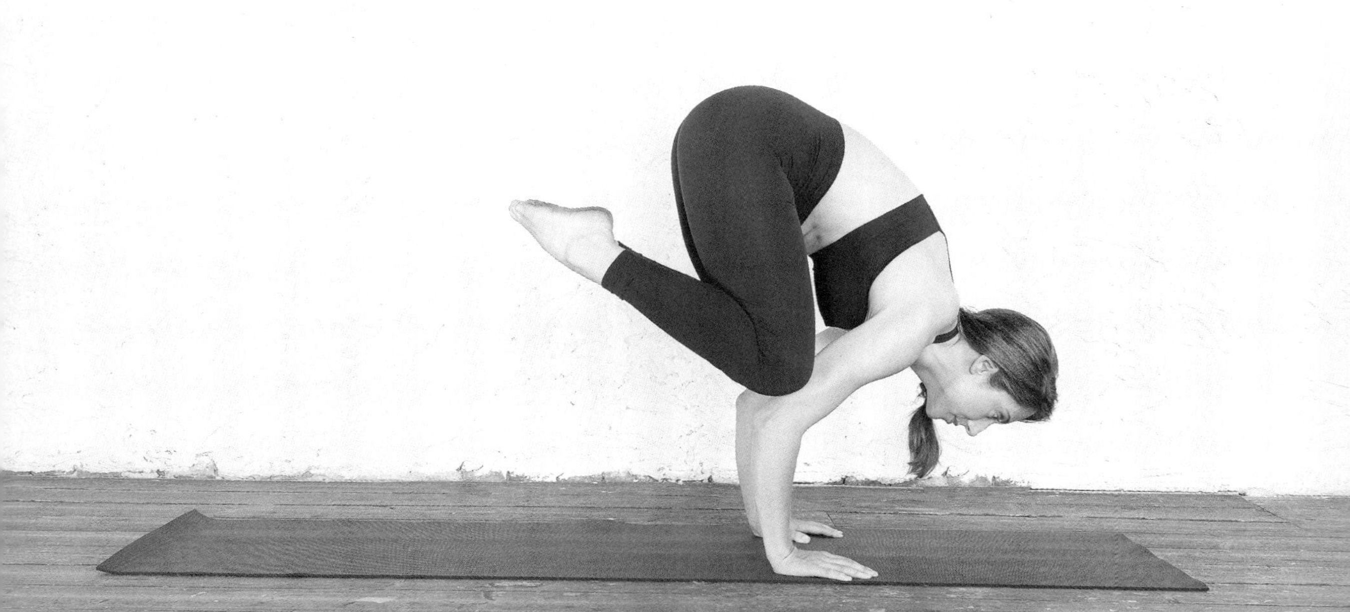

How to come into the pose

Stand on your mat, with your feet shoulder-width apart.

Bend forward, and as you do so, allow your knees to bend and place them against your upper arms, just above your elbows.

Maintaining the connection between your arms and knees, place your hands on the floor.

Look forward toward the floor in front of you and shift your weight onto your hands.

Lift your feet off the floor, one by one, and pull them up toward your hips.

If you are stable, press through your hands to straighten your arms as far as possible.

Hold the pose steadily as long as comfortable and breathe evenly.

Next pose

Rest in Child's Pose for 30–45 seconds, then continue to Triangle Pose or a variation thereof.

Alignment cues

Hands are parallel, fingers spread. Push the heels of your palms, your knuckles, and fingertips actively into the floor.

The back is rounded, the tailbone tucked in.

Keep the heels tucked in toward your buttocks, with your big toes toward each other.

Keep your head in a neutral position, looking at the floor in front of you. You can also lift your head slightly (making sure not to compress the back of your neck) and look forward.

Contraindications & cautions

The same contraindications and cautions apply as in Easy Crow Pose.

Modifications & Adjustments

If you feel tension in your wrists, you can place the heels of your hands on a folded blanket to relieve pressure.

If, initially, balancing is challenging, you can press your forehead against a cushion on the floor to practice the weight shift.

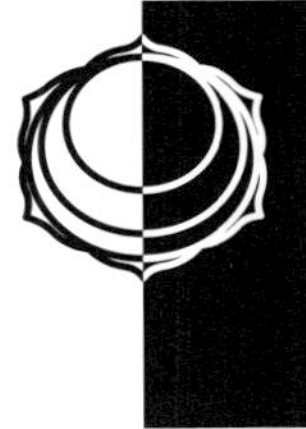

Bakasana
Crane Pose

How to come into the pose

Stand on your mat, with your feet shoulder-width apart.

Squat halfway down, allowing your knees to open shoulder-width apart and focus on keeping your lifted heels toward each other.

Then bend forward and place your knees as high up against your upper arms as comfortable, or in your armpits if possible.

Keep the connection between your arms and knees, and then place your hands on the floor.

Look forward to the floor in front of you and shift your weight to your hands.

Lift your feet off the floor, one by one, and pull them up toward your hips.

If you are stable, press through your hands to straighten your arms as far as possible.

Hold the pose steadily as long as is comfortable and breathe evenly.

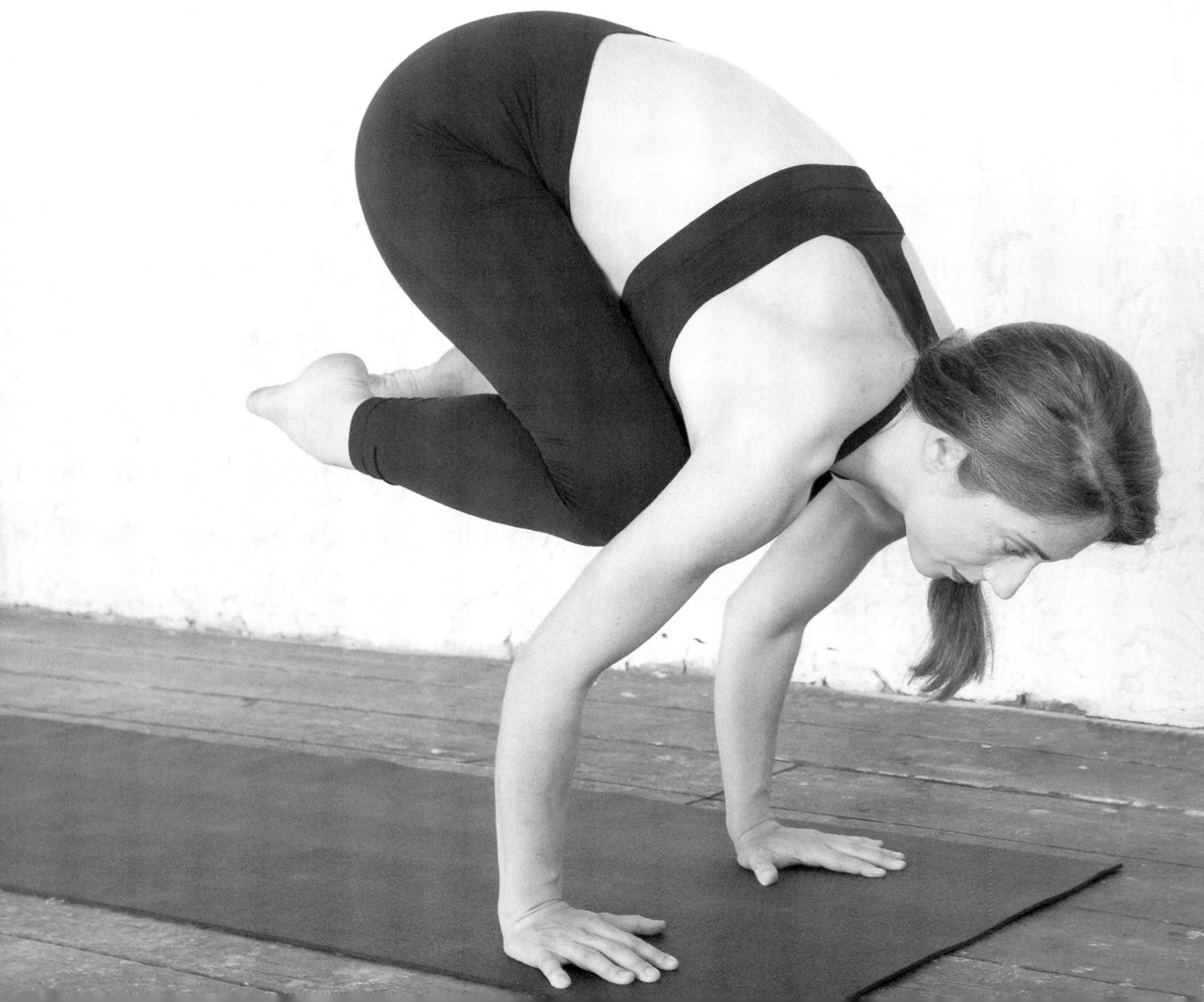

Next pose

Rest in Child's Pose for 30–45 seconds, then continue to Triangle Pose or a variation thereof.

Alignment cues

Hands are parallel, fingers spread. Push the heels of your palms, your knuckles, and fingertips actively down into the floor and try to straighten your arms as much as possible.

The back is rounded, the tailbone tucked in.

Keep the heels tucked in toward your buttocks, with your big toes toward each other.

Seen from the side, your shoulders are slightly in front of the wrists and arms are angled slightly forward.

The knees should be glued to the upper arms, high up near the armpits.

Keep your head in a neutral position, with your eyes looking at the floor in front of you. You can also lift your head slightly (making sure not to compress the back of your neck) and look forward.

Contraindications & cautions

The same contraindications and cautions apply as in Easy Crow Pose.

Modifications & Adjustments

If you feel pain in your wrists, you can place the heels of your hands on a folded blanket to relieve pressure.

If balancing on the balls of your feet is challenging as you set up for the pose, you can place a rolled blanket or a block underneath your heels.

If balancing is challenging initially, you can press your forehead against a cushion on the floor to practice the weight shift.

Variations

Eka Pada Bakasana A

One-Legged Crane Pose A

Start from Downward-Facing Dog Pose and walk your feet slightly closer to your hands. From here, lift your right leg up, bend your right knee, and place your right knee on top of your right elbow. Look forward and come up high on the toes of your left foot. Make sure to bend your arms, while pressing your elbows toward each other to create a strong platform. Lift your hips up and then gently hop or slide your left foot closer to you. Now, lean forward, engage your core, and lift your left foot off the mat. Lift your hips and your left foot up as high as you can and hold the pose for a few breaths.

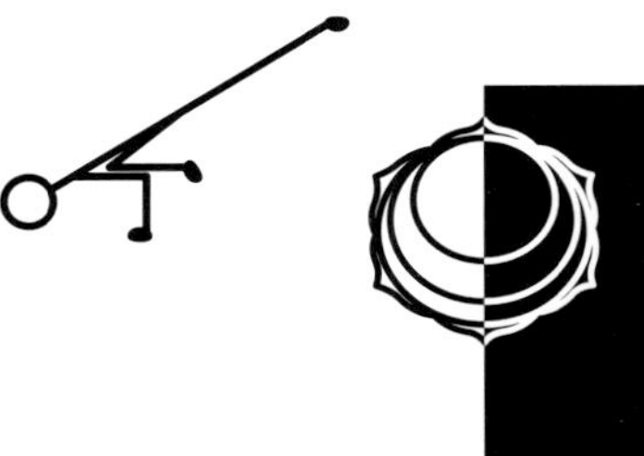

Eka Pada Bakasana B

One-Legged Crane Pose B

Come into a squatting position and place your right kneecap against your right armpit. Lift your hips up and walk your left leg forward in order to place your left shoulder underneath your left upper thigh. From there, bend your elbows and sit your hips back down. Lift your left foot off the floor. Now press through your hands, engaging your core, and lift your hips a bit higher. To properly align the position of your right leg, aim your right foot straight backward, as in Crane Pose.

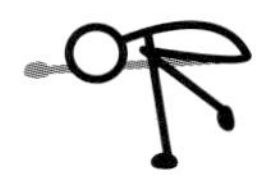

Parshva Kakasana
Twisted Crow Pose

How to come into the pose

Come into a squatting position, with your heels off the floor.

Keeping your knees and ankles together and your upper body straight, swivel your knees 90 degrees to your left.

Place your left upper arm (just above the elbow) against the outside of your right thigh, and your right upper arm (just above the elbow) to the side of your right hip, then place your hands on the floor.

Maintaining the connection between your elbows and your body, shift your weight to your hands.

Your right hip and knee should create a flat beam across the backs of both arms. Keep your knees together.

Press down through your right hip and lift both feet off the floor. Work toward bringing your feet and legs parallel to the floor.

Raise your chest and head to look forward toward the horizon.

Find your balance and hold the pose steadily as long as comfortable and breathe evenly.

Then release the pose and repeat the same on the other side.

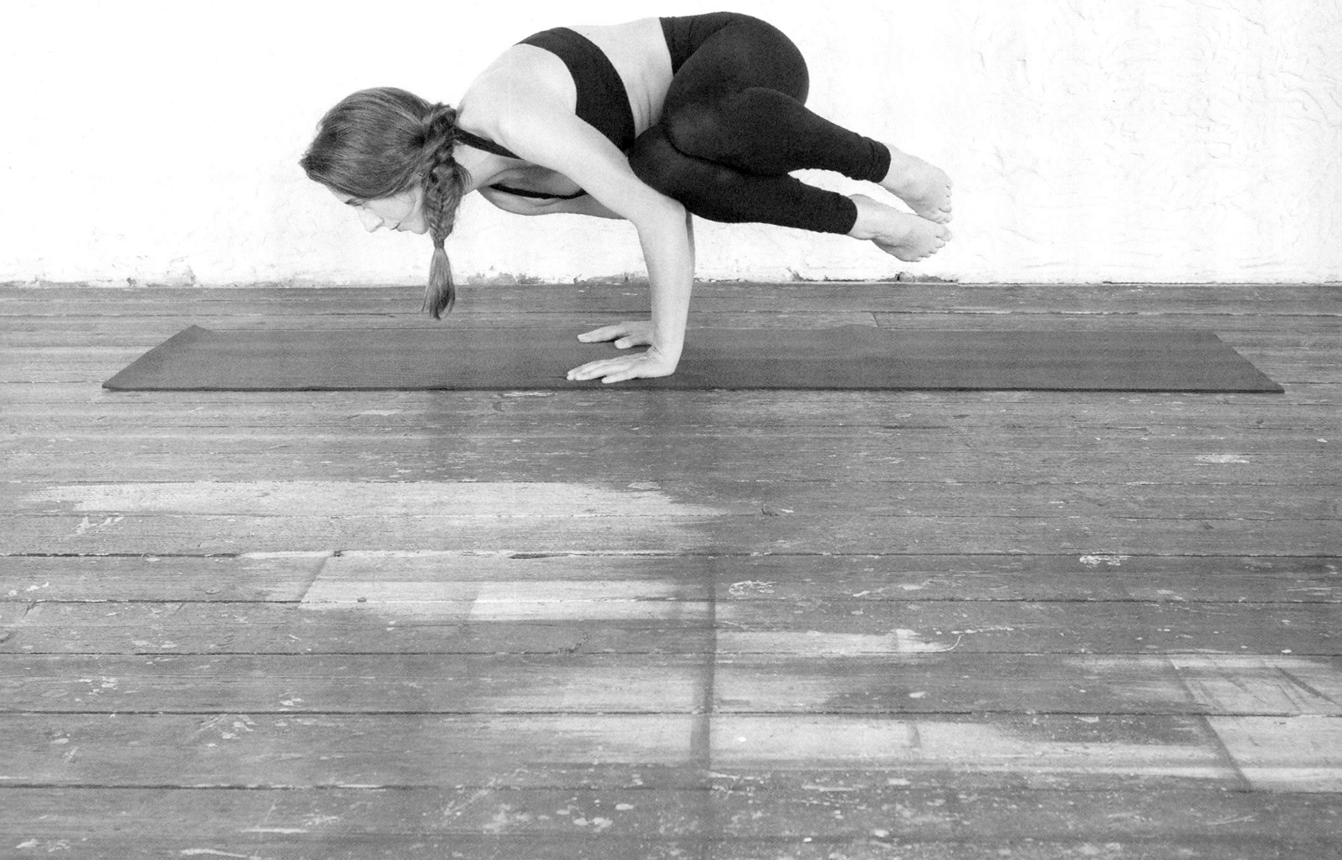

Next pose

Rest in Child's Pose for 30–45 seconds, then continue to Triangle Pose or a variation thereof.

Alignment cues

Arms are bent; your upper arms are almost parallel to the floor.

Hands are parallel, fingers spread and facing forward to the top of your mat. Push the root of your palms, your knuckles, and fingertips actively into the floor.

The lower thigh is resting on both upper arms.

Contraindications & cautions

The same contraindications and cautions apply as in Easy Crow Pose. Also be cautious in this pose if you have lower-back or spinal issues.

Modifications & Adjustments

If you feel tension in your wrists, you can place the heels of your hands on a folded blanket to relieve pressure.

If balancing is challenging initially, you can press the forehead against a cushion on the floor to practice the weight shift.

Variations

Parshva Kakasana I

Twisted Crow Pose I

Come into the pose as instructed on the left. Then, keeping the lower leg bent, extend the upper leg back and up.

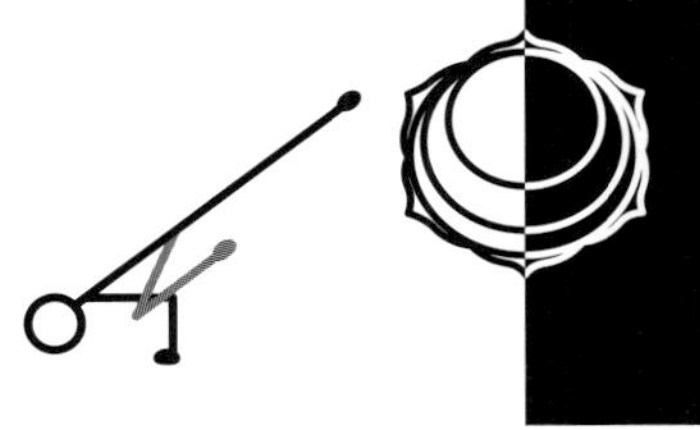

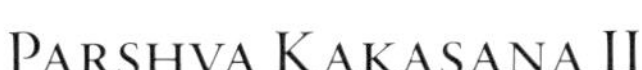

Parshva Kakasana II

Twisted Crow Pose II

Come into the pose as instructed on the left. Then, straighten the lower leg sideways and simultaneously extend the upper leg backward.

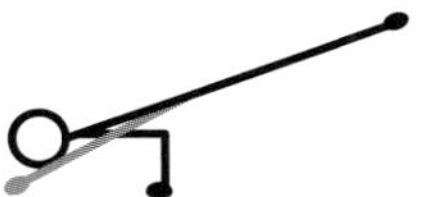

Dwi Pada Koundinyasana
Two-Legged Sage Koundinya Pose

How to come into the pose

Come into a squatting position, with your heels off the floor.

Keep your knees and ankles together, your upper body straight, and swivel your knees 90 degrees to your left.

Place your left upper arm (just above the elbow) against the outside of your right thigh, and then place your hands on the floor.

Maintaining your connection between your left upper arm and thigh, shift your weight forward toward your hands.

Lean forward and bend your elbows 90 degrees, so that your biceps are parallel to the floor and your forearms perpendicular. Your right hip and knee come parallel to the floor, knees together.

Now straighten your legs, keeping the inner edges of your feet close together.

Raise your chest and head to look forward toward the horizon.

Find your balance and breathe evenly. Then release the pose and repeat the same on the other side.

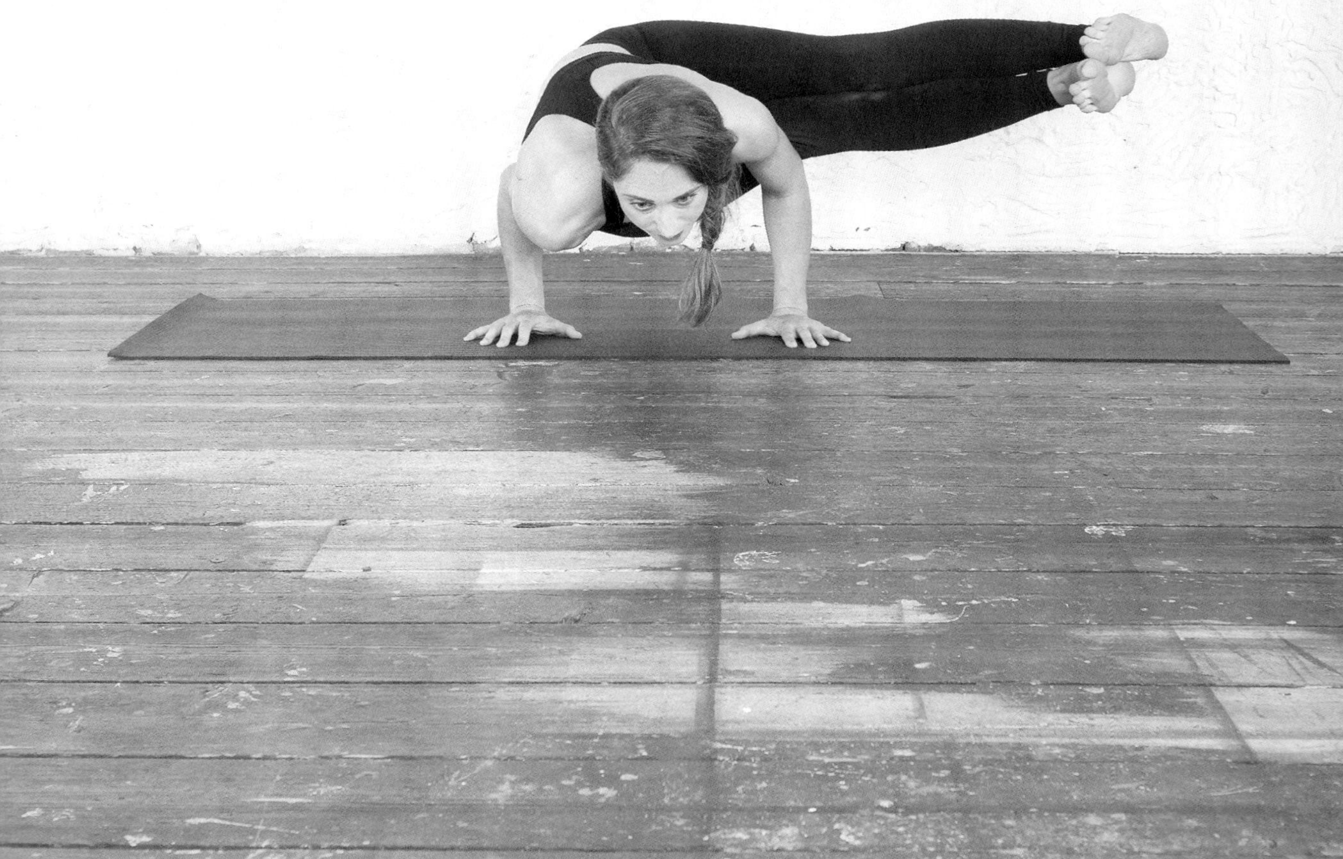

Next pose

Rest in Child's Pose for 30–45 seconds, then continue to Triangle Pose or a variation thereof.

Alignment cues

Hands are parallel, fingers spread and pointing forward. Push the heels of your palms and your knuckles and fingertips actively into the floor.

Arms are bent; your upper arms are almost parallel to the floor.

The legs are supported on one arm only, with the hips suspended between the arms. The opposite arm is free, but make sure to keep it hugged in toward you.

Make sure to keep the elbows over the wrists and let your shoulders drop down evenly in line with your elbows.

Activate your core and inner thighs to keep your legs straight and parallel to the floor.

Contraindications & cautions

The same contraindications and cautions apply as in Easy Crow Pose. Also be cautious in this pose if you have lower-back or spinal issues.

Modifications & Adjustments

If you feel tension in your wrists, you can place the heels of your hands on a folded blanket to relieve pressure.

If balancing is challenging initially, you can press your forehead against a cushion on the floor to practice the weight shift.

If straightening your legs is not accessible, keep them bent. This is often also taught as a version of Twisted Crow Pose.

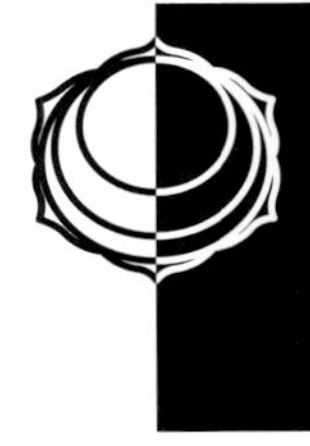

Mayurasana
Peacock Pose

How to come into the pose

Sit on your knees, with your hips on your heels.

Open your knees slightly wider than shoulder-width apart and bring your elbows to your lower abdomen.

Keep the connection between your elbows and abdomen and place your hands in between your knees, with your fingers pointing backward.

Allow your back to round, and place the top of your head on the floor.

Shift your weight toward your head and walk your feet as far back as possible; legs are straight and toes curled (pushing out through your heels). At this point, your abdomen might have slightly lifted off your elbows. That is no problem and will be corrected with the next step.

From here, lift your head off the floor and look forward. Let your abdomen rest steadily on your elbows and see if you can open your chest and lift your upper body just a little further away from the floor.

Then push with your toes and with control shift your weight forward until your legs come off the floor. Do not hop!

Hold the pose steadily as long as comfortable and breathe evenly.

To release the pose, place your feet and knees on the floor again and shift your hips toward your heels, then release the hands.

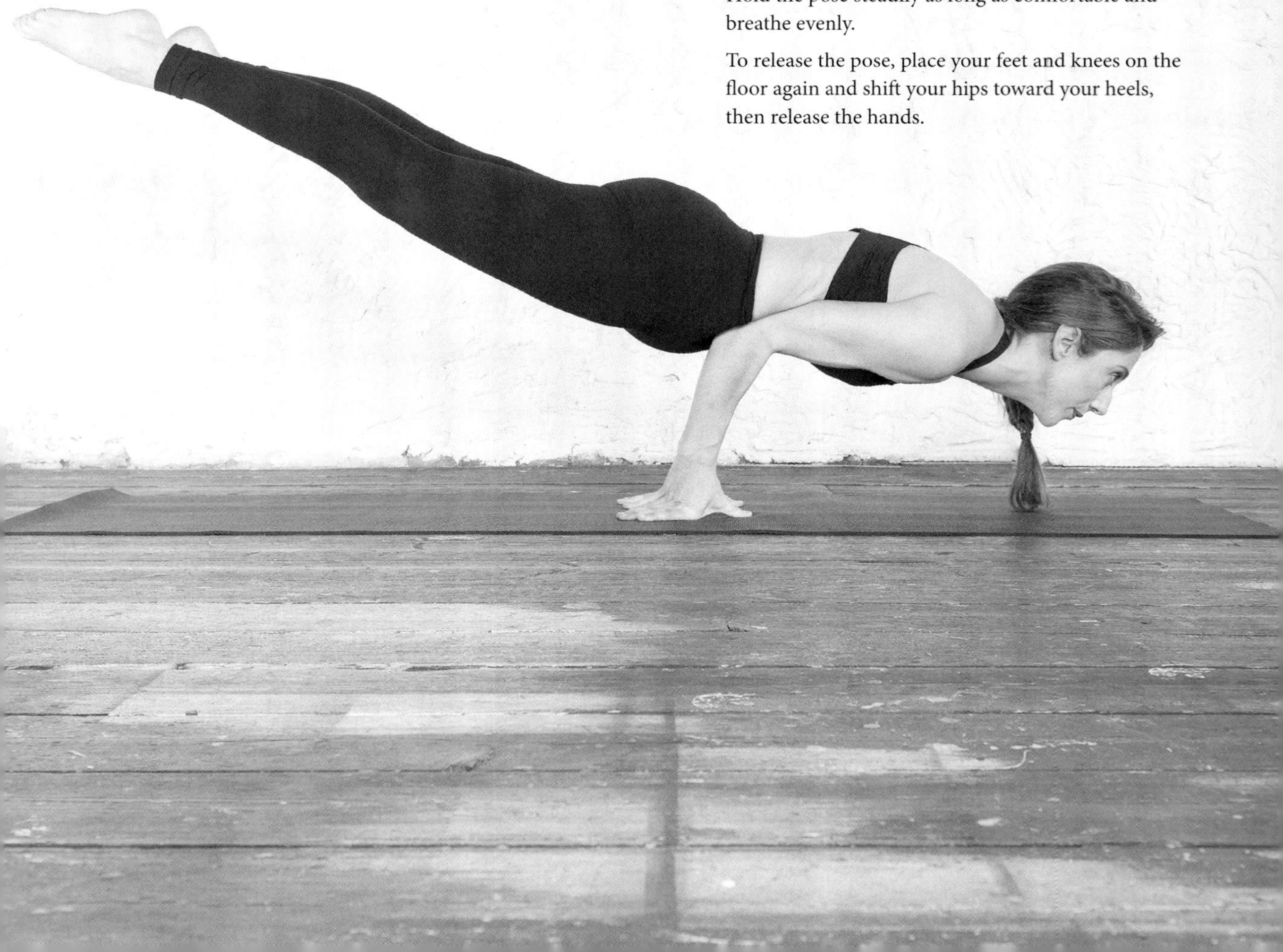

Next pose

Rest in Child's Pose for 30–45 seconds, then continue with Triangle Pose or a variation thereof.

Alignment cues

Focus on keeping your elbows together to keep them from slipping out. Your wrists can be slightly apart.

Avoid jumping your feet off the floor, but rather shift your weight forward until your feet gently come off the floor.

Think about lifting your chest off the floor, opening and leading with your sternum as you shift forward into the point of balance.

Contraindications & cautions

The same contraindications and cautions apply as in Easy Crow Pose. Also be cautious in this pose if you have any abdominal issues.

Modifications & Adjustments

According to your own preference, you can try out different hand positions (fingers pointing forward, fingers pointing sideways, making fists).

If you feel pain or tension in your wrists, you can place a folded blanket under the heels of your hands.

Variations

Ardha Mayurasana

Half Peacock Pose

Half Peacock Pose is a slightly easier version of the full pose, because you have the support of the chin. Follow the first six steps as described on the left. Then, instead of keeping your head off the floor, place your chin on the floor as you shift your weight forward. Firmly press it into the floor and lift your legs up toward the ceiling.

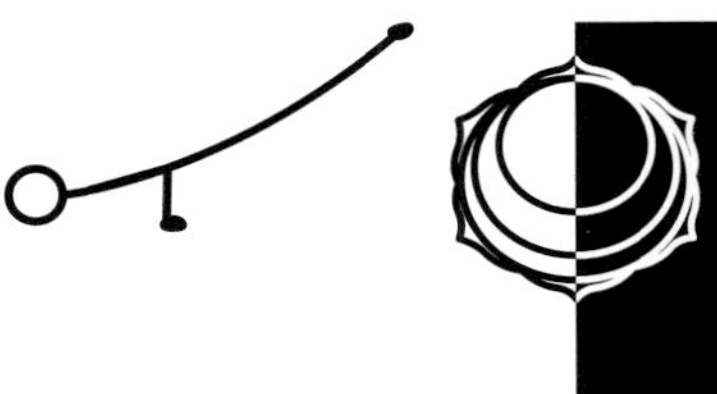

Padma Mayurasana

Lotus Peacock Pose

If Lotus Position is comfortable and easy, this pose actually is also easier than the version described on the left, because your body is more compact. Fold your legs into the Lotus Position and then come up on your knees. Then place your hands in front of you on the floor (wrists slightly apart, elbows together), placing your elbows against the upper abdomen, and then follow the further steps as described on the left.

Eka Pada Koundinyasana
One-Legged Sage Koundinya Pose

How to come into the pose

Come into Downward-Facing Dog Pose, but with your heels actively lifted and your core engaged.

As you shift your weight toward your hands, lift your left leg and bring your knee to the top of your left upper arm.

Keep shifting your weight forward and bend both arms. Hug your right elbow in and support your right lower abdomen on it.

Straighten out your left leg and then gently push off from your right leg, shifting your weight forward until your right foot also lifts off the floor.

Look forward to a spot approximately half a meter in front of you on the floor.

Hold the pose steadily as long as comfortable and breathe evenly.

To release the pose, place your right foot back on the floor, and step back into Downward-Facing Dog Pose. Then proceed to the other side.

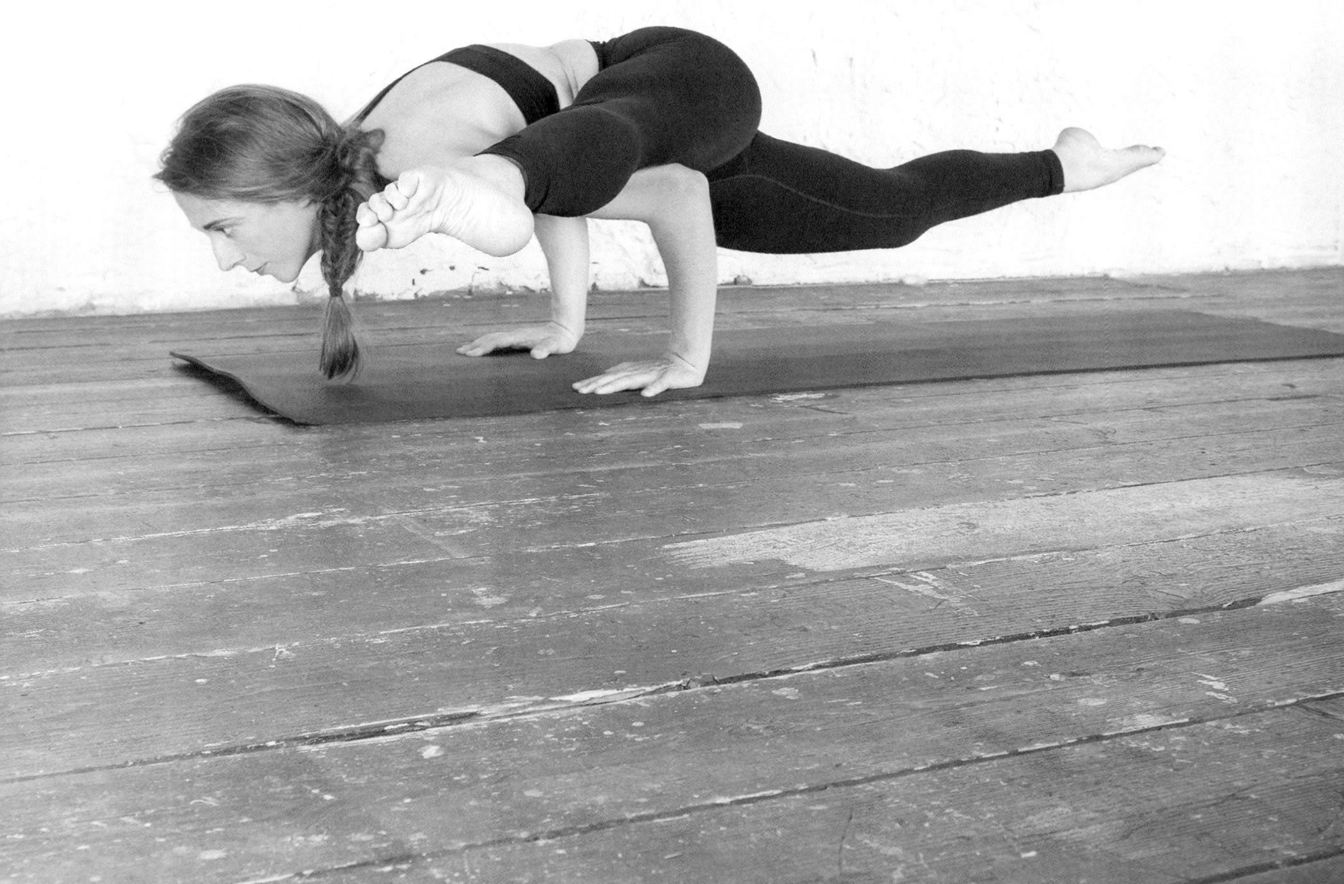

Next pose

Rest in Child's Pose for 30–45 seconds, then continue with Triangle Pose or a variation thereof.

Alignment cues

Hands are parallel, fingers spread. Push the heels of your palms and your knuckles and fingertips actively into the floor.

Upper arms are parallel to each other and to the floor, fingertips pointing forward.

Keep your chest open, collarbones wide, and shoulder blades drawn away from your ears.

Keep the fronts of your shoulders lifted, level, and not dipping below your elbows.

Contraindications & cautions

The same contraindications and cautions apply as in Easy Crow Pose. Also be cautious in this pose if you have any abdominal issues.

Modifications & Adjustments

If you feel tension in your wrists, you can place the heels of your hands on a folded blanket to relieve pressure.

If balancing is challenging initially, you can press your forehead against a cushion on the floor to practice the weight shift.

You can do this pose even if you have tight hamstrings. In this case, keep the forward-reaching leg slightly bent.

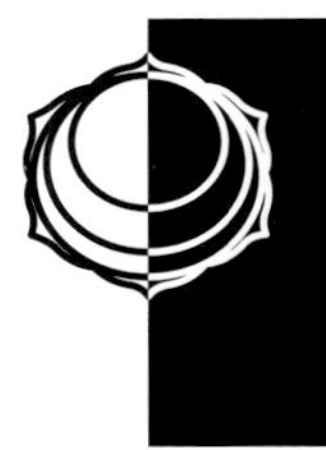

Ashtavakrasana
Eight-Angle Pose

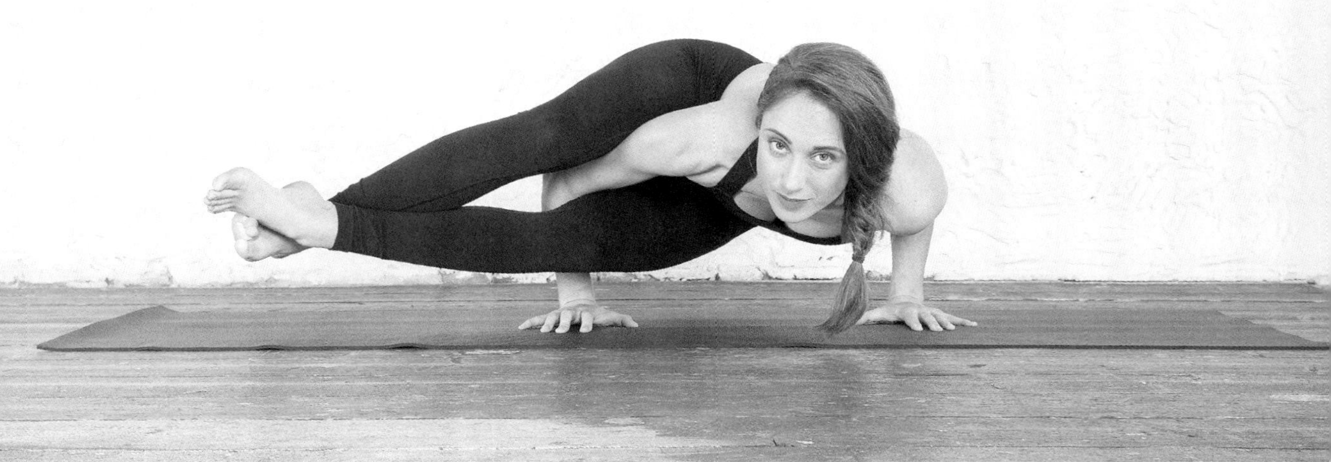

How to come into the pose

Start in a seated position, with your legs straight in front of you.

Bend your right knee inward toward your chest, then bring your right arm to the inside of your bent right leg.

Take hold of your right foot or ankle with your left hand and begin to bring the underside of your right knee in closely behind your right shoulder. Hook your right leg as firmly behind your right shoulder as you can.

Place your palms down on either side of your hips. Spread your fingers wide, keeping your chest lifted and your collarbone as broad as you can.

Maintaining the hug of your right leg around the shoulder and your palms planted on the floor, pick up your left leg and lightly cross your left ankle over your right.

Start to push your legs downward toward the floor so that your hips lift off the floor. Squeeze your legs firmly and extend them as straight as you can.

Now start to bend your elbows to about 90 degrees and lean your upper body forward. Press your left elbow in toward your waist and at the same time move your legs out to your right.

Hold the pose steadily as long as comfortable and breathe evenly.

To release the pose, place your feet and knees on the floor again and shift your hips toward your heels, then release the hands.

Next pose

Rest in Child's Pose for 30–45 seconds, then continue with Triangle Pose or a variation thereof.

Alignment cues

Hands are parallel, fingers spread. Push the heels of your palms, your knuckles, and fingertips actively into the floor.

Keep the tops of both shoulders lifted and level with one another.

Keep your gaze lifted slightly forward, without straining your neck.

Contraindications & cautions

The same contraindications and cautions apply as in Easy Crow Pose.

Modifications & Adjustments

If you feel tension in your wrists, you can place the heels of your hands on a folded blanket to relieve pressure.

If balancing is challenging initially, you can press your forehead against a cushion on the floor to practice the weight shift.

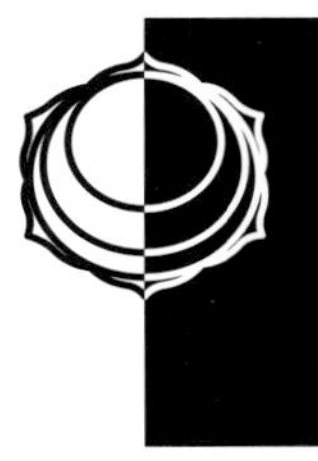

Eka Pada Galavasana
Flying-Pigeon Pose

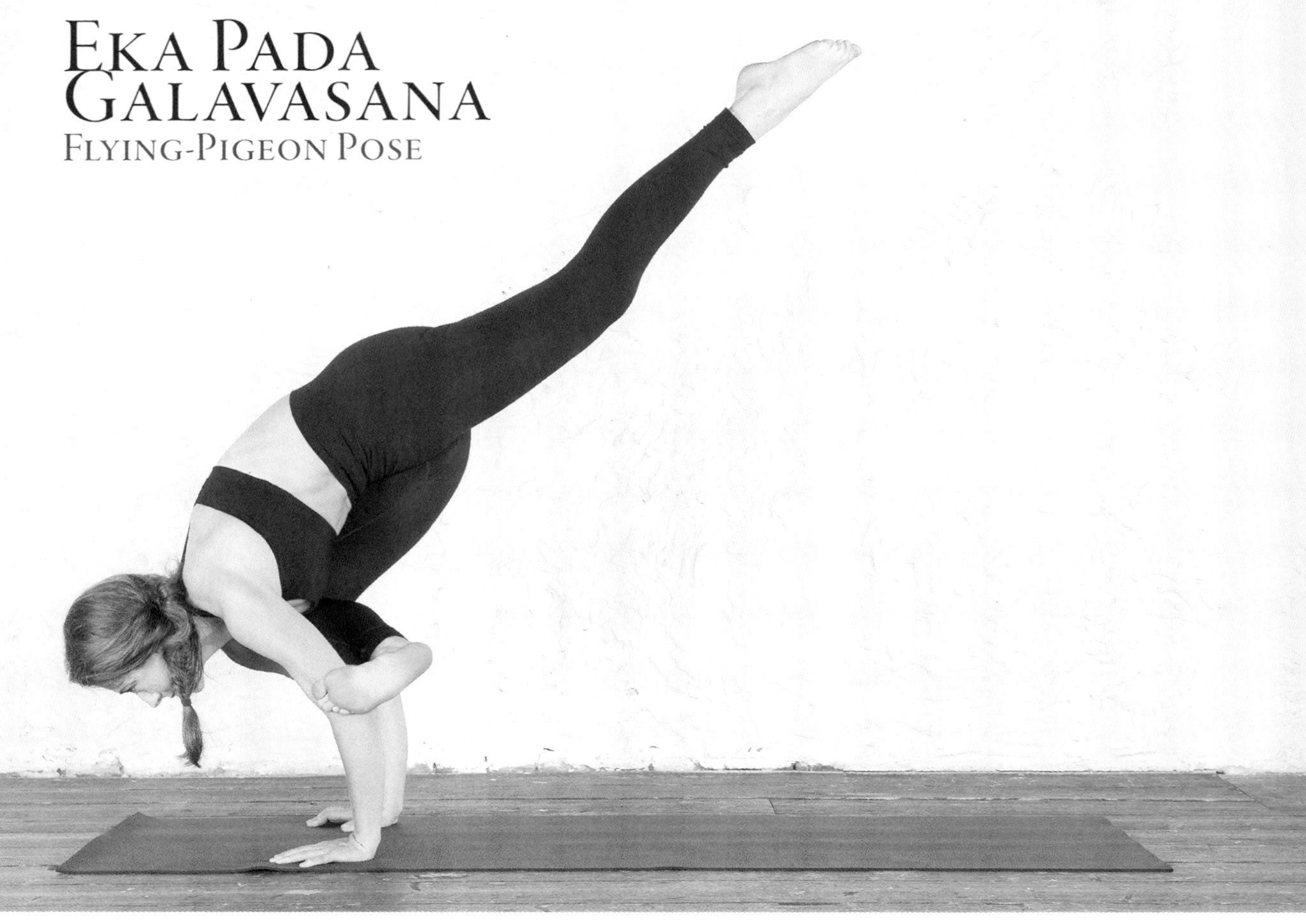

How to come into the pose

Stand on your mat, with your feet hip-width apart.

Place your right outer ankle on top of your left knee; your foot is flexed.

Bend your standing knee, lengthen your spine, and reach your arms toward the ceiling.

Fold forward and place both hands on the floor, in front of your shoulders. Lower your hips and draw your chest forward until your right knee connects to your right upper arm.

Lean forward slightly and wrap your right foot around the outside of your left triceps. Flex your foot strongly so that the top of your foot grips your outer arm.

Continue to shift forward, pushing your right knee against your right upper arm and bending your elbows until they are approaching a 90-degree angle. As you do so, lift your left leg back and upward.

Hold the pose steadily as long as comfortable and breathe evenly.

Then release the pose and repeat the same on the other side.

Next pose

Rest in Child's Pose for 30–45 seconds, then continue with Triangle Pose or a variation thereof.

Alignment cues

Engage your hamstrings and glutes to help lift, and keep your back leg up.

Press the floor away from you, draw your chest forward, and look forward to a point around half a meter in front of your fingertips.

Feel the opposition between your bent knee pressing into your upper arm and your extended foot reaching out and back.

Hands are parallel, fingers spread. Push the heels of your palms and your knuckles and fingertips actively into the floor.

Contraindications & cautions

The same contraindications and cautions apply as in Easy Crow Pose. Also be cautious in this pose if you have tight hips or knee issues.

Modifications & adjustments

If you feel tension in your wrists, you can place the heels of your hands on a folded blanket to relieve pressure.

This pose requires a considerable amount of hip rotation. If you feel strain in your front knee, do not proceed further.

The last step of straightening out the leg is the most challenging. Initially you can work on finding the balance with the back knee bent.

If initially balancing is challenging, you can press your forehead against a cushion on the floor to practice the weight shift.

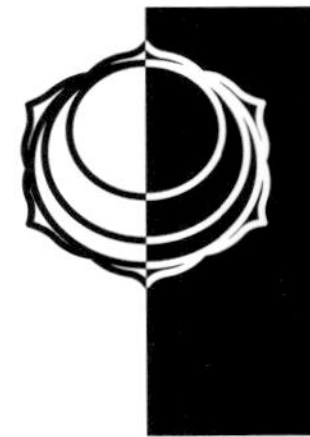

BHUJAPIDASANA
SHOULDER-PRESSING POSE

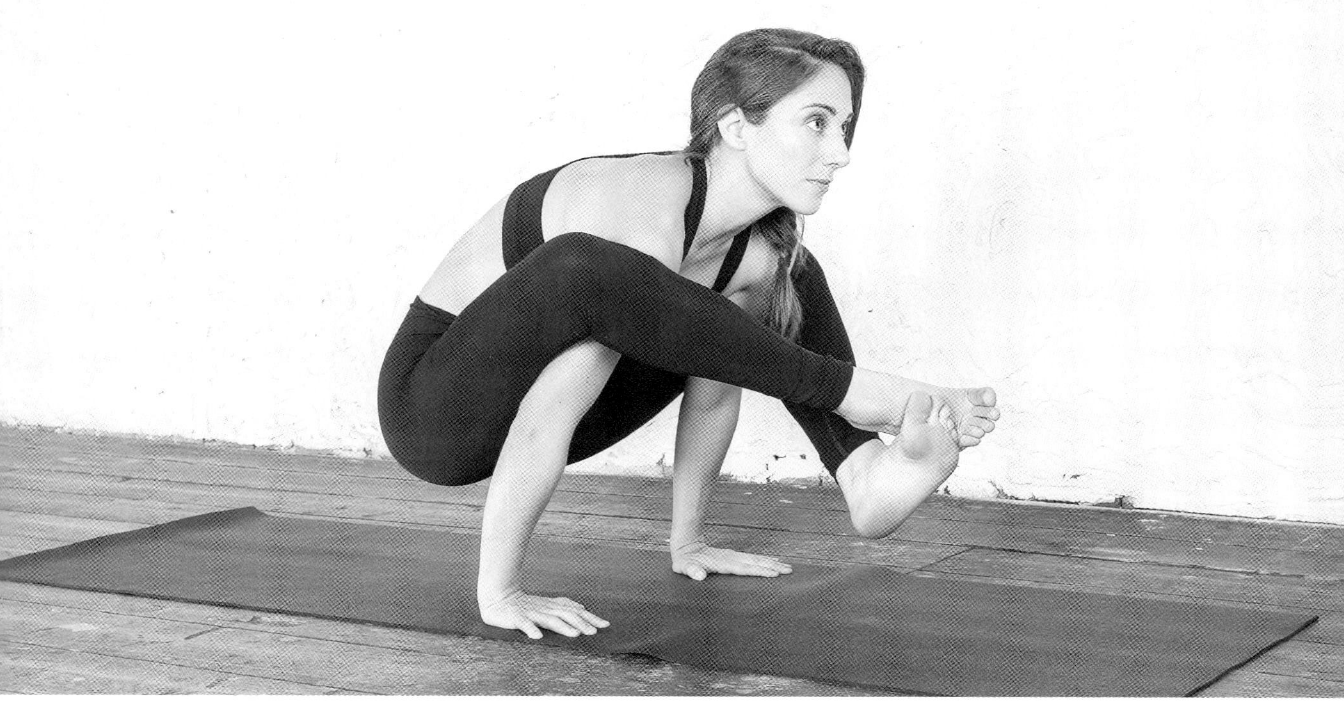

HOW TO COME INTO THE POSE

Squat, with your feet a little more than shoulder-width apart, knees wide.

Tilt your torso forward between your inner thighs. Then, keeping your torso low, raise your hips until your thighs become almost parallel to the floor.

Press your left upper arm and shoulder as closely as possible under the back of your left thigh, just above your knee, and place your left hand on the floor behind and just a little toward the outside of your left heel, fingers pointing forward.

Do the same on your right, then press your hands firmly against the floor and slowly begin to shift your weight backward.

Start to wiggle or walk your feet toward each other over the floor, and cross your right ankle over your left. As you continue to shift your weight backward, your feet will come off the floor.

Squeeze your outer arms with your inner thighs and look straight ahead.

Hold the pose steadily as long as is comfortable and breathe evenly.

Repeat the pose a second time with your left ankle on top.

Next pose

Rest in Child's Pose for 30–45 seconds, then continue with Triangle Pose or a variation thereof.

Alignment cues

Arms are slightly bent, fingers pointing forward.

Push the heels of your palms and your knuckles and fingertips actively into the floor.

Bring your awareness to where your upper arms and inner thighs touch. Squeeze your thighs in against your arms, while simultaneously pressing your arms out against your thighs.

Keep your hips lifted by engaging the pelvic floor and lower abdominals.

Keep your collarbones broad and shoulder blades drawn down toward your waist.

Contraindications & cautions

The same contraindications and cautions apply as in Easy Crow Pose. Also be cautious in this pose if you have lower-back or spinal issues.

Modifications & Adjustments

If you feel tension in your wrists, you can place the heels of your hands on a folded blanket to relieve pressure.

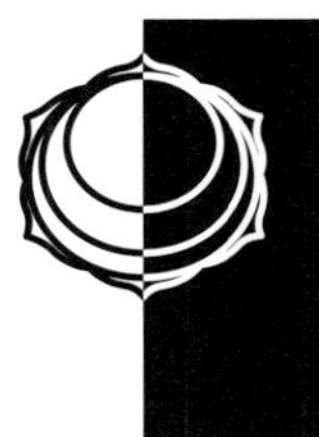

Variations

Bhujapidasana B

Shoulder-Pressing Pose B

Starting in classical Shoulder-Pressing Pose as explained on the left, breathe out, and move your shoulders forward, aiming your chin toward the floor. Keep lifting and engaging to avoid tumbling or dumping your weight forward. Slowly shift into the strength of your shoulders. Keep your feet lifted off the floor as they slide back behind the plane of your wrists. Hover your chin just above the floor and hold for a few breaths. Then slide your chest forward and upward to return to the starting position.

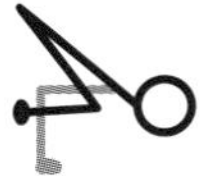

Tittibhasana
Firefly Pose

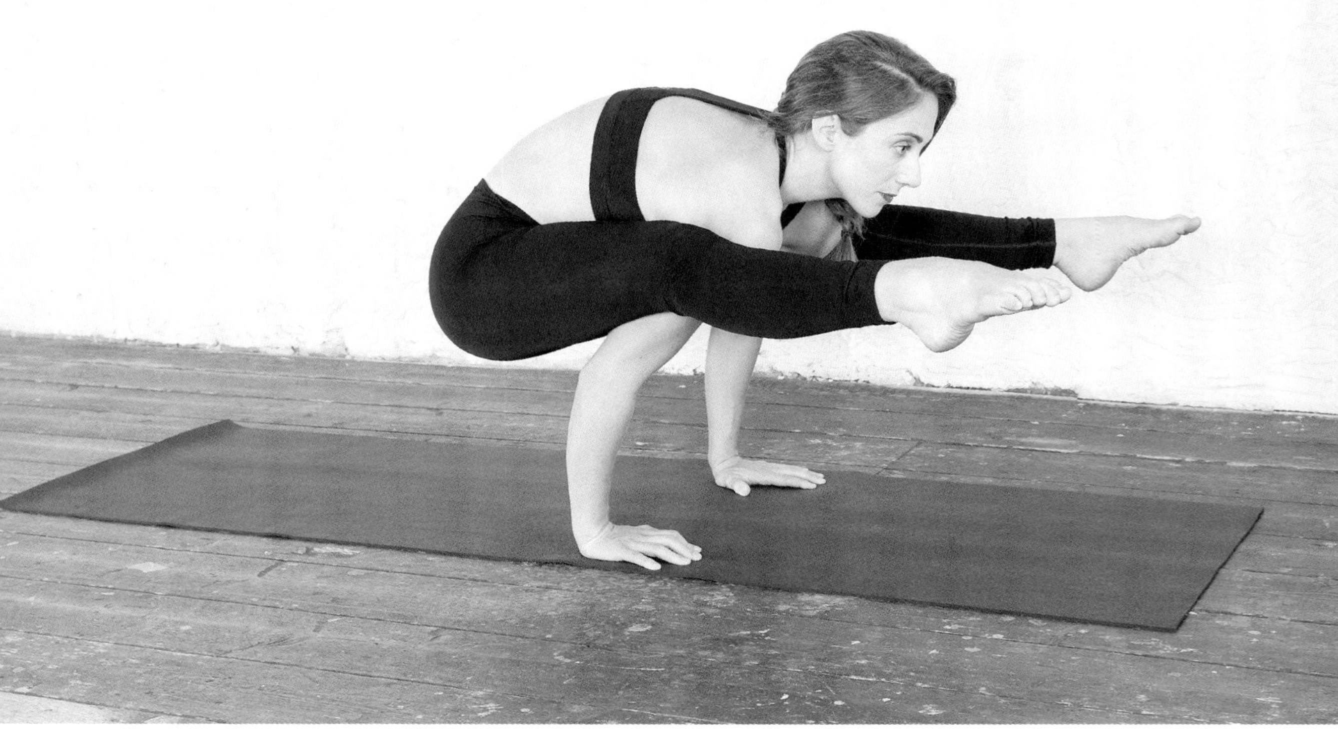

How to come into the pose

Stand on your mat, with your feet a little wider than your shoulders, and rotate your feet slightly outward.

Bend forward and tuck your shoulders behind your knees.

Place your hands behind your heels, with your fingers pointing forward.

Bend your knees and your elbows, sitting back so the weight of your pelvis comes onto your arms.

Squeeze your inner thighs against your outer arms, lift your feet, and straighten your legs. Focus on reaching your legs forward, parallel to the ground and look straight ahead.

Hold the pose steadily as long as comfortable and breathe evenly.

Next pose

Rest in Child's Pose for 30–45 seconds, then continue with Triangle Pose or a variation thereof.

Alignment cues

Arms are slightly bent, fingers pointing forward.

Push the heels of your palms and your knuckles and fingertips actively down into the floor.

Bring your awareness to where the upper arms and inner thighs touch. Squeeze your thighs in against your arms, while simultaneously pressing your arms out against your thighs.

Keep your hips lifted by engaging your pelvic floor and lower abdominals.

Focus on opening up your chest and keeping your collarbones broad and shoulder blades drawn down toward your waist.

Contraindications & cautions

The same contraindications and cautions apply as in Easy Crow Pose. Also be cautious in this pose if you have tight hamstrings or lower-back or spinal issues.

Modifications & Adjustments

If you feel tension in your wrists, you can place the heels of your hands on a folded blanket to relieve pressure.

If hamstrings are tight, you can keep your knees slightly bent.

Be careful of your back when you straighten your legs, making sure to respect your limits.

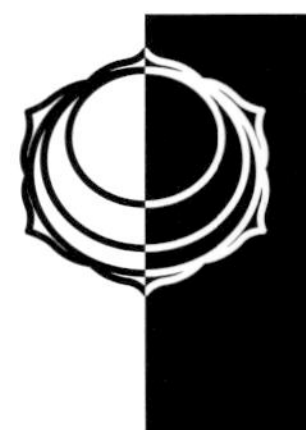

Variations

Utthita Tittibhasana

Lifted Firefly Pose

This variation of the Firefly Pose is quite challenging and requires truly flexible hamstrings and back as well as a strong core. Start by coming into Firefly Pose as explained on the left, with your legs parallel to the floor and your hips lifted. From here, engage your core and start to lower your hips toward the floor, while extending your arms and reaching with your feet upward. Your hips are hovering over the floor, your chest is lifted, and your gaze is straight ahead or diagonally upward.

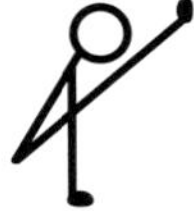

Maksikanagasana
Grasshopper Pose

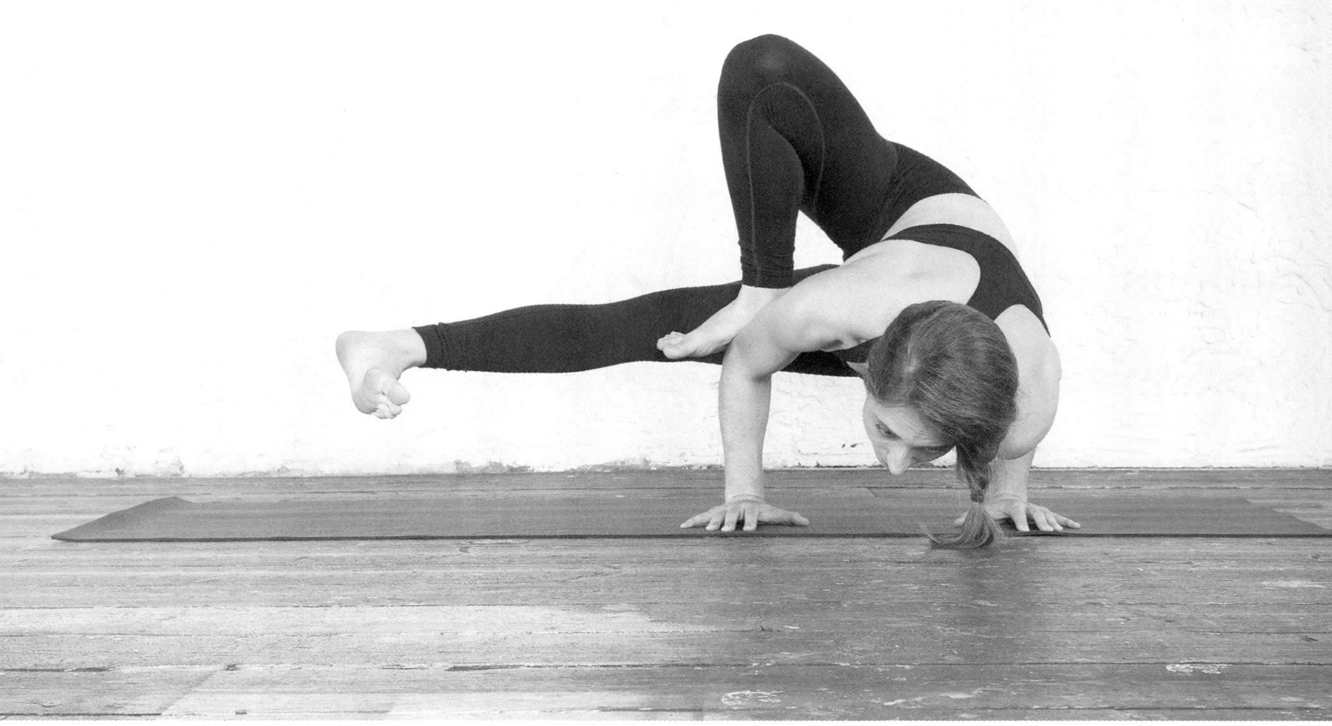

How to come into the pose

Come into a standing position.

Shift your weight to your left leg and cross your right ankle above your left knee so that your right shin is parallel to the floor.

Bend your left knee to about a 90-degree angle, as if you were sitting in a chair, and twist your upper body toward your left.

Place the arch of your right foot as close as possible to your right armpit, or at least on the mid-upper arm. Lower both palms to the floor, fingertips pointing forward.

Slightly lift your hips and shift your weight toward your hands. Your right arm supports your right foot. At the same time, extend your left leg parallel to the floor, pushing out through the heel.

Look at a point on the floor slightly in front of you and breathe evenly. After releasing the pose, repeat on the other side.

Next pose

Rest in Child's Pose for 30–45 seconds, then continue with Triangle Pose or a variation thereof.

Alignment cues

Elbows are bent at approximately a 90-degree angle.

Fingers are pointing forward. Make sure to push the heels of your palms, and your knuckles and fingertips, actively into the floor.

Keep your collarbones broad and shoulder blades drawn down toward your waist.

Firmly press the sole of your foot against your upper arm and at the same time push out through the heel of the extended leg.

Contraindications & cautions

The same contraindications and cautions apply as in Easy Crow Pose. Also be cautious in this pose if you have tight hips or knee issues.

Modifications & adjustments

You can also enter the pose from Tip Toe Pose, with one ankle crossed over the opposite knee. This is ideal if you are afraid of toppling over or falling on your nose when starting from a standing position.

If you feel tension in your wrists, you can place the heels of your hands on a folded blanket to relieve pressure.

If initially balancing is challenging, you can press your forehead against a cushion on the floor to practice the weight shift.

This pose requires quite some external rotation in the hip of the bent leg. If you feel strain in your knee or your foot keeps slipping off the arm, back off and work toward more hip opening before attempting the pose again.

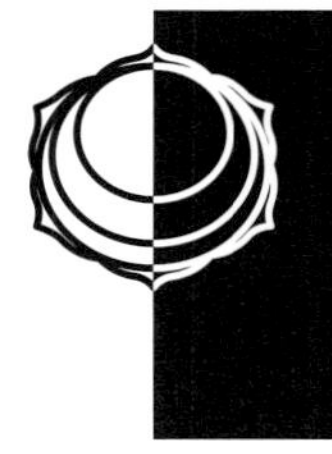

Tolasana
Scale Pose

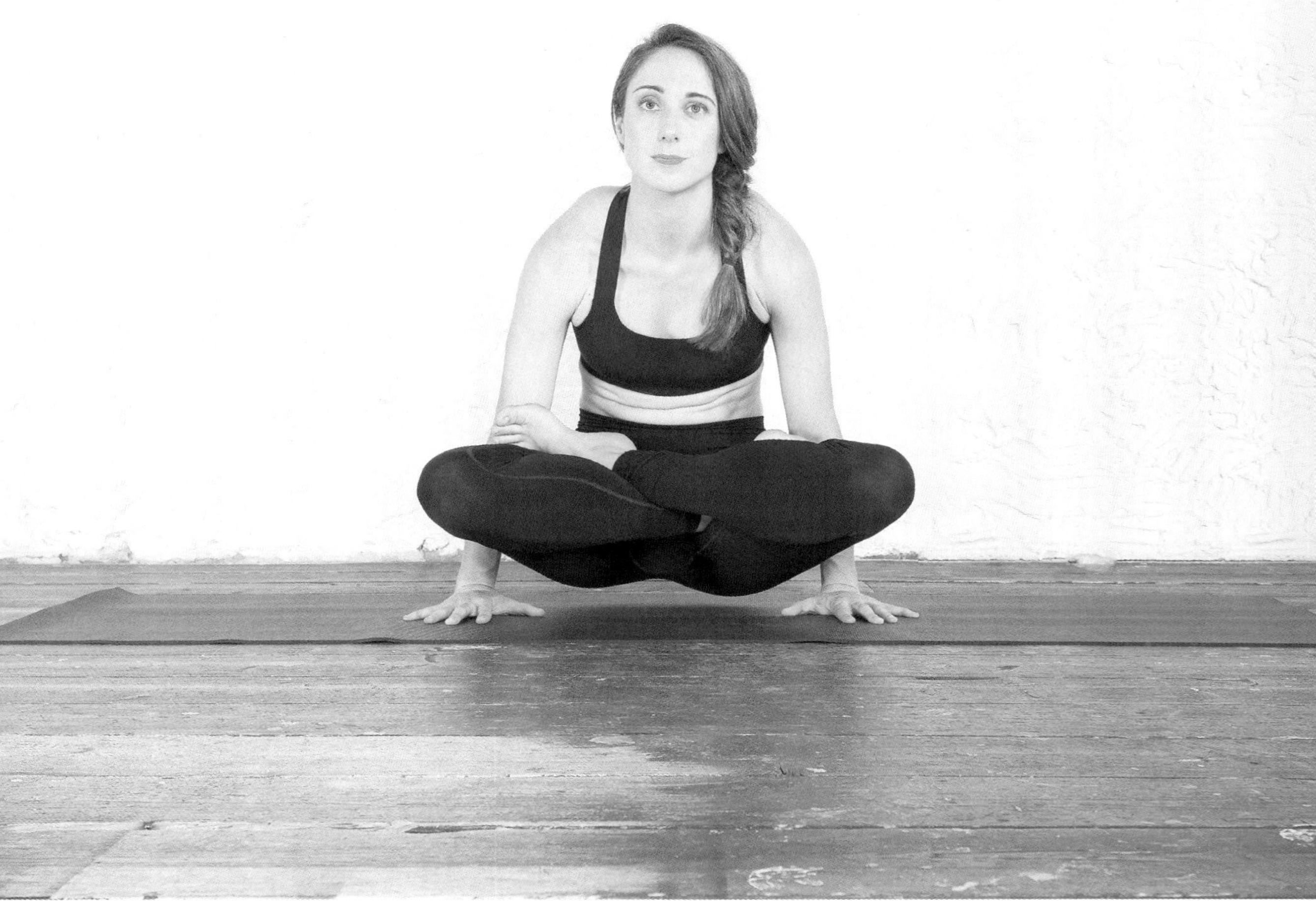

How to come into the pose

Sit with your legs straight in front of you.

Fold your legs into Lotus Pose and place the palms on the floor beside your hips.

Breathe out, push your hands against the floor, contract your abdominal muscles, and lift your legs and buttocks away from the floor.

Look straight ahead, hold the pose steadily as long as comfortable, and breathe evenly.

To release the pose, lower your legs and buttocks on an exhalation, change the cross of your legs, and repeat for the same length of time.

Next pose

Rest in Child's Pose for 30–45 seconds, then continue with Triangle Pose or a variation thereof.

Alignment cues

Because Lotus Pose is the foundation for Scale Pose, it is important to get the alignment correct in Lotus Pose first. If you are unable to come into Lotus Pose, sit with your legs crossed in Easy Sitting Pose instead. Draw your knees in toward your chest and lift your hips up. Your feet can initially remain on the floor or on a block for support. You can also cross your top leg into Half Lotus Pose and perform the pose as described on the left.

Fingers are pointing forward. Make sure to push the heels of your palms and your knuckles and fingertips actively into the floor.

Keep your shoulder blades wide and drawn away from your ears.

Contraindications & cautions

The same contraindications and cautions apply as in Easy Crow Pose. Also be cautious in this pose if you have tight hips or knee issues.

Modifications & adjustments

If you feel tension in your wrists, you can place the heels of your hands on a folded blanket to relieve pressure.

Variations

Lolasana
Pendant Pose

Come to sit on your knees, with your hips on your heels. Place your hands on the floor next to your knees, and lift your pelvis off your feet. Now cross your ankles, lean forward, and, with an exhalation, push firmly down with your hands and lift both feet off the floor. Move your shoulder blades apart to lift your body as high as possible and, at the same time, draw yourself into as tight a ball as you can by pulling your heels up and curling your trunk. Then, once you are balanced, gradually lift your head and gaze forward.

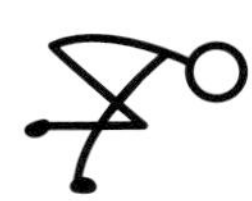

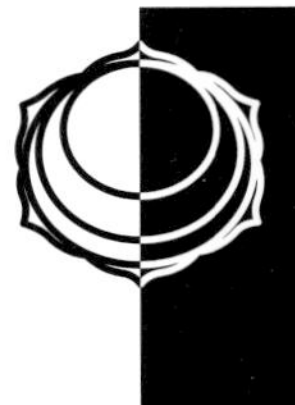

Kukkutasana
Rooster Pose

Start in Lotus Pose, then insert your arms between your thighs and calf muscles all the way to your elbows. Now place your palms on the floor, with your fingers spread wide and pointing forward. Shift your weight onto your hands and lift your hips up and off the floor. Balancing on your hands, look forward and breathe evenly.

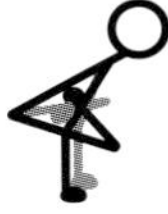

Pincha Mayurasana
Forearm Stand

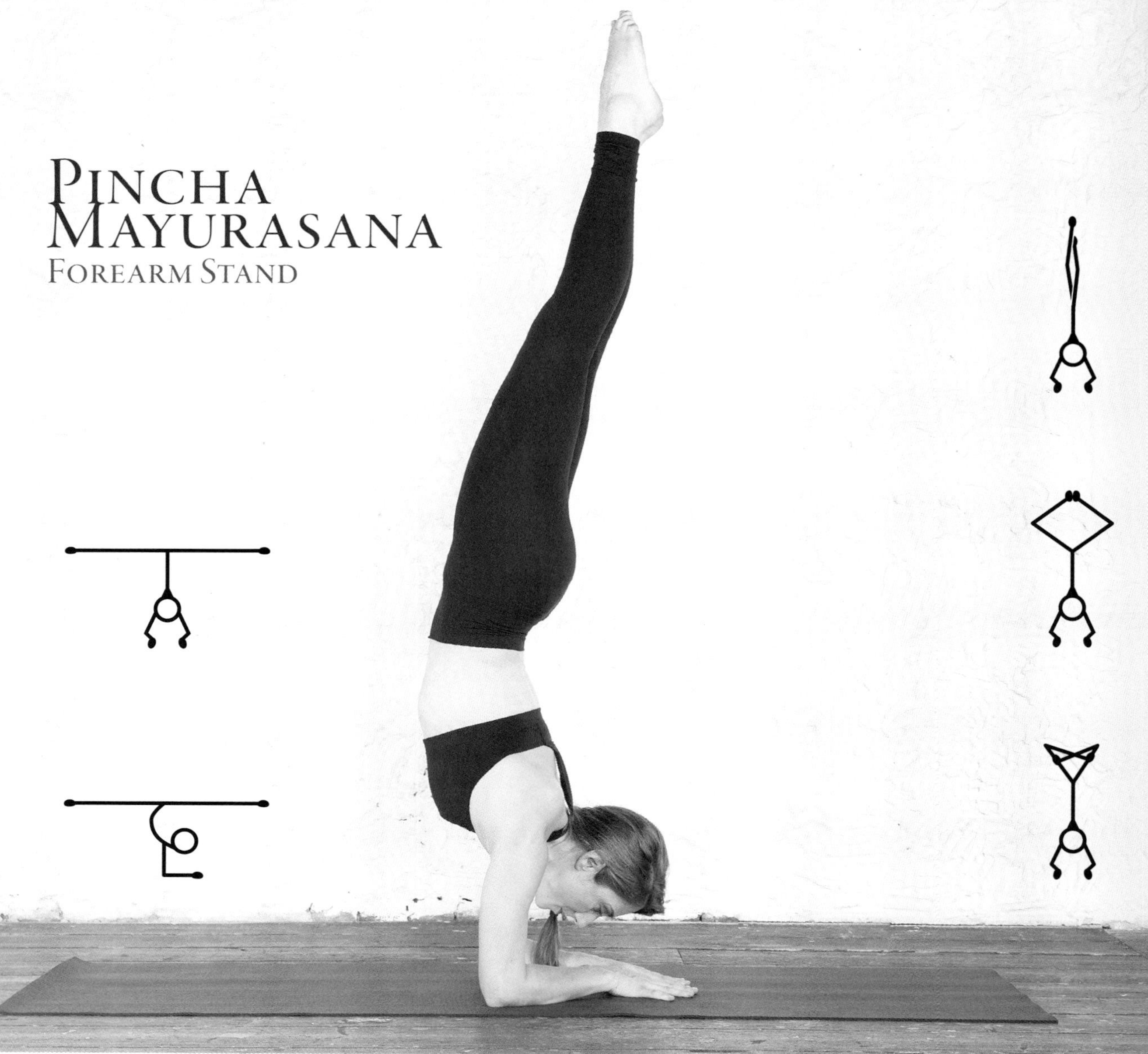

How to come into the pose

Sit on your knees with your hips on your heels and hold on to your opposite elbows. Then place your forearms on the floor.

Keeping your elbows where they are, place your hands flat on the floor until your upper arms are parallel to each other.

Fingers spread out, looking slightly forward or between your hands, curl your toes, push your hips toward the ceiling, and straighten your legs.

Walk your feet toward your chest until your shoulders are almost above your elbows.

Make sure to push your forearms firmly into the floor and push your shoulders away from your ears.

Lift one leg straight up to the ceiling. Push off from the other leg, and with a gentle hop follow with the other leg so that you are standing on your forearms. Point your feet toward the ceiling, breathe evenly, and focus your eyes on a point on the floor.

Bring one leg at a time down, with control, to release the pose.

Next pose

Rest in Child's Pose for 30–45 seconds, then continue with Triangle Pose or a variation thereof.

Alignment cues

Once in the pose, keep your core and legs active. Do not fall into an arch, but try to simply keep your spine in its natural curve.

Do not allow yourself to sink in with your arms. Firmly push your elbows against the floor and keep your shoulders lifted away from your ears.

Look in between your hands or slightly forward, without straining your neck.

Contraindications & cautions

The same contraindications and cautions apply as in Easy Crow Pose.

Modifications & Adjustments

Initially, this pose needs to be practiced with the support of a teacher, who helps you come up, and stay up, and release safely. Once you have gained some confidence there, you can build up further with the support of a wall. Maintain an approximately one-hand distance between the wall and your fingertips. Kick your legs up against the wall, and then start to push away from the wall, with one leg initially, to find the balance point. Make sure not to just lean against the wall, but stay active in your core and work toward finding balance.

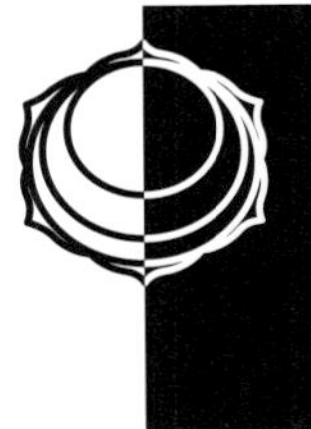

Variations

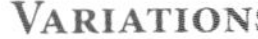

Vistrit Pada Pincha Mayurasana

Forearm Stand with Leg Variations

Once you are able to stand steady and still in Forearm Stand, you can implement some leg variations to increase control and coordination.

Vrischikasana
Scorpion Pose

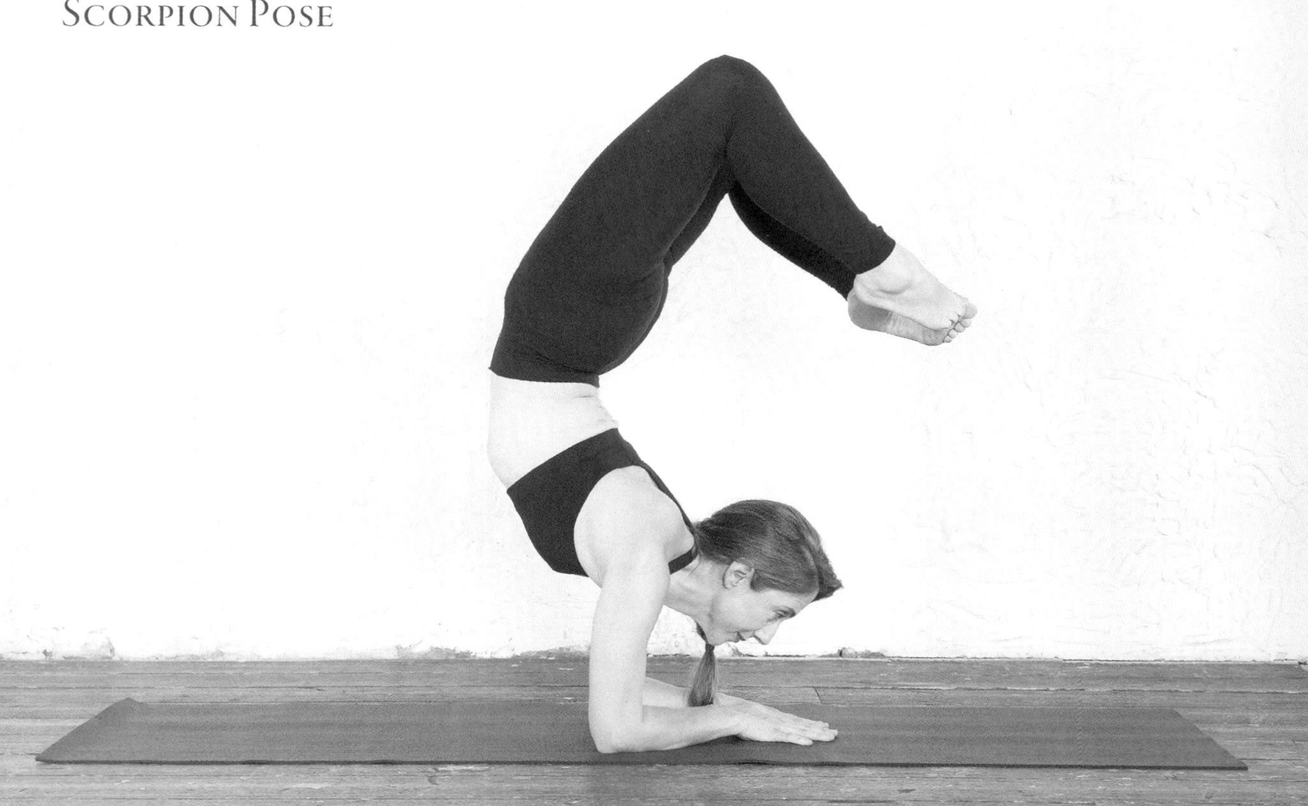

How to come into the pose

Sit on your knees with your hips on your heels and hold on to your opposite elbows. Then place your forearms on the floor.

Keeping your elbows where they are, place your hands flat on the floor until your upper arms are parallel to each other.

Fingers spread out, looking slightly forward or between your hands, curl your toes, push your hips toward the ceiling, and straighten your legs.

Walk your feet toward your chest until your shoulders are almost above your elbows. Make sure to push your forearms firmly down into the floor while pushing your shoulders away from your ears.

Lift one leg straight up toward the ceiling. Push off from the other leg, and with a gentle hop follow with the other leg so you are standing on your forearms.

Once you are in a stable forearm balance, start to bend your knees, arch your back, and reach with your feet toward your head.

Hold the pose steadily as long as comfortable and breathe evenly.

Bring down one leg at a time, with control, to release the pose.

Next pose

Rest in Child's Pose for 30–45 seconds, then continue with Triangle Pose or a variation thereof.

Alignment cues

Do not allow yourself to sink in with your arms. Firmly push your elbows against the floor and keep your shoulders lifted away from your ears.

Reach with your feet toward your head and at the same time open your chest and look upward, reaching with your head toward your feet as well.

Make sure not to strain your neck or hang in your lower back; keep your core active and spine in an active arch.

Contraindications & cautions

The same contraindications and cautions apply as in Easy Crow Pose. Also be cautious with this pose if you suffer from neck, lower-back, or spinal issues.

Modifications & Adjustments

Initially, this pose needs to be practiced with the support of a teacher, who helps you come up, and stay up, and release the pose safely. Once you have gained some confidence there, you can build up further with the support of a wall. Maintain a distance of approximately the length of your forearm between the wall and your fingertips. Kick your legs up against the wall, bend your knees, and rest your toes against the wall. Then start to push away from the wall, with one leg initially, to find your balance. Make sure not to just lean against the wall, but keep your whole body active and work toward the balance point.

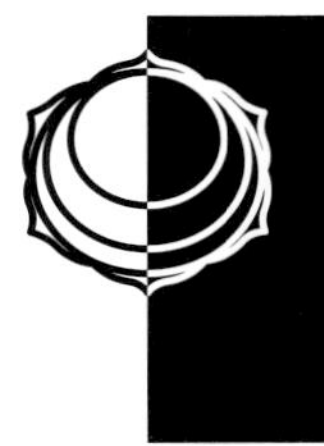

Adho Mukha Vrkshasana
Handstand Pose

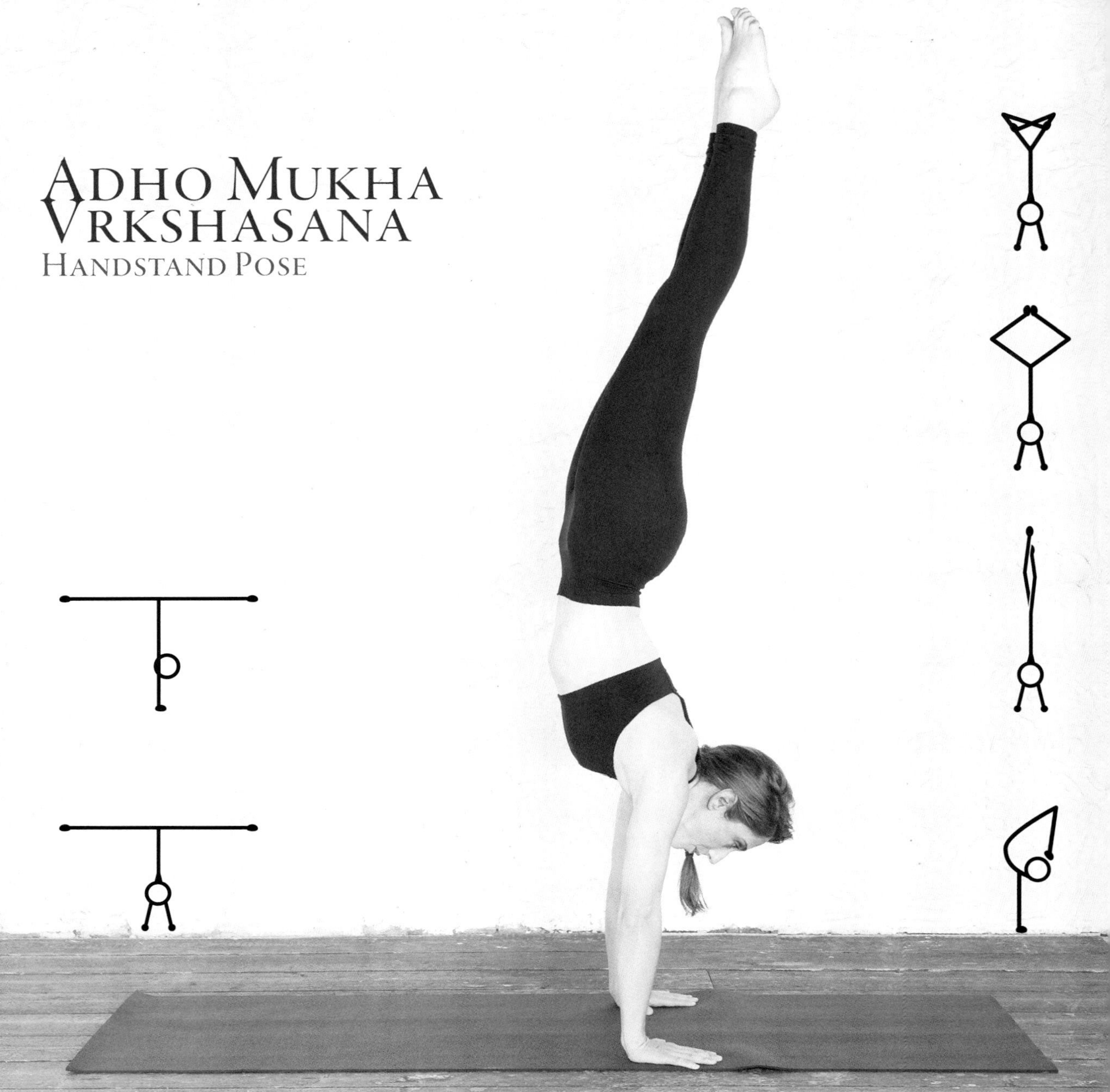

How to come into the pose

Start from Downward-Facing Dog Pose, with your hands in line with your shoulders, fingers spread and actively pushing into the floor.

Now walk your feet inwards as close as you can toward your chest, while keeping your arms completely straight and your shoulder blades drawn away from your ears. Engage your core and suck in your navel toward your spine as you do so.

Look slightly forward, keeping your core engaged and lifting one leg up toward the ceiling.

Push off from the other leg, and with a gentle hop follow with that leg so that you are standing on your hands.

Squeeze your inner thighs together, point your feet up toward the ceiling, and focus on a point on the floor in front of you.

Hold the pose steadily as long as comfortable and breathe evenly.

Bring one leg at a time down, with control, to release the pose.

Next pose

Rest in Child's Pose for 30–45 seconds, then continue with Triangle Pose or a variation thereof.

Alignment cues

Once in the pose, keep your core and legs active. Do not fall into an arch, but try to simply keep your spine in its natural curve.

Do not allow yourself to sink in with your arms. Keep your arms straight and your shoulder blades lifted away from your ears.

Push the heels of your palms, your knuckles, and fingertips actively down into the floor.

Look in between your hands or slightly forward, without straining your neck.

Contraindications & cautions

The same contraindications and cautions apply as in Easy Crow Pose.

Modifications & adjustments

If your shoulders are tight, turn your index fingers out slightly; otherwise arrange them parallel to each other.

Initially, this pose needs to be practiced with the support of a teacher, who helps you to come up, and stay up, and release the pose safely. Once you have gained some confidence there, you can build up further with the support of a wall. Maintain a 1- to 2-inch distance between the wall and your fingertips. Kick your legs up against the wall and then start to push away from the wall, with one leg initially, to find the balance point. You can also press the back of your head against the wall and focus on keeping your body completely straight. Make sure not to just lean against the wall, but to remain active in your core and legs and work toward the balance point.

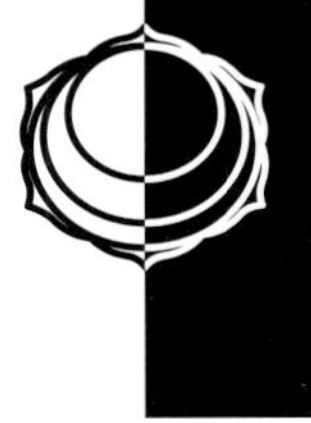

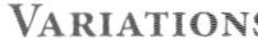

Variations

Vistrit Pada Adho Mukha Vrkshasana

Handstand Pose with Leg Variations

Once you are able to stand steadily and still in Handstand Pose, you can implement some leg variations to increase control and coordination.

VASHISHTASANA
SIDE PLANK POSE

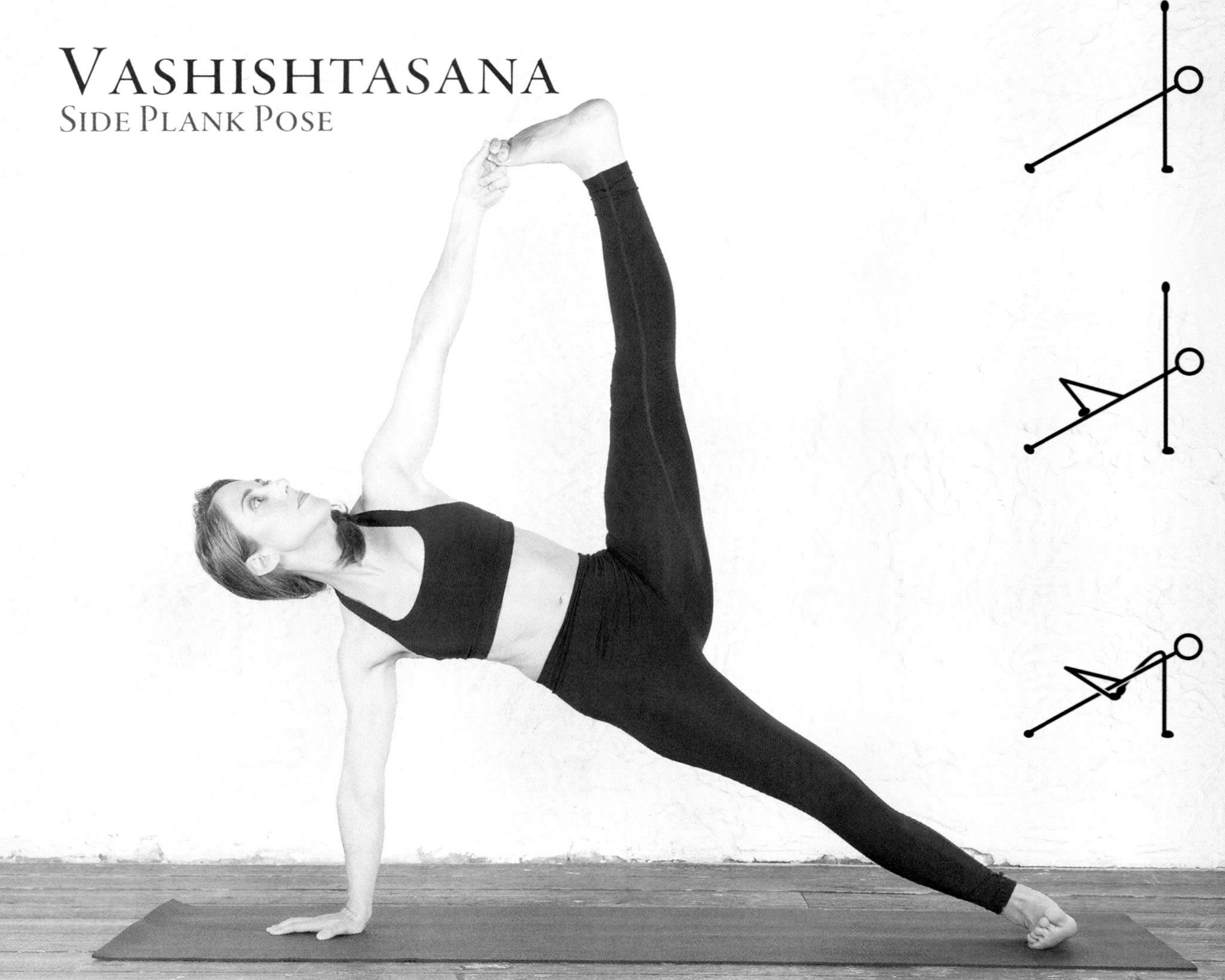

HOW TO COME INTO THE POSE

Come into a high plank position, with your wrists below your shoulders, legs straight and feet together.

Start to lift your left arm off the floor and at the same time rotate your body so that your left shoulder comes above your right.

Stack your left foot on top of your right and support the weight of your body on the outer right foot and right hand.

Bend your left knee and draw your thigh toward your torso. Now reach inside the bent leg and use the index and middle fingers of your top hand to grab your big toe.

Hold on tightly, then stretch your left leg perpendicularly toward the ceiling.

Look up toward the ceiling and find your balance.

Hold the pose steadily as long as comfortable and breathe evenly.

Then release the pose and repeat on the other side.

Next pose

Rest in Child's Pose for 30–45 seconds, then continue with Triangle Pose or a variation thereof.

Alignment cues

Fingers of the supporting hand are pointing toward the front of the mat. Make sure to push the heel of your palm, your knuckles, and fingertips actively into the floor.

The wrist of the supporting arm is straight below your shoulder. Keep your triceps firmly engaged.

Make sure to balance on the outer edge of your lower foot. To do so, flex your foot and push out through the heel.

Create opposition between your upper foot and hand to maintain your balance.

Keep your collarbones broad and shoulder blades drawn down toward your waist.

Keep your whole body engaged and align your entire body into one long diagonal line from the heels to the crown.

Contraindications & cautions

Most contraindications and cautions apply as in Easy Crow Pose. This is a great alternative for anyone who should not be doing inverted postures (for example, if suffering from hypertension or inflammation in the head region).

Modifications & adjustments

If balancing is challenging, start with the Easy Side Plank as described on the right. You may even rest your upper foot in front of your lower foot on the floor for extra support and balance.

If your wrists are hurting or you feel any lack of strength in your arms, you can set up the pose on your elbows. In this case, instead of placing your hand on the floor, place your elbow below your shoulder, with your hand pointing out toward the side of the mat.

Variations

Sukha Vashishtasana

Easy Side Plank

Follow the instructions on the left but skip the step where you lift your upper leg up and hold on to the big toe. Keep your feet stacked on top of each other, upper arm reaching up toward the ceiling, and look upward along the arm.

Eka Pada Vashishtasana

One-Legged Side Plank

Follow the instructions for Easy Side Plank, as described above. Once you are in Easy Side Plank, lift your upper leg and place it against the inside of the opposite leg.

Kasyapasana

Half Bound-Lotus Side Plank

Start in a seated position, with your legs extended in front of you. Come into Half Lotus with your right leg, and wrap your right arm behind your back in order to take hold of your foot. Now place your left hand on the floor in line with your hip and about 30 centimeters from your pelvis, fingertips pointing to the back of your mat. Externally rotate your arm, and draw your shoulder blade down your back. Begin to lean onto your left arm and start to straighten your left leg in the opposite direction. Simultaneously start to lift your hips. If you're able to lift your hips and maintain the bind, take a few breaths before you open the right side of your chest toward the ceiling. To release, let go of your foot, lower your hips to the floor, and gently release the Lotus leg. Then repeat on the other side. (Caution: Do not use any force and attempt this only if you are experienced in folding safely into Half Lotus.)

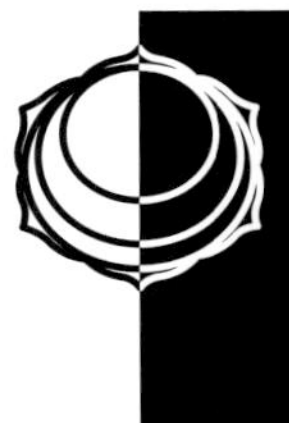

Vishvamitrasana
Pose Dedicated to the Sage Vishvamitra

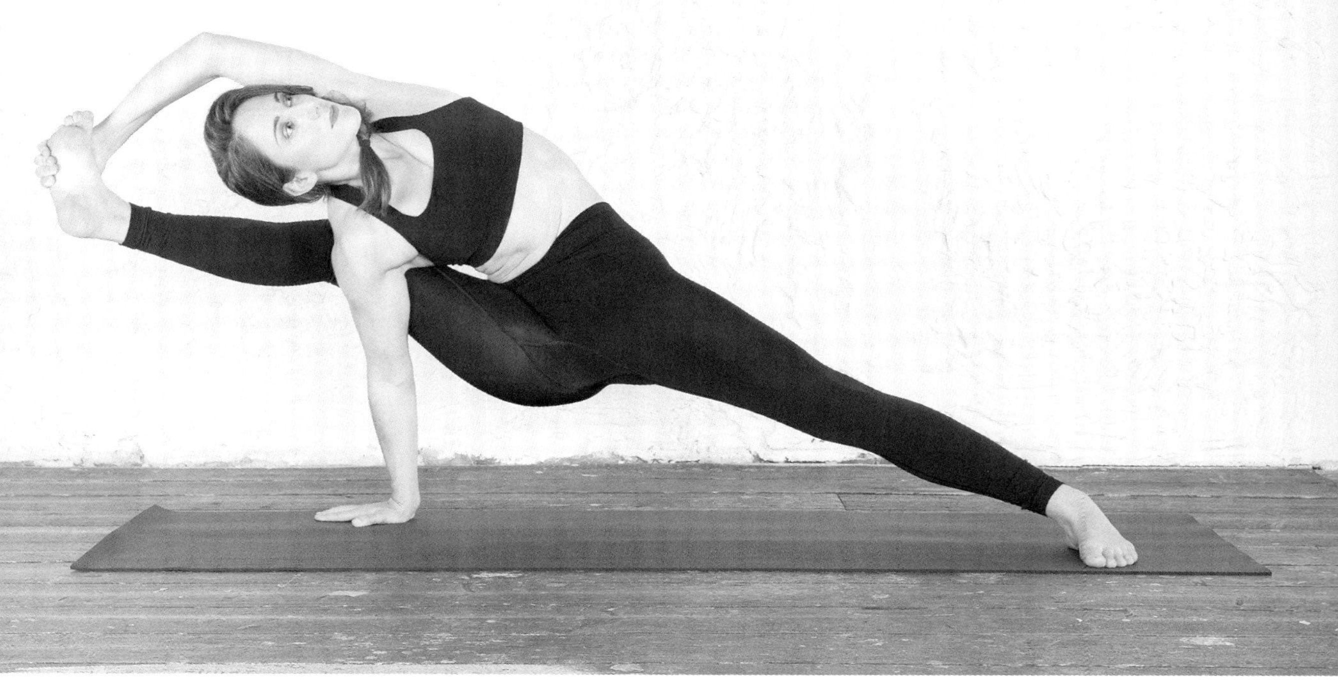

How to come into the pose

Start in a wide stance, with your right foot toward the front of your mat, and your back foot turned slightly inward.

Bend your front knee and press your right shoulder against your inner right knee. Drop your right shoulder underneath your front knee, press your right arm in behind your shin, and place your right hand outside your foot on the floor.

Press your back foot into the floor and start to shift your weight slightly to your right and into your right arm.

Lean onto your right hand until your right foot lifts off the floor. Then hold the outside edge of your right foot with your left hand.

Extend your right leg straight, squeezing your inner thigh against your arm in order to keep it from slipping toward the floor.

Now reach your top elbow toward the ceiling and roll your chest open. Look up toward the ceiling and hold the pose steadily as long as comfortable, breathing evenly.

Then release the pose and repeat on the other side.

Next pose

Rest in Child's Pose for 30–45 seconds, then continue with Triangle Pose or a variation thereof.

Alignment cues

Fingers of the supporting hand are pointing toward the front of the mat. Make sure to push your palm, knuckles, and fingertips actively down into the floor.

The wrist of the supporting arm is straight below your shoulder. Keep your triceps firmly engaged.

Gently externally rotate your arm so the elbow crease and biceps turn toward the front of your mat, and draw your shoulder blade down your back.

Bring your awareness to where the upper arms and inner thighs touch. Squeeze your thighs in against your arms, while simultaneously pressing your arms out against your thighs.

Increase your stability by working your back leg strongly, as though you were doing a standing pose.

Contraindications & cautions

Most contraindications and cautions apply as in Easy Crow Pose. This is a great alternative for anyone who should not be doing inverted postures (for example, if suffering from hypertension or inflammation in the head region).

Modifications & adjustments

This posture requires considerable hamstring flexibility, especially because of holding on to the upper foot. An easier modification is lifting the front foot off the floor and stretching it out as far as possible, while reaching the top hand toward the ceiling.

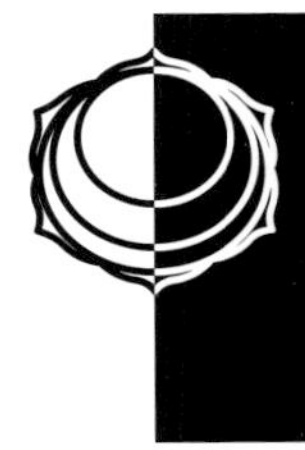

Sukha Kakasana (Easy Crow Pose) Alternatives

MALASANA
GARLAND POSE

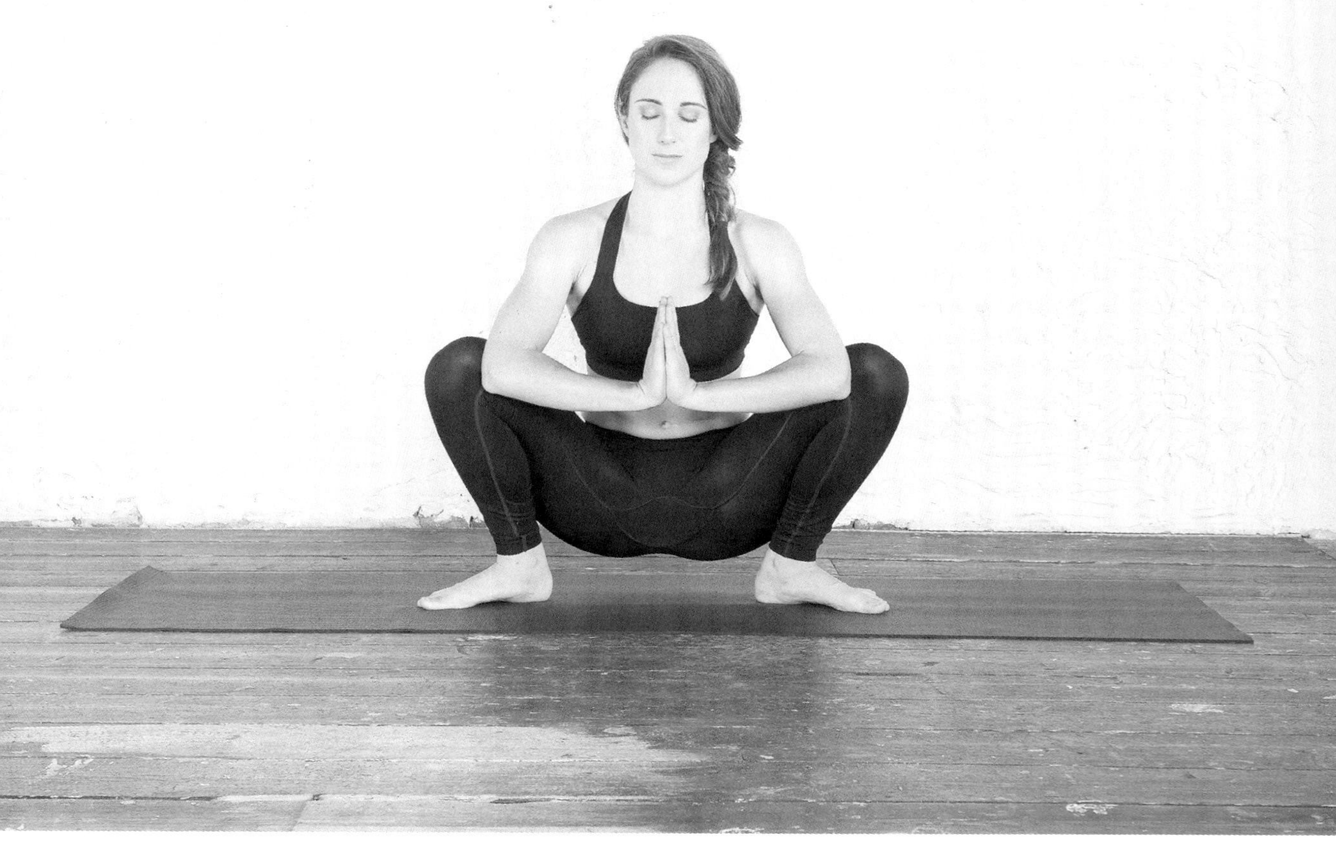

HOW TO COME INTO THE POSE

Squat with your feet hip- or shoulder-width apart, while keeping your heels on the floor.

Separate your thighs slightly wider than your torso.

Breathe out, lean your torso forward, and fit it snugly between your thighs.

Press your elbows against your inner knees, bringing your palms together, and create opposition between your knees and elbows.

Lengthen your front torso and look straight ahead.

Hold the pose steadily as long as comfortable, breathing evenly.

Next pose

Continue with Triangle Pose or a variation thereof.

Alignment cues

Keep your heels on the floor if you can. Otherwise, support them on a folded mat.

Straighten your spine and lengthen your front torso.

Draw your shoulder blades down and away from your ears and keep the back of your neck elongated.

Contraindications & cautions

This is a great alternative for anyone who should not be doing hand balancing or inverted postures (for example, if suffering from hypertension or inflammation in the head region). However, be cautious if you have any knee issues.

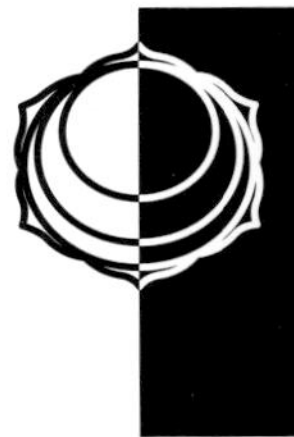

Variations

Baddha Malasana

Bound Garland Pose

From Garland Pose, reach your arms and chest forward and wrap your upper arms around your shins. Clasp your hands behind your heels or hold on to your ankles, then release your head and pelvis down toward the floor as much as possible.

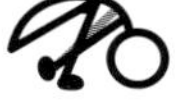

Prapadasana

Tip Toe Pose

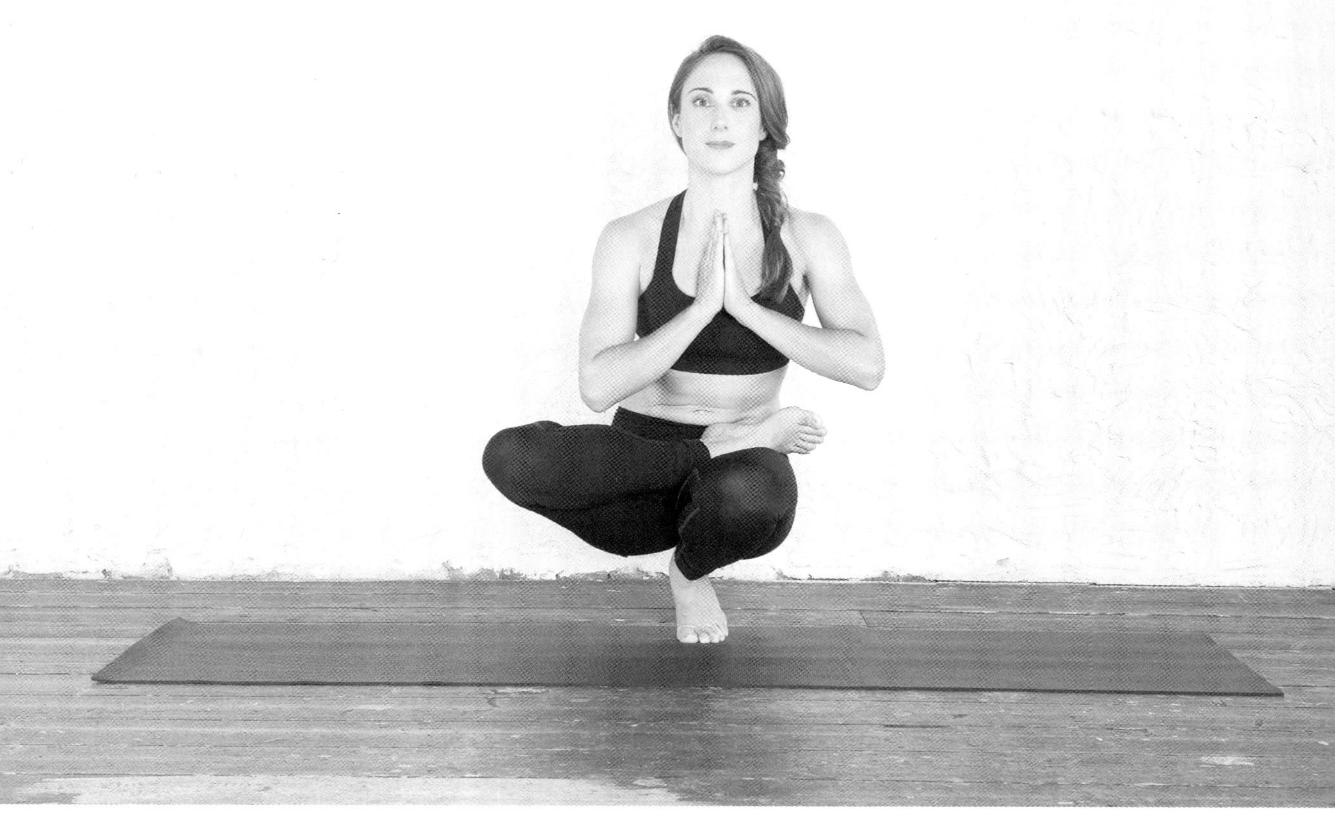

How to come into the pose

Start in a standing position, with your feet hip-width apart.

From here, bend your knees and then cross your right ankle over your left knee.

Fold forward and take your fingertips to the floor.

Come high onto the ball of your left foot and bring your buttocks to rest on your left heel.

Look forward, lift your torso, and look at a steady point at eye level.

Bring your hands together at the center of your chest and breathe evenly to maintain your balance.

Hold the pose steadily as long as comfortable, then release the pose and repeat on the other side.

Next pose

Continue with Triangle Pose or a variation thereof.

Alignment cues

Keep the upper foot firmly flexed to protect your knee.

When you sit on your heel, you will have to experiment a bit on where to place it exactly. Most people are able to press the heel against the tailbone or center it in the perineum area to distribute the weight between both sitting bones. Some people find they must keep the heel to one side in order to find their balance.

Contraindications & cautions

This is a great alternative for anyone who should not be doing hand balancing or inverted postures (for example, if suffering from hypertension or inflammation in the head region) but still wants to work on core awareness and balance. Be cautious in this pose if you have tight hips or knee or ankle issues.

Variations

Dwi Pada Prapadasana I

Two-Legged Tip Toe Pose I

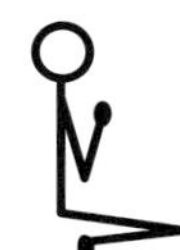

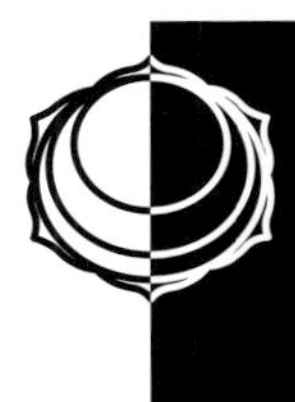

Come into a squat, with your feet together and your heels lifted off the floor. Allow your hips to rest on your heels, and squeeze your feet, knees, and inner thighs together. Bring your hands in front of your chest, palms together, and look straight ahead.

Dwi Pada Prapadasana II

Two-Legged Tip Toe Pose II

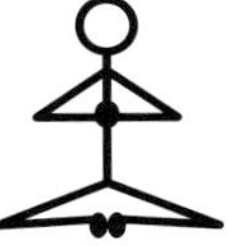

Come into a squat, with your feet together and your heels lifted off the floor. Allow your hips to rest on your heels. Now keep your heels together and open your knees to the side. Bring your hands in front of your chest, palms together, and look straight ahead.

VATAYANASANA
HORSE POSE

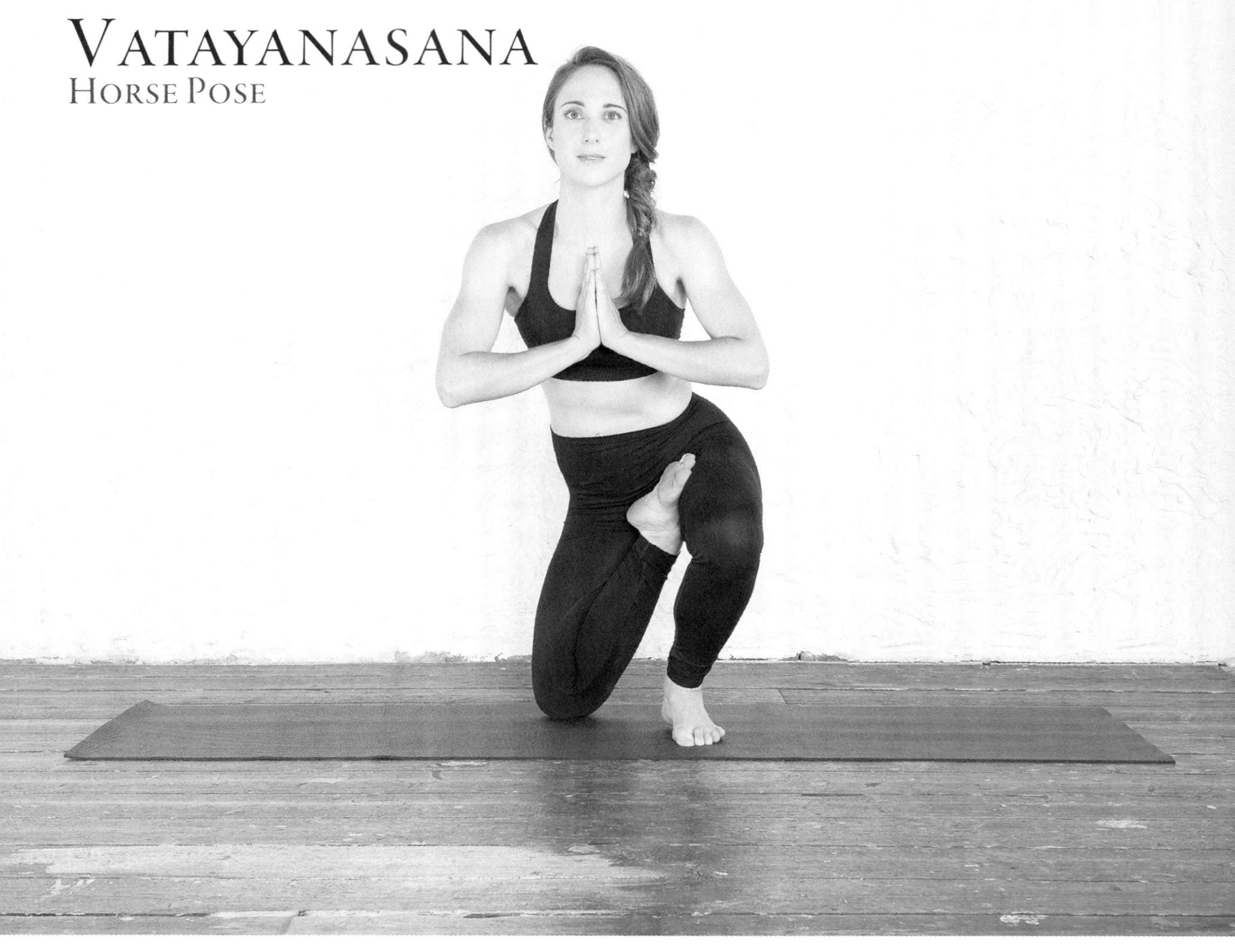

HOW TO COME INTO THE POSE

Come into a seated position, with your legs straight in front of you. Then bring your right leg into a Half Lotus position, so that the heel of your right foot is touching your left groin. (Caution: If you cannot fold into a Lotus position easily and without forcing your leg or knee, do not continue with this pose.)

Bend your left knee and place your left foot on the floor. Lift your hips up and rest the folded right knee on the floor.

Press your weight down into the floor through your left heel and right knee.

Bring your palms together in front of your chest and look straight ahead.

Hold the pose steadily as long as comfortable and breathe evenly.

Then release the pose, shake your legs out in front of you, and repeat on the other side.

Next pose

Continue with Triangle Pose or a variation thereof.

Alignment cues

Press both your knee and heel firmly into the floor.

Bring your heel as close as possible to the knee that is in the Lotus position, with the toes pointing out sideways.

Contraindications & cautions

This is a slightly challenging alternative for anyone who should not be doing hand balancing or inverted postures (for example, if suffering from hypertension or inflammation in the head region). As it requires Half Lotus Pose, it is advised to be cautious if you have tight hips or knee or ankle issues.

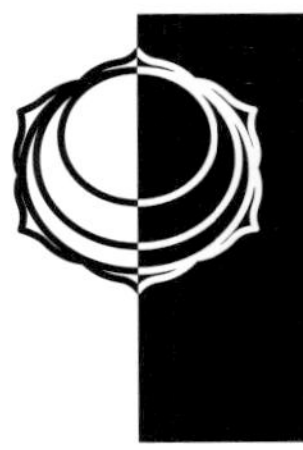

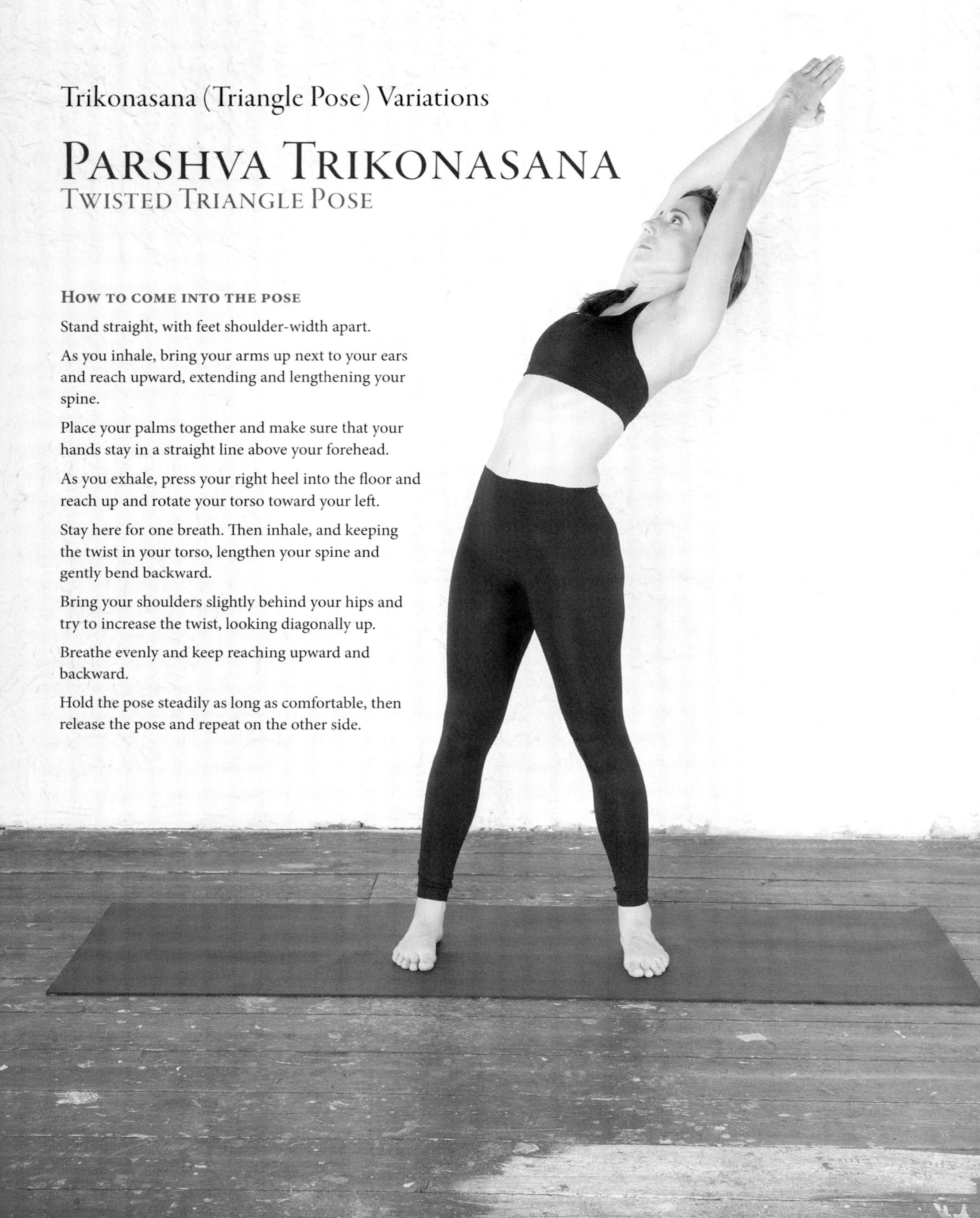

Trikonasana (Triangle Pose) Variations

Parshva Trikonasana

Twisted Triangle Pose

How to come into the pose

Stand straight, with feet shoulder-width apart.

As you inhale, bring your arms up next to your ears and reach upward, extending and lengthening your spine.

Place your palms together and make sure that your hands stay in a straight line above your forehead.

As you exhale, press your right heel into the floor and reach up and rotate your torso toward your left.

Stay here for one breath. Then inhale, and keeping the twist in your torso, lengthen your spine and gently bend backward.

Bring your shoulders slightly behind your hips and try to increase the twist, looking diagonally up.

Breathe evenly and keep reaching upward and backward.

Hold the pose steadily as long as comfortable, then release the pose and repeat on the other side.

Next pose

Continue with Tree Pose or a variation thereof.

Alignment cues

Keep the feet parallel and both legs engaged and rotating externally.

Make sure not to collapse at the rib cage, but keep reaching backward and upward.

The shoulders will lift up, but make sure to keep the back of your neck elongated.

Contraindications & cautions

- Lower-back issues and spinal issues
- Hamstring and groin issues

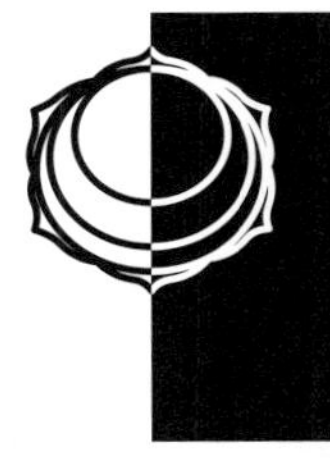

Utthita Trikonasana
Extended Triangle Pose

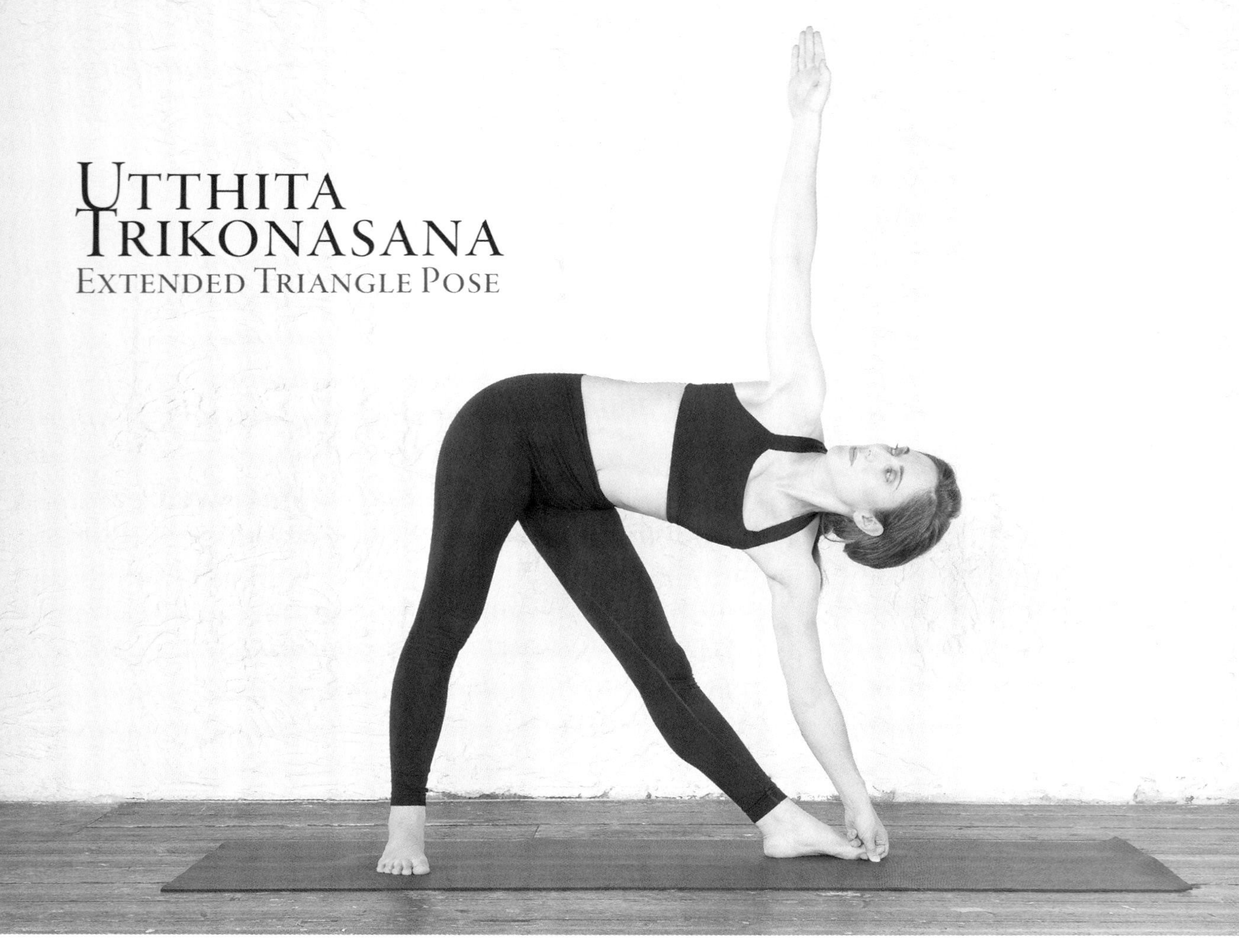

How to come into the pose

Stand on your mat with your feet wide and parallel (just about below your elbows when your arms are extended sideways).

Raise your arms parallel to the floor and reach them actively out to the sides, shoulder blades wide, palms facing downward.

Turn your left foot out to your left at 90 degrees, keeping the heels in one line.

Breathe out and extend your torso to your left, directly over your left leg.

Rest your left hand on your shin or ankle, or hold the big toe of your left foot, whatever is possible without distorting the sides of your torso.

Stretch your right arm toward the ceiling, in line with the tops of your shoulders. Look up along your right arm toward the ceiling, with the back of your neck elongated.

Breathe evenly and keep reaching upward and backward.

Hold the pose steadily as long as comfortable.

To release the pose, reach out through your right hand and bring your upper body upright again. Bring your feet parallel to each other, take a few breaths, and then proceed on the other side.

Next pose

Continue with Tree Pose or a variation thereof.

Alignment cues

Make sure that you are bending from the hip joint, not your waist, and that you keep the two sides of your torso elongated.

Keep both legs engaged and rotated externally.

Allow the hip of the back leg to come slightly forward, and focus on lengthening your entire spine, from the tailbone up and out through the crown of your head.

Broaden your shoulders by sending energy through your arms and out from the fingertips. At the same time, draw your shoulder blades downward toward your waist.

Keep your back foot firmly grounded and make sure to equally distribute your weight on both feet.

Contraindications & cautions

- Lower-back issues and spinal issues
- Hamstring and groin issues

Modifications & adjustments

If you have tight hamstrings or groin, a block as support under your lower hand brings great relief in this pose.

If your neck feels tight or painful, look down toward the floor instead of upward.

Similarly, if you feel dizzy easily, you might prefer to keep your gaze toward your lower hand.

If initially balancing is challenging in this pose, you can keep a small gap between your heels (so as not to align heel to heel) and look downward toward the floor.

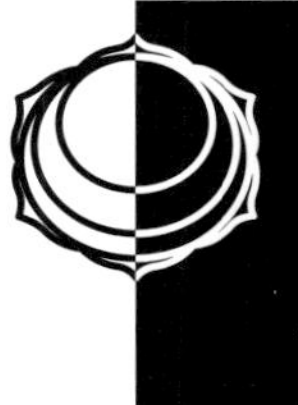

Variations

Utthita Trikonasana II

Extended Triangle II

Start in a wide stance with your feet parallel (just about below your elbows when your arms are extended sideways). Raise your arms parallel to the floor and reach them actively out to the sides, shoulder blades wide, palms facing downward. Reach out with your left hand and sweep it overhead; at the same time place your right palm on your right outer thigh. Bend over to your right, bringing your upper body and left arm as horizontal as possible.

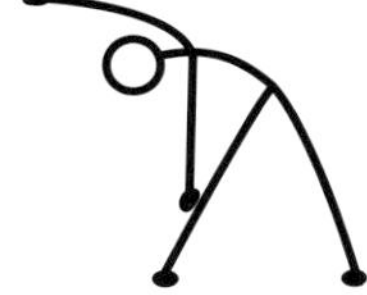

Parivrtta Trikonasana

Revolved Triangle Pose

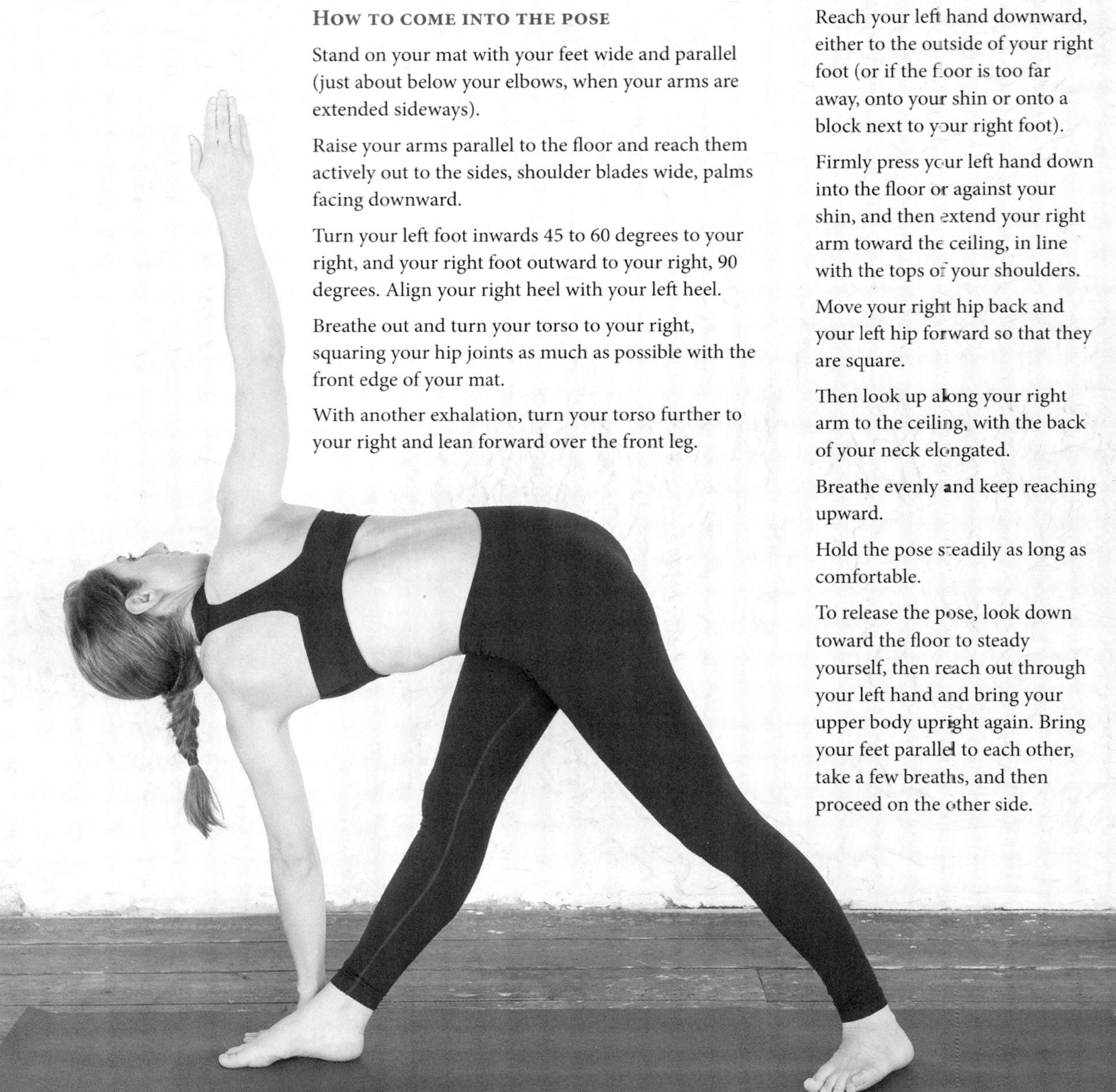

How to come into the pose

Stand on your mat with your feet wide and parallel (just about below your elbows, when your arms are extended sideways).

Raise your arms parallel to the floor and reach them actively out to the sides, shoulder blades wide, palms facing downward.

Turn your left foot inwards 45 to 60 degrees to your right, and your right foot outward to your right, 90 degrees. Align your right heel with your left heel.

Breathe out and turn your torso to your right, squaring your hip joints as much as possible with the front edge of your mat.

With another exhalation, turn your torso further to your right and lean forward over the front leg.

Reach your left hand downward, either to the outside of your right foot (or if the floor is too far away, onto your shin or onto a block next to your right foot).

Firmly press your left hand down into the floor or against your shin, and then extend your right arm toward the ceiling, in line with the tops of your shoulders.

Move your right hip back and your left hip forward so that they are square.

Then look up along your right arm to the ceiling, with the back of your neck elongated.

Breathe evenly and keep reaching upward.

Hold the pose steadily as long as comfortable.

To release the pose, look down toward the floor to steady yourself, then reach out through your left hand and bring your upper body upright again. Bring your feet parallel to each other, take a few breaths, and then proceed on the other side.

Next pose

Continue with Tree Pose or a variation thereof.

Alignment cues

Make sure that you are bending from the hip joint, not your waist, and that you are keeping the two sides of your torso elongated.

Keep both your legs engaged and rotated externally.

Allow the hip of the back leg to drop slightly toward the floor and focus on lengthening your entire spine from the tailbone upward and outward, through the crown of your head.

Broaden your shoulders by sending energy through your arms and out from the fingertips. At the same time, draw your shoulder blades downward toward your waist.

Contraindications & cautions

- Lower-back issues and spinal issues
- Hamstring and groin issues
- Hypertension: Keep your head elevated above heart level by using a block underneath your lower hand
- Abdominal issues

Modifications & adjustments

If you have tight hamstrings or groin, a block as support under your lower hand brings great relief in this pose.

If initially balancing is challenging in this pose, you can keep a small gap between your heels (so as not to align heel to heel) and look downward toward the floor.

If your neck feels tight or painful, look downward toward the floor instead of upward.

Similarly, if you feel dizzy easily you might prefer to keep your gaze toward your lower hand.

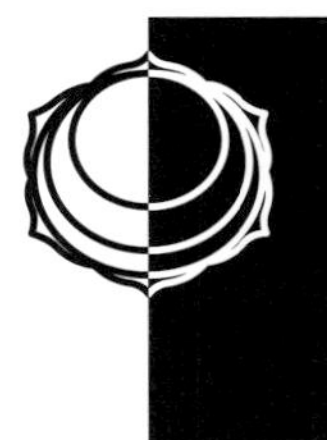

ARDHA CHANDRASANA
HALF MOON POSE

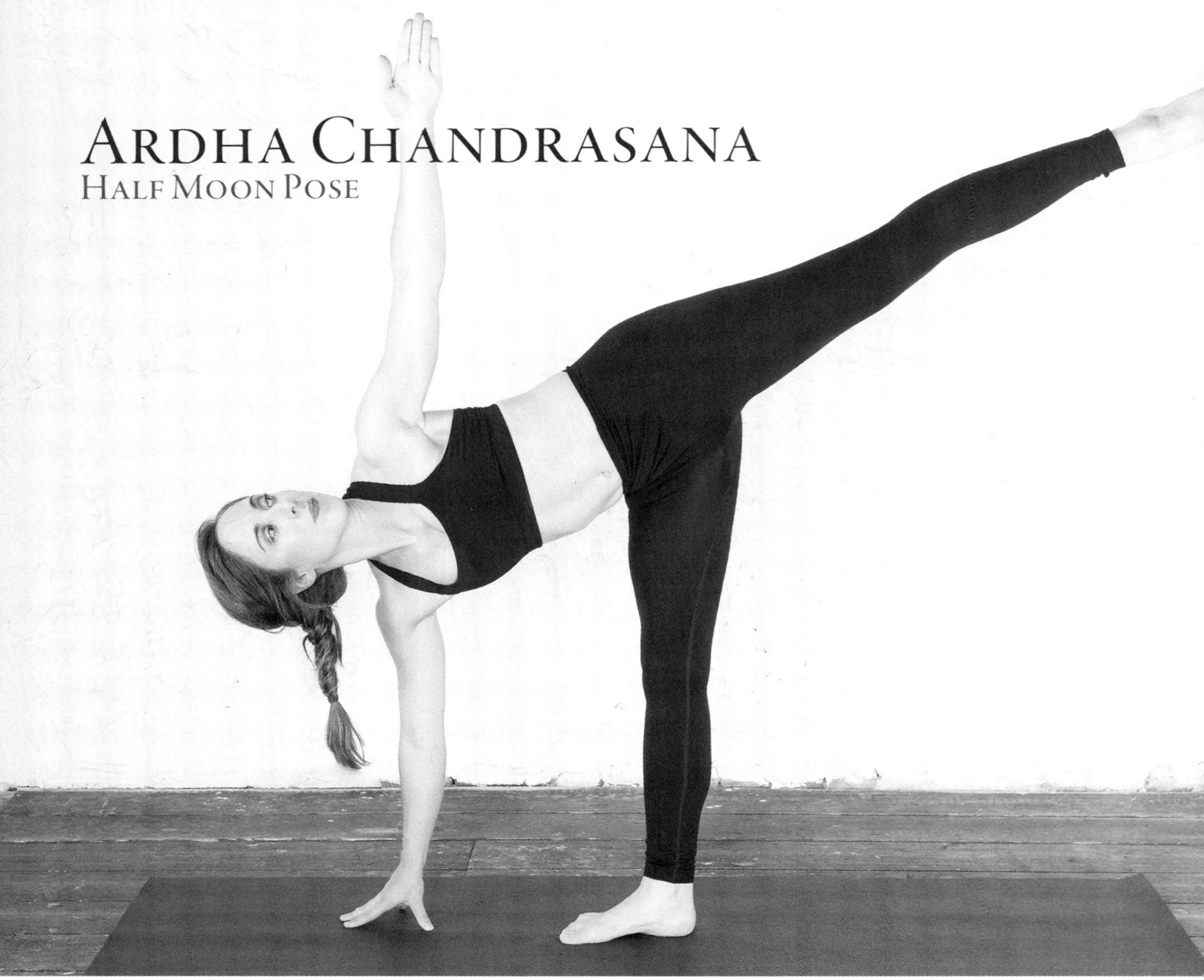

HOW TO COME INTO THE POSE

Perform Extended Triangle Pose to your right side, with your left hand resting on your left hip.

Breathe in, bend your right knee, and slide your left foot about 15 to 30 centimeters forward along the floor. At the same time, reach your right hand forward to the floor beyond the little-toe side of your right foot, at least 12 inches in front of your right foot.

Breathe out, press your right hand and right heel firmly downward into the floor, and straighten your right leg, simultaneously lifting your left leg parallel (or a little above parallel) to the floor.

Push out actively through your left heel to keep the raised leg strong.

Bear your body's weight mostly on the standing leg. Press the lower hand lightly to the floor, using it to intelligently regulate your balance.

Now raise the top arm perpendicular to the floor. Imagine there is a wall in front of you, and press the top hand actively into this pretend wall.

Then, if your balance is steady, slowly lift your head to gaze upward at the raised hand.

Breathe evenly and keep reaching out through your back foot, hand, and crown of your head. upward and backward.

Hold the pose steadily as long as comfortable, then release and repeat on the other side.

Next pose

Continue with Tree Pose or a variation thereof.

Alignment cues

Lift the inner ankle of the standing foot strongly upward, as if drawing energy from the floor into the standing groin.

Press your shoulder blades firmly against your back torso and elongate your spine, pressing out through the raised heel and the crown of your head.

Contraindications & cautions

- Hamstring and groin issues
- Hypertension: Keep your head elevated above heart level by using a block underneath your lower hand

Modifications & adjustments

Be careful not to lock (and so hyperextend) the standing knee. Keep your leg active and make sure your kneecap is aligned straight forward and is not turned inwards.

For people with tight hamstrings or groins, a block as support under your lower hand brings great relief in this pose.

Keep rotating your upper torso, aiming to bring the top shoulder right above the lower shoulder.

If your neck feels tight or painful, look downward toward the floor instead of upward. You can also keep your upper hand against your waist, instead of extending it up toward the ceiling.

Similarly, if you feel dizzy easily you might prefer to keep your gaze toward your lower hand.

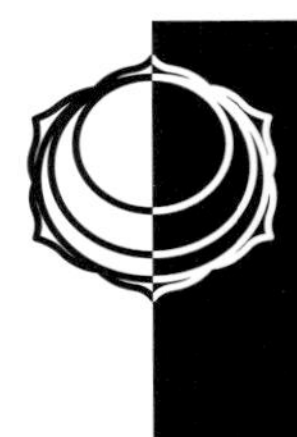

Variations

Ardha Chandra Chapasana

Sugarcane Pose

From Half Moon Pose, bend your top knee, reach your upper hand back, and catch the top of your foot. Once you are holding on to your foot, expand your chest and look up toward the ceiling.

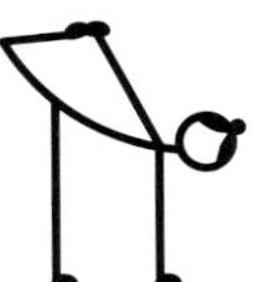

UTTHITA PARSHVAKONASANA
EXTENDED SIDE-ANGLE POSE

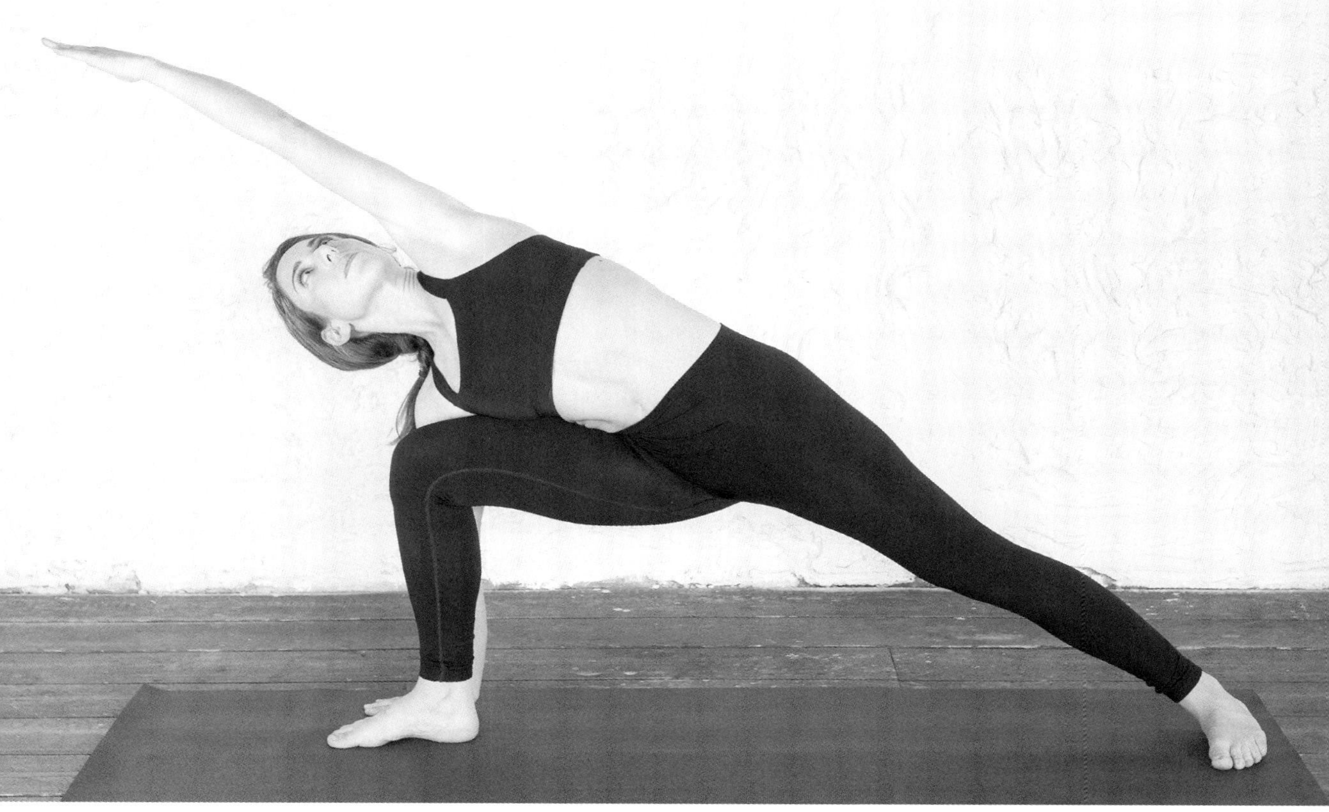

HOW TO COME INTO THE POSE

Stand on your mat, with your feet wide and parallel (just about below your wrists when your arms are extended sideways).

Raise your arms parallel to the floor and reach them actively out to the sides, shoulder blades wide, palms facing downward.

Turn your left foot inwards slightly toward your right and your right foot outwards toward your right, 90 degrees. Align your right heel with your left heel.

Breathe out, bend your right knee to about 90 degrees, and extend your torso toward your right, directly over your right leg.

Rest your right hand on the floor, along the outer edge of your right foot.

Extend your left arm straight up toward the ceiling, then turn your left palm to face toward your head, and with an inhalation reach the arm over the back of your left ear, palm facing the floor.

Turn your head to look toward your left elbow, and breathe evenly.

Hold the pose steadily as long as comfortable.

To release the pose, reach out through your left hand and bring your upper body upright again. Bring your feet parallel to each other, take a few breaths, and then proceed on the other side.

Next pose

Continue with Tree Pose or a variation thereof.

Alignment cues

The kneecap of your bent leg is slightly behind or right above the center of your ankle. Maintain an angle of at least 90 degrees. Ideally, the inside of your bent thigh should be parallel to the long edge of your mat.

Actively push your bent knee back against the inner arm.

Keep your back heel firmly grounded down into the floor.

Stretch from your back heel all the way through the fingertips of your extended arm, lengthening the entire side of your body. At the same time, try to create as much length along the other side of your torso as well.

Draw your shoulder blades downward toward the waist and keep the back of your neck elongated.

Contraindications & cautions

Hamstring or groin issues

Modifications & adjustments

If you have tight hamstrings or groin, a block as support under your lower hand brings great relief in this pose. Instead of a block, you can also simply rest your forearm on the top of the front thigh.

If your neck feels tight or painful or if you feel dizzy easily or have high blood pressure, look straight ahead, with the sides of your neck lengthened evenly, or look down at the floor.

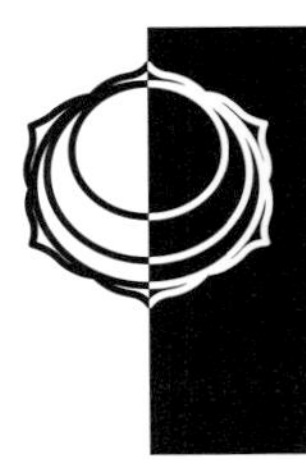

Parivrtta Parshvakonasana
Revolved Side-Angle Pose

How to come into the pose

Stand on your mat, with your feet wide and parallel (just about below your wrists when your arms are extended sideways).

Raise your arms parallel to the floor and reach them actively out to the sides, shoulder blades wide, palms facing downward.

Turn your left foot in, 45 to 60 degrees to your right, and your right foot out to your right, 90 degrees. Align your right heel with your left heel.

Breathe out, bend your right knee to about 90 degrees, and turn your torso to your right, squaring your hip joints as much as possible with the front edge of your mat.

With another exhalation, turn your torso further to your right and lean forward over the front leg.

Reach your left hand downward, to the outside of your right foot.

Firmly press your left hand into the floor, keep rotating your upper body, and then reach your right arm along your right ear, palm facing the floor.

Turn your head to gaze to your right elbow, and breathe evenly.

Hold the pose steadily as long as comfortable. To release the pose, look downward toward the floor to steady yourself, then reach out through your left hand and bring your upper body upright again. Bring your feet parallel to each other, take a few breaths, and then proceed on the other side.

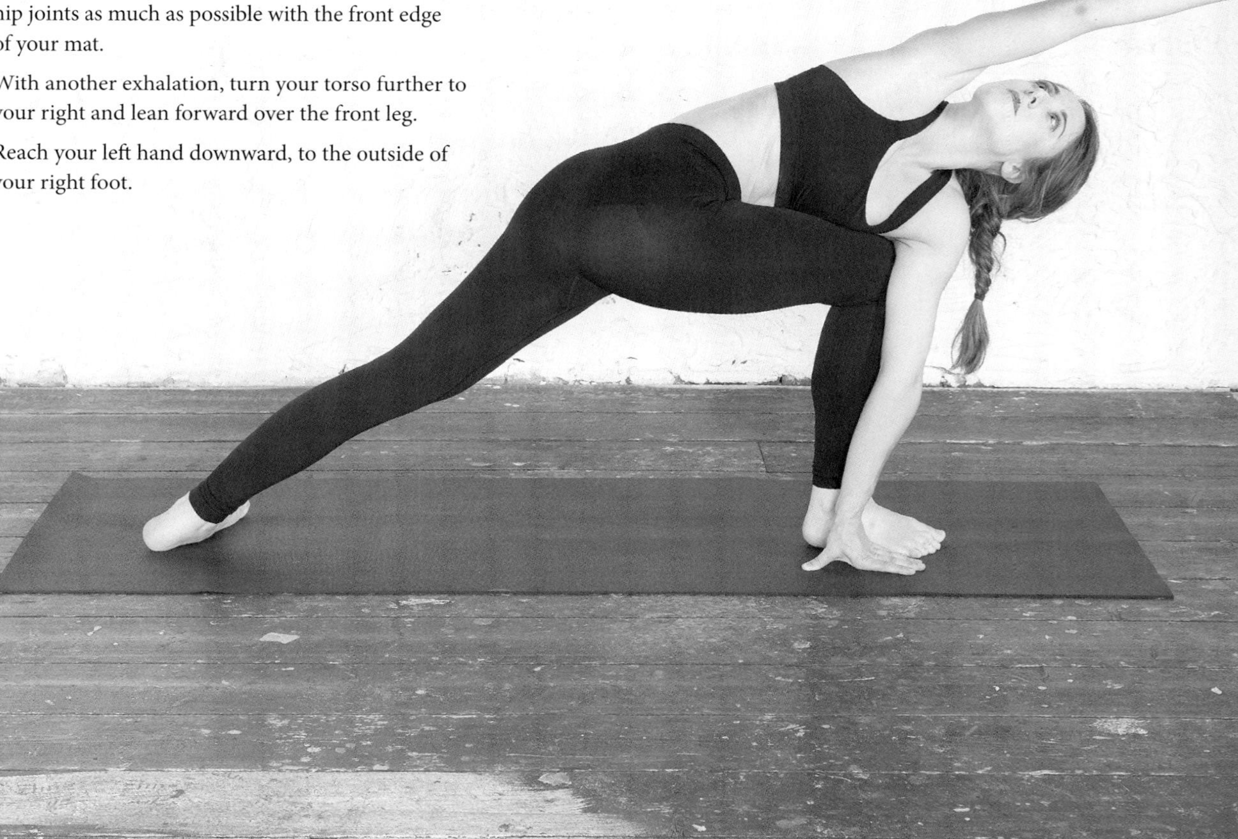

Next pose

Continue with Tree Pose or a variation thereof.

Alignment cues

The kneecap of the bent leg is slightly behind or right above the center of the ankle. Maintain an angle of at least 90 degrees. Ideally, the inside of your bent thigh should be parallel with the long edge of your mat.

Keep the back heel firmly grounded into the floor.

Stretch from your back heel all the way through your extended arm's fingertips, lengthening the entire side of your body. At the same time, try to create as much length along the other side of your torso as well.

Draw your shoulder blades downward toward the waist and keep the back of your neck elongated.

Contraindications & cautions

- Lower-back issues and spinal issues
- Hamstring and groin issues
- Hypertension: Keep your head elevated above heart level by using a block underneath your lower hand
- Abdominal issues

Modifications & adjustments

This is quite an intense pose. It requires a deep twist and quite some flexibility in your legs and groin. To make it slightly easier you have two options:

- You can press the bent elbow against the outside of the bent knee, but do not straighten the arm. Then bend the top elbow and press your palms together.
- You can also allow your back heel to lift off the floor or even place the back knee on the floor and then go for the deep twist, placing your hand on the floor at the outer edge of your front foot.

If your neck feels tight or painful or if you feel dizzy easily or have high blood pressure, look straight ahead, with the sides of your neck lengthened evenly, or look down at the floor.

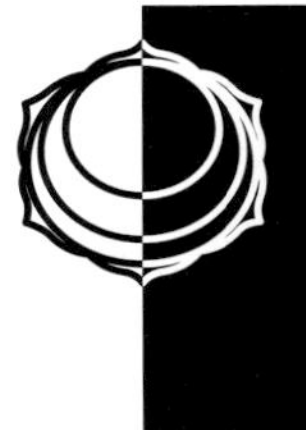

Trikonasana (Triangle Pose) Alternatives

Parshvottanasana

Intense Side-Stretch Pose

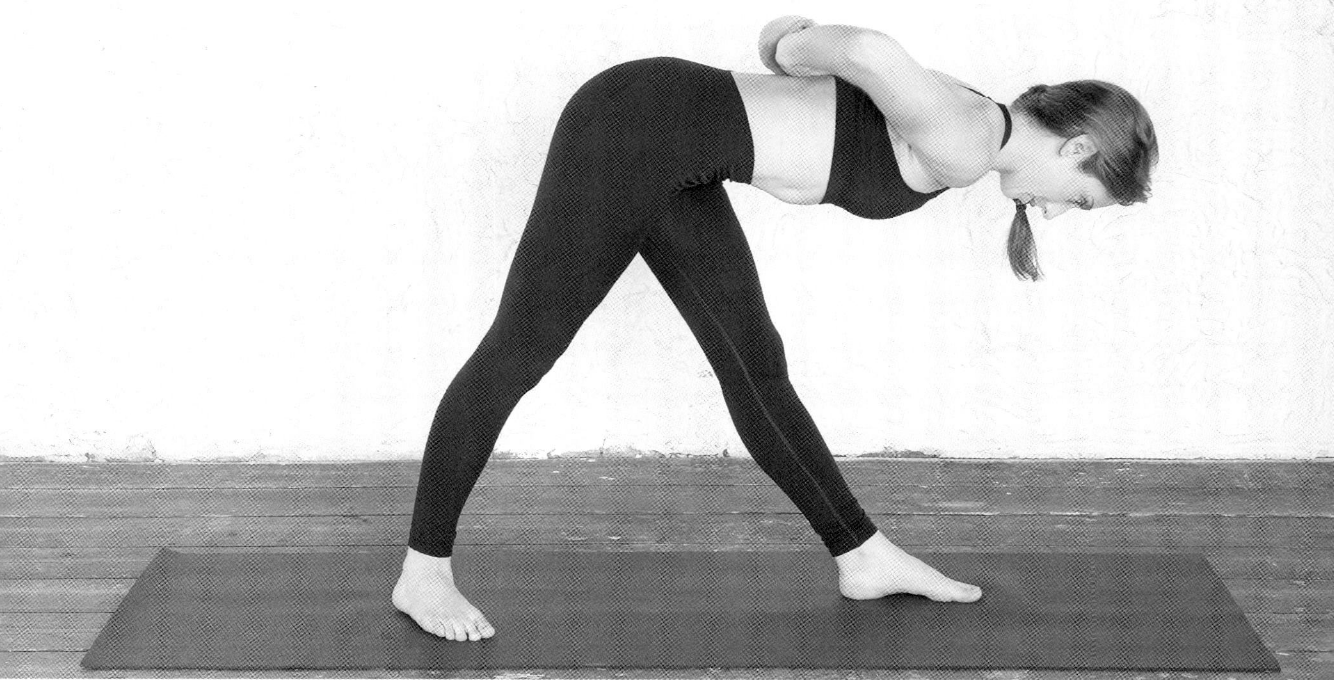

How to come into the pose

Stand on your mat, with your feet wide and parallel (just about below your elbows, when your arms are extended sideways).

Raise your arms parallel to the floor and reach them actively out to the sides, shoulder blades wide, palms facing downward.

Turn your right foot 45 to 60 degrees to your left and your left foot out to your left, 90 degrees. Align your left heel with your right heel.

Breathe out and turn your torso to your left, squaring your hip joints as much as possible with the front edge of your mat.

Bring your palms together behind your shoulder blades, as high up as possible (in the Reverse Prayer position).

Breathe in to lift your chest, breathe out, then elongate your spine forward as you fold from your hips.

Reach with your chin toward your left shin and hold steadily as long as comfortable, breathing evenly.

To release the pose, reach out through the crown of your head and bring your upper body upright again. Bring your feet parallel to each other, release your arms, and take a few breaths before proceeding on the other side.

Next pose

Continue with Tree Pose or a variation thereof.

Alignment cues

Keep your spine elongated, reaching in opposition with your tailbone and crown of your head.

Keep both your legs engaged and rotated externally.

Allow the hip of the back leg to drop slightly toward the floor and focus on lengthening your entire spine, from your tailbone up and out through the crown of your head.

Keep your collarbones wide, pressing your palms against each other and rolling your shoulders backward.

Contraindications & cautions

- Lower-back issues and spinal issues: Support your hands against a block on the floor or a wall in front of you and keep your torso parallel to the floor
- Hamstring and groin issues
- Hypertension: Support your hands against a block on the floor or a wall in front of you and keep your torso parallel to the floor
- Shoulder or wrist issues

Modifications & adjustments

If bringing your palms together is challenging, simply cross your arms behind your back, parallel to your waist. Hold each elbow with the opposite hand.

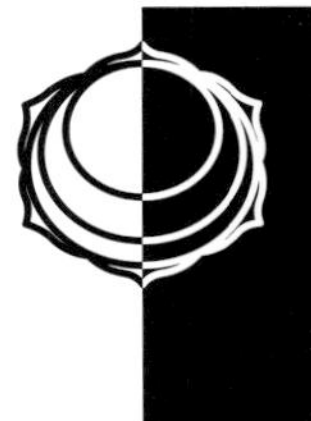

Variations

Parshvottanasana II
Intense Side-Stretch Pose II

Follow the first few steps as explained on the left. Instead of bringing your hands behind your back, simply place them on the floor next to your feet and fold forward, nose reaching toward your knee or shin. Keep both legs straight. If reaching the floor is not accessible you can support your hands against your front shin.

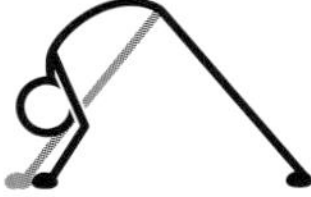

PRASARITA PADOTTANASANA A

WIDE-LEGGED FORWARD BEND A

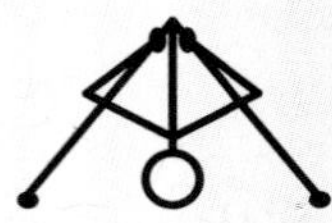

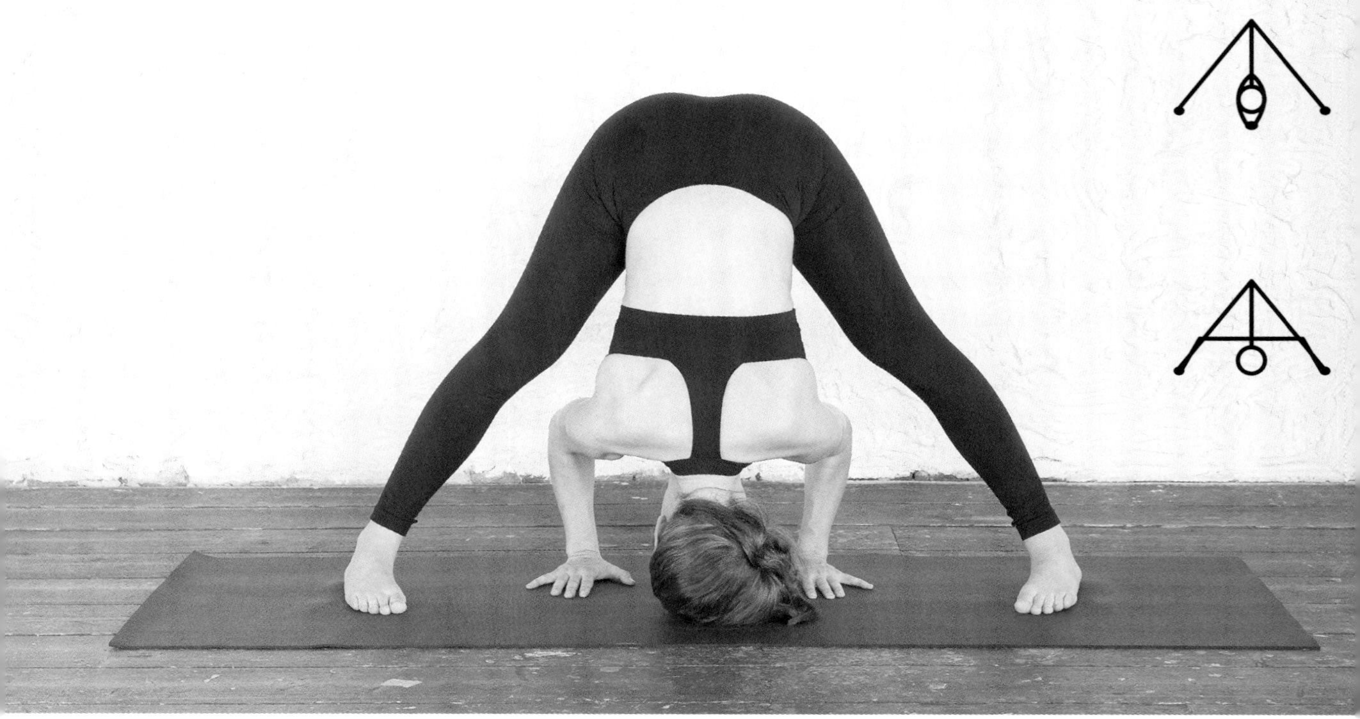

HOW TO COME INTO THE POSE

Stand on your mat, with your feet wide and parallel (a little wider than your elbows, when your arms are extended sideways).

Place your hands on your waist, breathe in, and lift your chest, making the front of your torso slightly longer than the back.

Breathe out, and, maintaining the length of the front torso, lean your torso forward from the hip joints. As your torso approaches being parallel to the floor, press your fingertips onto the floor directly below your shoulders.

Bring your head up, keeping the back of your neck elongated, and direct your gaze forward or upward toward the ceiling.

Then breathe out and bend your elbows and lower your torso and head into a full forward bend.

Walk your hands back until your forearms are perpendicular to the floor.

Hold the pose steadily as long as comfortable and breathe evenly.

To come out of the pose, lift your chest and straighten your arms. Bring your hands to your waist again, and, reaching out through the crown of your head, come up all the way into an upright position.

Next pose

Continue with Tree Pose or a variation thereof.

Alignment cues

Make sure your outer feet are parallel to each other. Keep your legs active and your weight evenly distributed across the bottom of each foot.

Widen your shoulder blades across your back and draw your shoulders away from your ears.

Make sure as you move down that you keep your front torso as long as possible. If possible rest the crown of your head on the floor.

Your neck is an extension of your spine, so keep it lengthening as you move more deeply into the pose.

Contraindications & cautions

- Lower-back issues and spinal issues: Support your hands against a block on the floor or a wall in front of you and keep your torso parallel to the floor
- Hamstring and groin issues
- Hypertension: Support your hands against a block on the floor or a wall in front of you and keep your torso parallel to the floor

Modifications & adjustments

If hamstrings and buttocks are very tight, bend your knees a little so there is not too much pressure on your lower back. When you bend your knees, keep your legs active and do not allow your knees to drop inwards.

Variations

Prasarita Padottanasana B

Wide-Legged Forward Bend B

Instead of placing your palms on the floor as you bend forward, keep your hands firmly on your waist. Widen the chest and pull the elbows toward each other as you reach out through the crown of your head toward the floor.

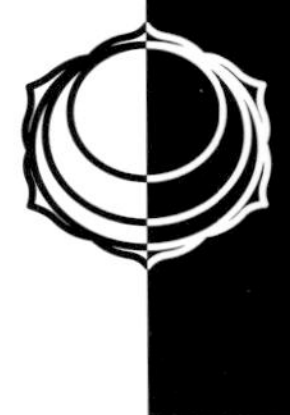

Prasarita Padottanasana C

Wide-Legged Forward Bend C

Before bending forward, clasp your arms behind your back, palms facing inward. Straighten your arms, push your hands away, and fold forward. Reach with the crown of your head toward the floor and allow your arms to gently drop over your head toward the floor.

Prasarita Padottanasana D

Wide-Legged Forward Bend D

As you bend forward, clasp your big toes with 2 fingers of each hand. Keep your wrists and elbows lifted as you reach with the crown of your head toward the floor.

UTTANASANA
STANDING FORWARD-BEND POSE

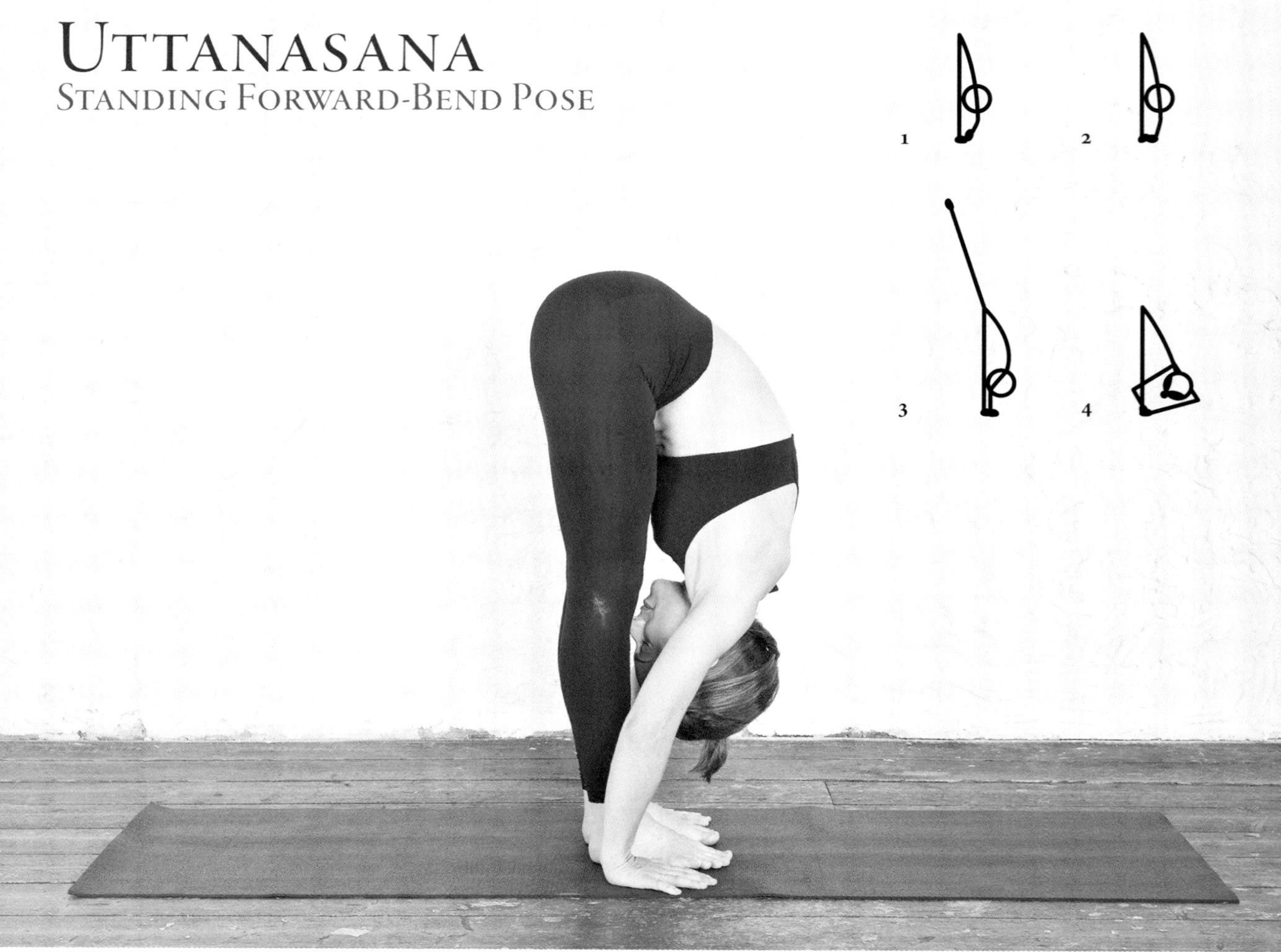

HOW TO COME INTO THE POSE

Stand on your mat, with your feet together or hip-width apart.

Breathe out and bend forward from the hip joints, not from your waist.

With your knees straight, bring your palms or fingertips to the floor slightly in front of or beside your feet.

With each inhalation in the pose, lift and lengthen the front torso just slightly; with each exhalation release a little more fully into the forward bend.

Hold steadily as long as comfortable and breathe evenly.

To come out of the pose, bend your knees until your torso touches your thighs. Then press your heels into the floor and roll your spine upward, vertebra by vertebra. Your shoulders and head come up last.

Next pose

Continue with Tree Pose or a variation thereof.

Alignment cues

Focus on lengthening the front torso as you move more fully into the pose.

Press your heels firmly into the floor and lift your sitting bones toward the ceiling. Turn the tops of your thighs slightly inward.

Let your head hang from the root of your neck, which is deep in the upper back, between your shoulder blades.

Contraindications & cautions

- Hypertension
- Lower-back and spinal issues

Modifications & adjustments

Classically this pose is performed with feet together. To create more space to move into this pose, you can keep your feet hip-width apart.

Instead of placing your palms on the floor you can also hold the backs of your ankles. If this is not possible, cross your forearms and hold your elbows.

If your hamstrings are tight or you feel strain in your lower back, bend your knees slightly.

Variations

1 - Padangusthasana

Big-Toe Pose

After bending forward, hold on to your big toes. With an inhalation, straighten your arms and lift your front torso away from your thighs, making your back as concave as possible. Then breathe out and lengthen down and forward, bending your elbows out to the sides. Draw your shoulder blades away from your ears and reach with the crown of your head toward the floor.

2 -Padahastasana

Hand-Under-Foot Pose

After bending forward, slide your hands underneath the soles of your feet, with the backs of your hands against the floor. With an inhalation, straighten your arms and lift your front torso away from your thighs, making your back as concave as possible. Then breathe out and lengthen down and forward, bending your elbows out to the sides. Draw your shoulder blades away from your ears and reach with the crown of your head toward the floor.

3 - Eka Pada Uttanasana

One-Legged Standing Forward Bend

Come into a Standing Forward Bend, with your feet hip-width apart. Place your right hand in between your feet on the floor and your left hand along the outer edge of your left foot. Shift your weight to your left foot, and, with an inhalation, raise your right leg up toward the ceiling. Firmly press your hands into the floor, reach up and out through the ball of your right foot, and reach with your nose toward your left knee or shin. Release your right foot down to the floor and repeat on the other side.

4 - Parivrtta Uttanasana

Revolved Standing Forward Bend

From Standing Forward Bend, hold on to your right big toe with your left hand and hold your left big toe with your right hand (right arm is crossing above your left arm). Breathe in and lengthen your spine, gently pulling your crown toward the floor. Breathe out and twist your upper body to your right. Look under your right arm to the ceiling, and reach with your left elbow toward the outside of your right knee or shin. To come out of the pose, bring your upper body back to the center, release your hands, and slowly roll upward. Repeat the same on the other side, with your left arm above your right arm, twisting to your left.

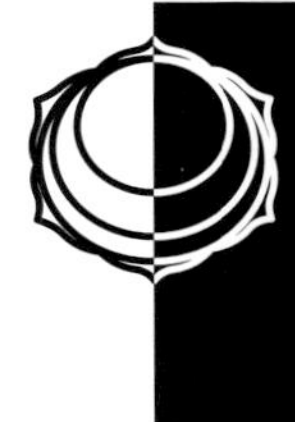

Ardha Baddha Padmottanasana

Half Bound-Lotus Standing Forward Bend

How to come into the pose

Start in a standing position, with your feet hip-width apart.

Shift your weight firmly downwards onto your left foot.

Moving slowly, bend your right knee up toward your chest. Raise your right foot, and gently bring your right heel to rest as high as you can on the front of your left thigh or hip, into a Half Lotus Position. The sole of your foot should be facing the ceiling, and the top of your foot should rest on your leg or hip. (Caution: Do not use any force, and attempt this only if you are experienced in folding safely into Half Lotus.)

Gently allow your right knee to drop toward the floor, until eventually it will be parallel to the other knee.

Hold on to your right foot with your left hand. Lengthen your spine. Inhale, and reach your right arm toward the ceiling. Then reach it behind your back and clasp your right toes with your right hand.

Inhale and lift your left arm straight upward. Exhaling, fold forward, hinging at your hips. Place your left hand on the floor. Draw your chin toward your chest and concentrate on bringing your forehead to your shin.

Hold the pose steadily as long as comfortable and breathe evenly.

To release the pose, breathe in, bend your left leg, and press down firmly through your left foot as you lift your torso back to an upright position. Unbind your right arm, then gently release your foot to the floor.

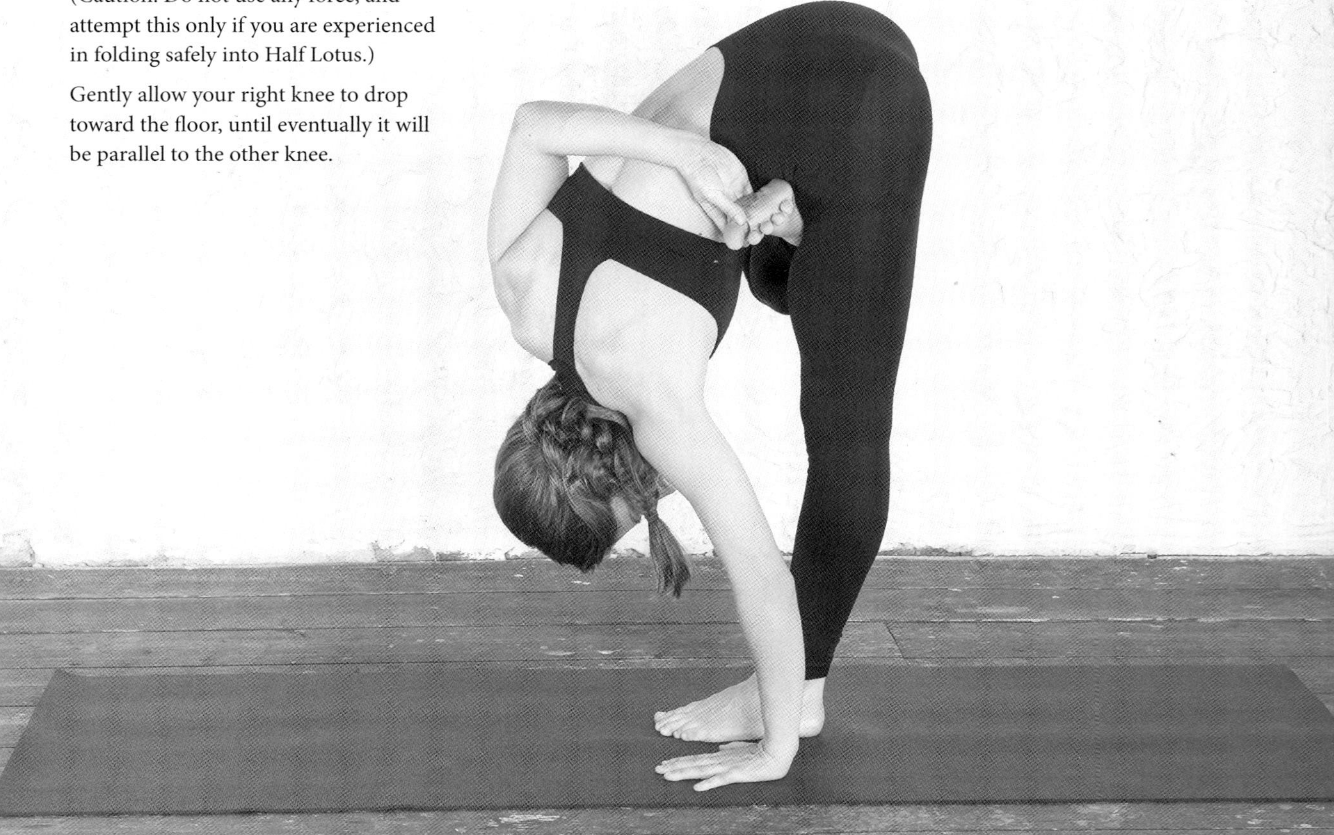

Next pose

Continue with Tree Pose or a variation thereof.

Alignment cues

You should not feel any strain or pain in your knee; if you do, back off a little or release the pose entirely.

Elongate your spine by reaching out through the crown of your head and drawing your shoulder blades away from your ears.

Keep your neck relaxed and your shoulders parallel to the floor.

Contraindications & cautions

- Knee or hamstring issues
- Hypertension
- Lower-back and spinal issues
- Abdominal issues

Modifications & adjustments

If you cannot clasp the toes of your foot with the same-side hand, catch hold with the opposite hand and then reach behind your back to hold the elbow. In this case, do not bend forward.

Keep the standing leg straight. If the standing leg bends when you fold forward, practice the upright version until you have built up enough strength to fold with a straight leg.

If you cannot touch your fingers or your palm to the floor, place your hand on a block.

If coming into Half Lotus is not accessible, simply cross the right ankle over the top of your left knee (push out through the heel). Now, bending your standing knee, fold your upper body forward with your hands in front of your chest in Prayer position.

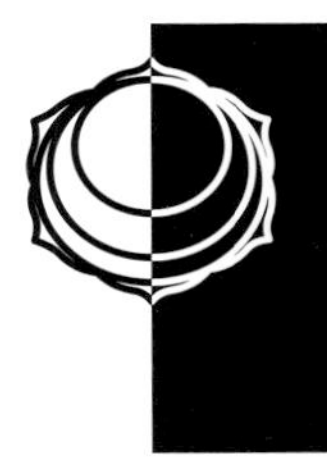

Chapter 17

Variations for the Root Chakra

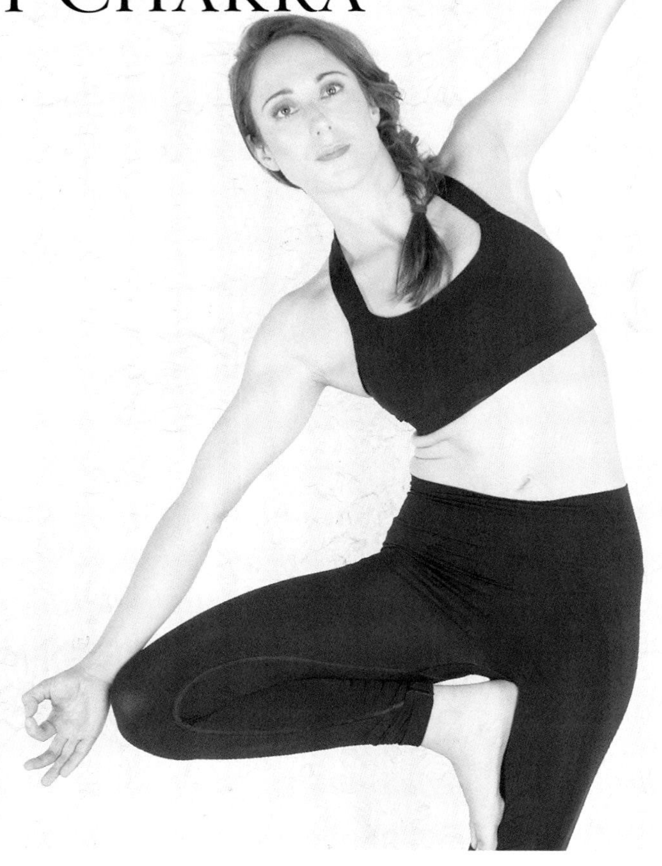

Vrkshasana (Tree Pose) Variations

Parshva Vrkshasana
Bending Tree Pose

How to come into the pose

Stand straight, with your feet together.

Shift your weight to your left foot, and with the help of your right hand, place your right foot high up along your left inner thigh.

Spread your arms sideways, slightly below shoulder level, keeping your palms facing forward.

Breathe in, elongate your spine, and reach out through your fingertips.

Breathe out and start to bend your torso sideways, keeping your arms in the fixed position.

Keep tilting until your right arm rests lightly on the top of your right knee.

Look at a point in front of you and breathe evenly.

Hold the pose steadily as long as comfortable, then, to release the pose, lead with your left hand to bring your torso back to center, release your arms and legs, and proceed to the other side.

Next pose

Continue with Mountain Pose or a variation thereof.

Alignment cues

Your foot should ideally be placed against the opposite inner thigh.

The knee of the upper foot is pointing sideways, rotating the leg in the hip joint without lifting your hip upward.

As you tilt to the side, aim to keep both sides of your torso elongated.

Keep the back of your neck elongated and shoulder down toward your waist.

Contraindications & cautions

The same contraindications and cautions apply as in Tree Pose.

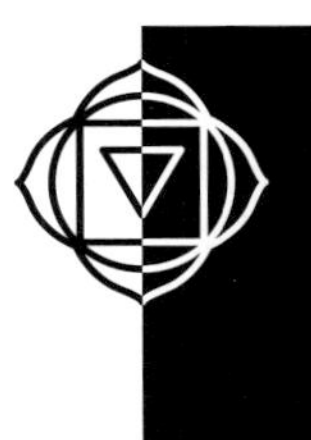

Ardha Padma Vrkshasana
Half-Lotus Tree Pose

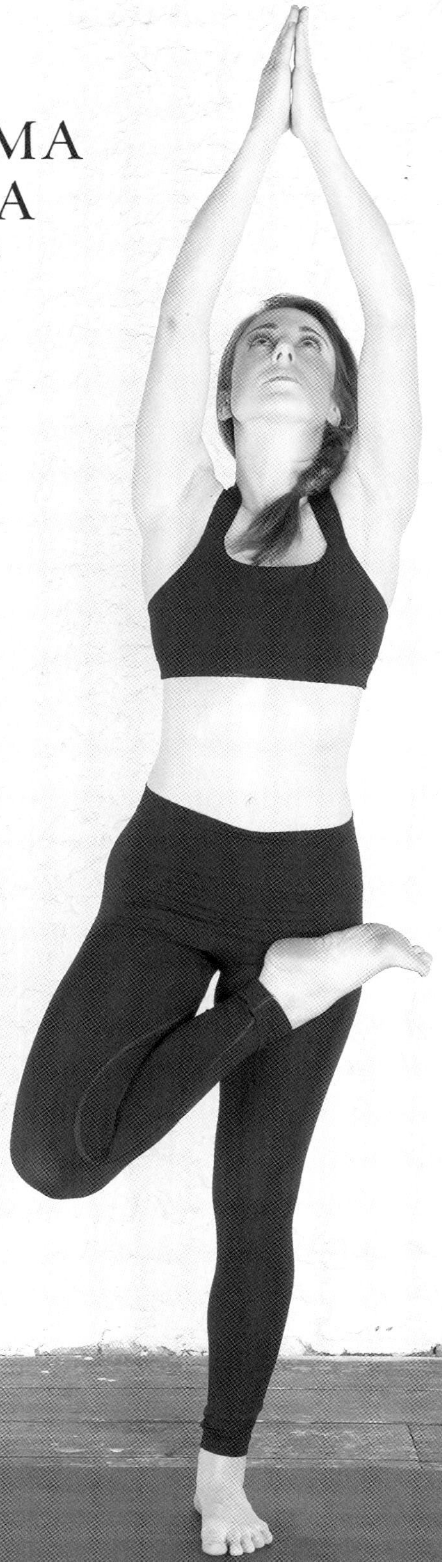

How to come into the pose

Start in a standing position, with your feet hip-width apart.

Shift your weight down firmly onto your left foot and the floor.

Moving slowly, bend your right knee upward toward your chest. Raise your right foot and gently bring your right heel to rest as high as you can on the front of your left thigh or hip, into a Half Lotus position. The sole of your foot should be facing the ceiling, and the top of your foot should rest on your leg or hip. (Caution: Do not use any force and attempt this only if you are experienced in folding safely into Half Lotus.)

Gently allow your right knee to drop toward the floor, until eventually it will be parallel to the other knee.

Bring your hands in front of your chest, in the Prayer position. Once you are stable here, raise your hands up toward the ceiling, keeping them in line with your forehead.

Look up toward your hands or gaze at a focal point at your eye level and breathe evenly.

Hold the pose steadily as long as comfortable.

To release, bring your hands down to your chest, unwind your right foot, and come into a standing position on both feet again. Then repeat on the other side.

Next pose

Continue to Mountain Pose or a variation thereof.

Alignment cues

Make sure to generate the rotation at your hip joint as you fold your leg into Half Lotus position. Do not torque your knee!

Elongate your spine. You can imagine that you are trying to touch the ceiling with your skull.

Do not keep the raised foot in place by sticking out your buttocks. Instead, release your tailbone toward the floor and maintain alignment through your spine.

Do not force the knee of the raised foot backward. Avoid any strain or pull in your knee region.

Contraindications & cautions

The same contraindications and cautions apply as in Tree Pose. Also be cautious in this pose if you have tight hips, or knee or ankle issues.

Modifications & adjustments

If your foot does not reach the upper thigh of the opposite leg or keeps slipping down, you have to work on your hip rotation first. Do not try to keep your foot up by sticking your buttocks out or forcing your knee down. Rather, cradle your lower leg and find your balance like that.

If a standing-leg cradle is also not accessible, practice the classical Tree Pose with your foot pressing against the opposite inner leg.

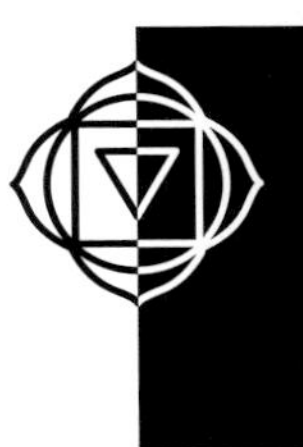

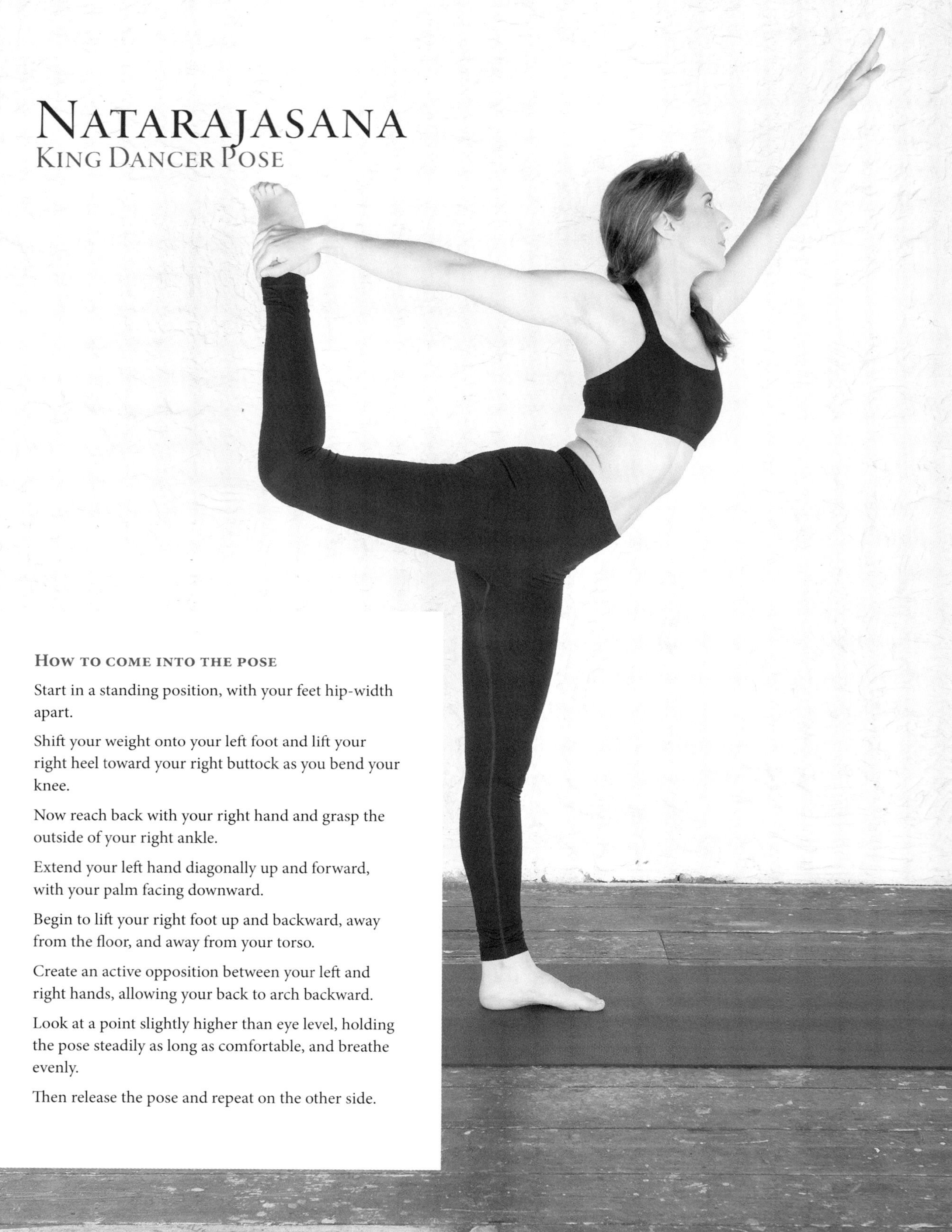

Natarajasana
King Dancer Pose

How to come into the pose

Start in a standing position, with your feet hip-width apart.

Shift your weight onto your left foot and lift your right heel toward your right buttock as you bend your knee.

Now reach back with your right hand and grasp the outside of your right ankle.

Extend your left hand diagonally up and forward, with your palm facing downward.

Begin to lift your right foot up and backward, away from the floor, and away from your torso.

Create an active opposition between your left and right hands, allowing your back to arch backward.

Look at a point slightly higher than eye level, holding the pose steadily as long as comfortable, and breathe evenly.

Then release the pose and repeat on the other side.

Next pose

Continue with Mountain Pose or a variation thereof.

Alignment cues

Aim to keep your hips square. Imagine that you want to keep the inner sides of your knees parallel to each other.

Avoid dipping your upper body forward, but rather aim to create a standing backbend, with your upper body as upright as possible.

Keep the elbow of the arm that is holding your foot straight, and push your foot into your hand. This will allow you to lift up higher into the backward arch.

Keep your core and legs engaged to avoid too much compression in your lower back.

Contraindications & cautions

The same contraindications and cautions apply as in Tree Pose. Also be cautious in this pose if you have spinal issues, pelvic instability, or groin issues.

Variations

Vistrit Natarajasana

Extended King Dancer Pose

Start as described on the left, but instead of holding on to the outside of the right ankle, hold on to the inside. Raise your opposite hand up and then start to push your right foot into your hand. Allow your right shoulder to release backward, extending your back leg as much as you can up toward the ceiling. At the same time, allow your upper body to tip forward until it is almost parallel to the floor. Keep pushing your back foot up toward the ceiling and reach forward and outward with your left hand.

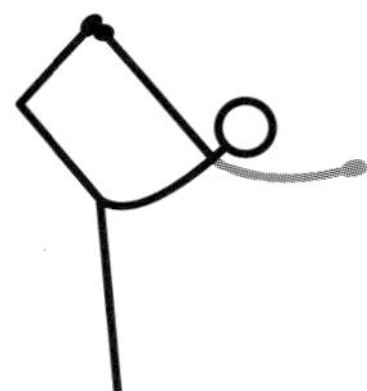

Purna Natarajasana

Full King Dancer Pose

Perform the first two steps as described on the left. Then turn your right arm actively outward so that the palm faces away from the side of your torso. Now bend the elbow and grip your big toe with the first 2 fingers and the thumb. As you breathe in, lift your right leg upward, and bring your thigh parallel to the floor. At the same time, rotate your right shoulder in such a way that the bent elbow swings around and upward, pointing toward the ceiling. Extend your left hand diagonally up in front of you.

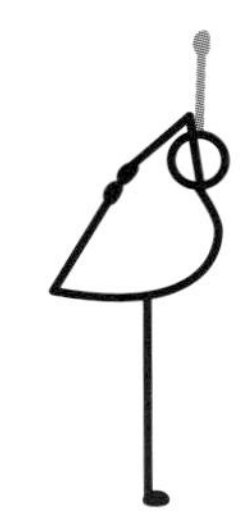

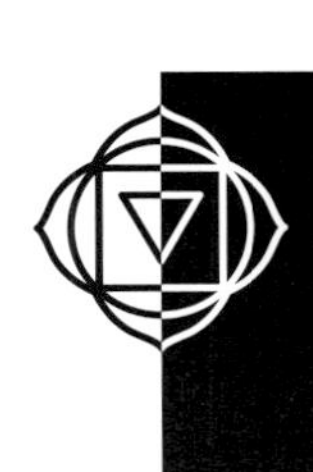

Garudasana
Eagle Pose

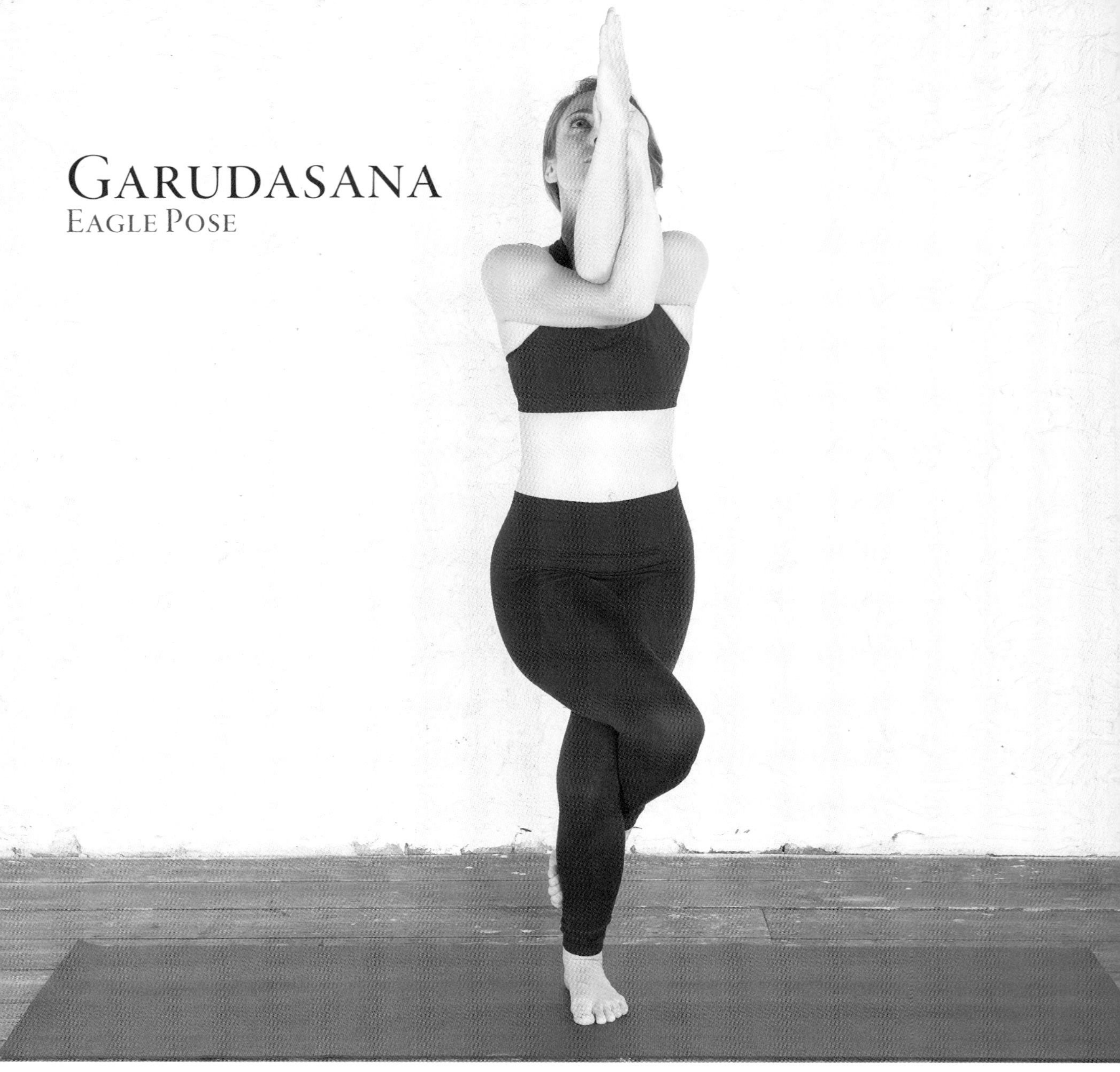

How to come into the pose

Stand on your mat, with your feet hip-width apart.

Bend both knees slightly, then lift your right foot upward and balance on your left foot.

Now cross your right thigh over your left. Point your right toes toward the floor, press your foot back, and then hook the top of your foot behind your lower left calf.

Stretch your left arm straight forward, parallel to the floor.

Now wrap your right arm from below around your left arm and bring your palms against each other, as parallel as possible.

Bring your forearms perpendicular to the floor.

Hold the pose steadily for as long as comfortable, while looking at your hands or a focal point straight in front of you and breathing evenly.

Then unwind your legs and arms and come into an easy standing position again. Repeat for the same length of time with your arms and legs reversed.

Next pose

Continue with Mountain Pose or a variation thereof.

Alignment cues

Keep your shoulder blades wide and drawn toward your waist.

Come as low as you can, without sticking your buttocks out, but aiming for a shoulder-over-hips and hips-over-ankle alignment.

Contraindications & cautions

The same contraindications and cautions apply as in Tree Pose. Also be cautious in this pose if you have tight hips, spinal issues, or pelvic instability.

Modifications & adjustments

If crossing your foot behind your calf is not accessible, simply cross your legs at your thighs, without hooking your foot.

If balancing is challenging, cross your legs at your thighs and press the big toe of the raised-leg foot against the floor to help maintain your balance.

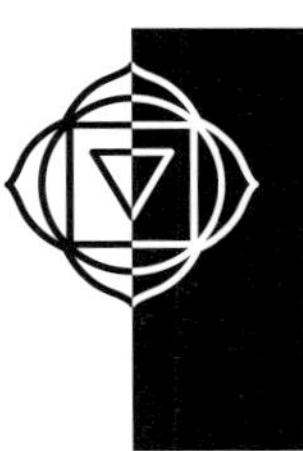

Utthita Hasta Padangusthasana

Extended Hand-to-Big-Toe Pose

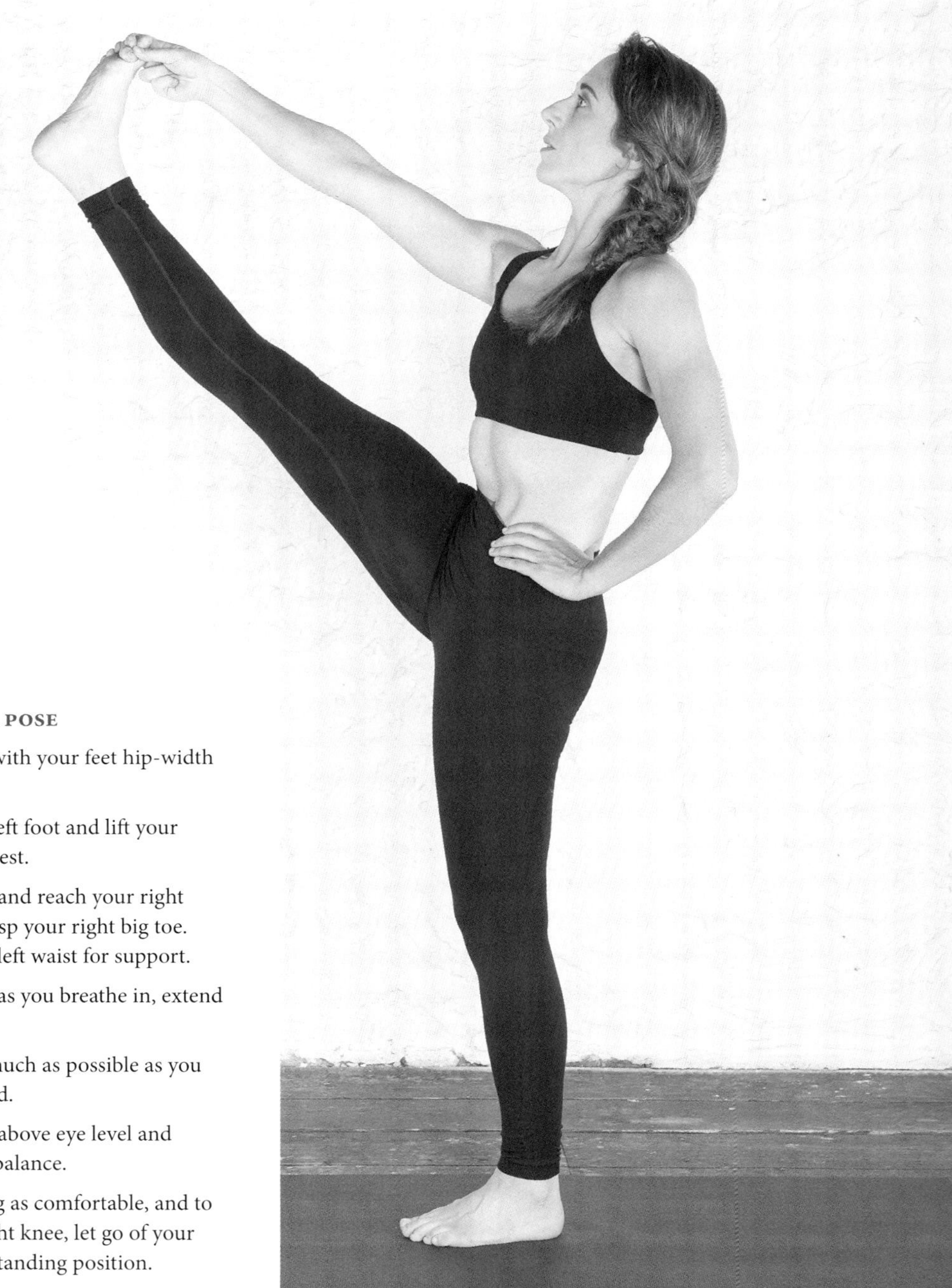

How to come into the pose

Start in a standing position, with your feet hip-width apart.

Shift your weight onto your left foot and lift your right knee up toward your chest.

Hug your knee to your chest and reach your right arm outside your thigh to clasp your right big toe. Place your left hand on your left waist for support.

Firm your standing leg, and, as you breathe in, extend your right leg forward.

Straighten your right leg as much as possible as you push your foot into your hand.

Look at a focal point slightly above eye level and breathe steadily to maintain balance.

Hold the pose steadily as long as comfortable, and to release slightly bend your right knee, let go of your toes, and come into an easy standing position.

Next pose

Continue with Mountain Pose or a variation thereof.

Alignment cues

Create opposition by also clasping your toe around your fingers.

Ideally, both legs should be straight. The standing leg should definitely be straight and firm, without hyperextending your knee (locking your knee).

Keep your back straight, shoulders back, and neck elongated.

Use your other hand to firmly grasp your waist for extra stabilization.

Make sure to keep both hips squared forward.

Contraindications & cautions

The same contraindications and cautions apply as in Tree Pose. Also be cautious in this pose if you have tight hips, spinal issues, or pelvic instability.

Modifications & adjustments

If you cannot keep your back straight, bend the knee of your lifted leg until you can.

If your grip around the toe is uncomfortable or not steady, you can also hold the side of your foot.

Variations

Utthita Hasta Padangusthasana A

Extended Hand-to-Big-Toe Pose A

Follow the instructions on the left. Once you are steady in the pose, fold your torso forward toward your lifted leg. Reach with your chin toward your shin, and keep your neck elongated, shoulders drawn away from your ears.

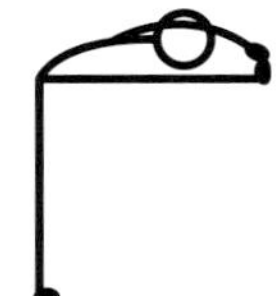

Utthita Hasta Padangusthasana B

Extended Hand-to-Big-Toe Pose B

Follow the basic instructions as described on the left. Once you are steady and comfortable, swing your right leg out to your right side. Keep your fingers locked around your big toe. Turn your head to your left and gaze out at the horizon, beyond your left shoulder.

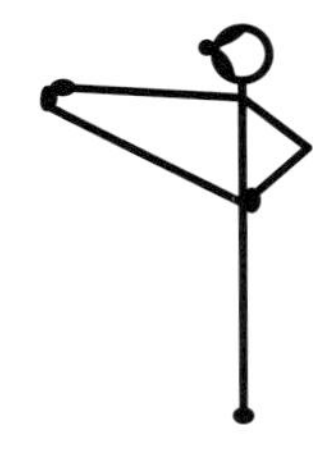

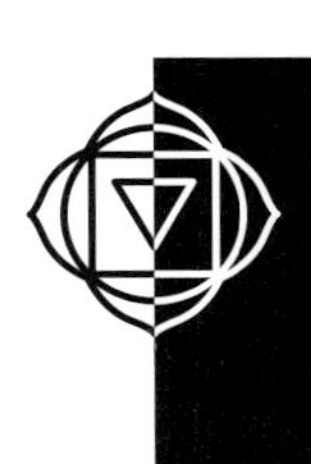

Tuladandasana
Balancing-Stick Pose

How to come into the pose

Start in a standing position, with your feet hip-width apart.

Breathe in and raise your arms to the ceiling, palms facing toward each other.

Step forward with your right foot.

Now slowly transfer all your weight onto your right foot as you begin to lift your left foot off the floor. Focus on keeping your spine straight at all times.

Continue to raise your left leg straight into the air behind you as you bend forward.

Look at a point below you on the floor, keeping the back of your neck elongated and reaching out through your fingertips and the heel of the foot of the back leg.

Hold the balance and breathe evenly, then release and come back to an easy standing position before proceeding to the other side.

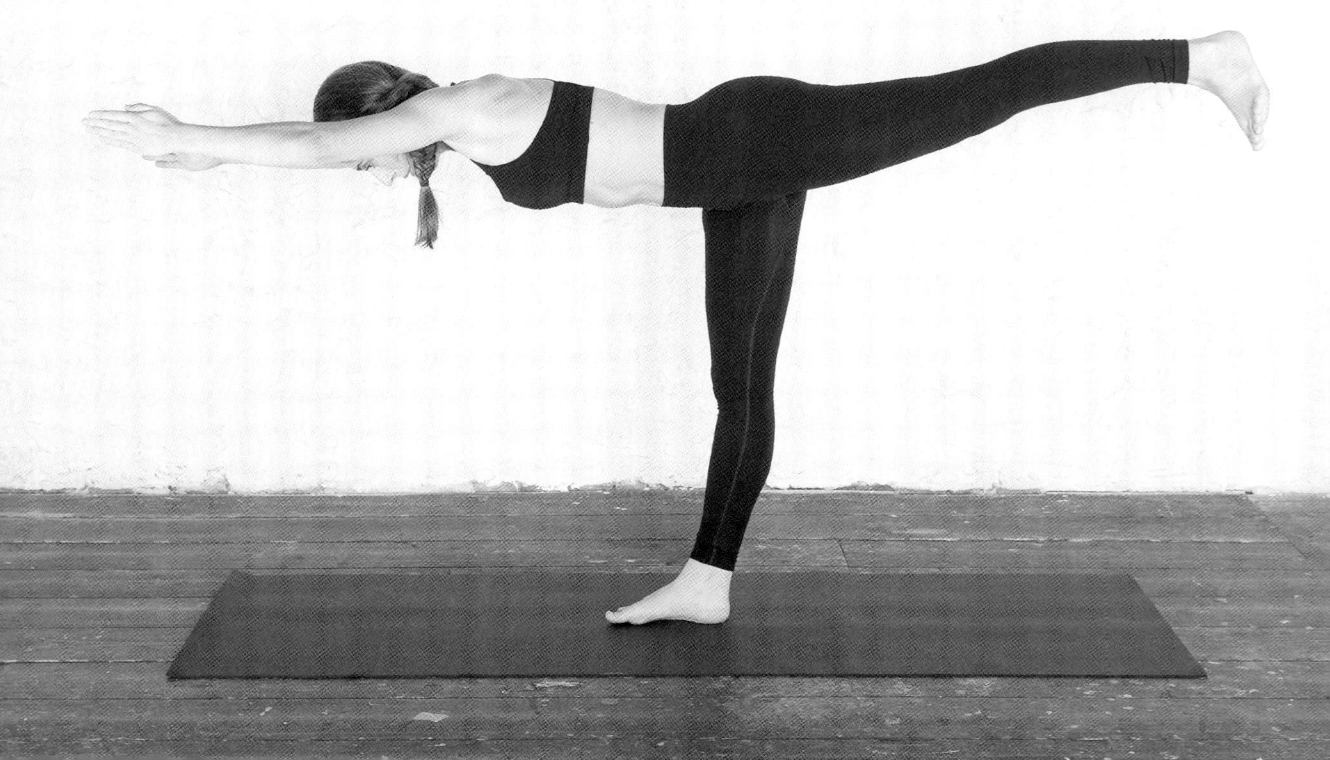

Next pose

Continue to Mountain Pose or a variation thereof.

Alignment cues

Keep your neck elongated and shoulder blades drawn down your back toward your waist.

Your arms, torso, and raised leg should be positioned relatively parallel to the floor. If your pelvis tilts, release the hip of the raised leg toward the floor until the two hip joints are even and parallel to the floor.

Keep your weight distributed evenly over the entire sole of the standing foot.

Keep the front part of your standing leg active to prevent your knee from locking or hyperextending.

Activate the back leg and extend it strongly toward the wall behind you; reach just as actively in the opposite direction with your arms.

Contraindications & cautions

The same contraindications and cautions apply as in Tree Pose.

Modifications & adjustments

You can also keep your hands folded in front of your chest, in Prayer position, or your arms alongside your body. In this case create the opposition between the heel of the back leg's foot and the crown of your head.

If balancing is challenging, use a chair or the wall as a balancing support underneath your hands.

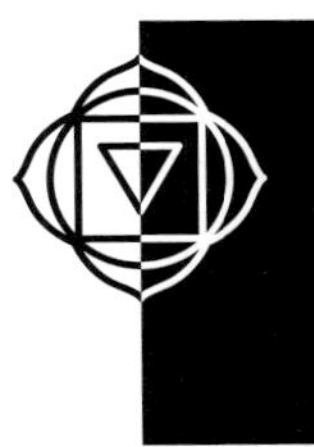

Svarga Dvijasana
Bird of Paradise Pose

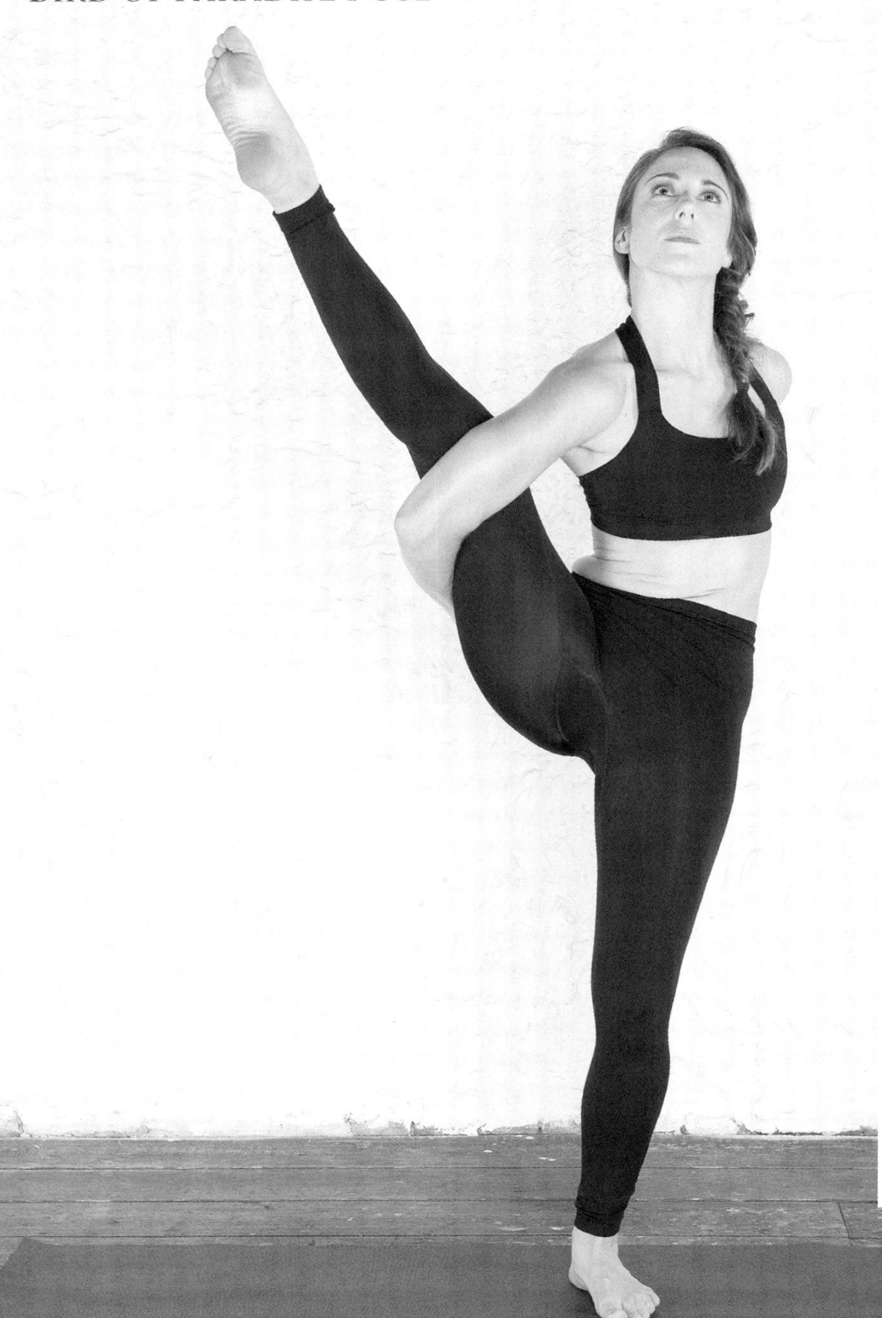

How to come into the pose

Start in Standing Forward Bend, with your feet shoulder-width apart and your right heel lifted.

Now hold your right calf with your right hand and slide your right shoulder behind your right knee.

Keep your shoulder in this position, then wrap your right hand behind your back, with your palm facing the ceiling. Take your left hand behind your back and clasp your hands.

Shift your weight to your left foot and pause there for a moment, with your right toe touching the floor lightly.

Then breathe in and start to slowly straighten your left leg and lift your torso into an upright position. Keep your right knee bent as you pull yourself upward.

Once you are stable in the upright position, gently extend your right leg as far as possible.

Look at a point just above your eye level and breathe evenly.

Hold the pose steadily as long as comfortable, then gently bend your right leg again, release your grip, and come into an easy standing position. From here fold forward again and repeat on the other side.

Next pose

Continue with Mountain Pose or a variation thereof.

Alignment cues

Keep your standing leg straight and active, without locking your knee.

Keep your primary focus on finding a firm and stable balance with your standing leg. As a further step only, explore your other leg's capacity to straighten out. It is okay to keep the upper leg bent.

Work on bringing your spine into a straight-upright position, with your collarbones wide and chest open.

Contraindications & cautions

The same contraindications and cautions apply as in Tree Pose. Also be cautious in this pose if you have shoulder issues, tight hamstrings, groin issues, lower-back issues, or pelvic instability.

Modifications & adjustments

If you cannot reach your hands to bind, use a strap to connect.

If finding the balance is challenging, practice with your back close to a wall.

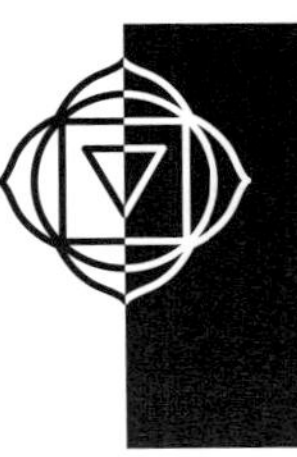

Vrkshasana (Tree Pose) Alternatives

VIRABHADRASANA I

WARRIOR POSE I

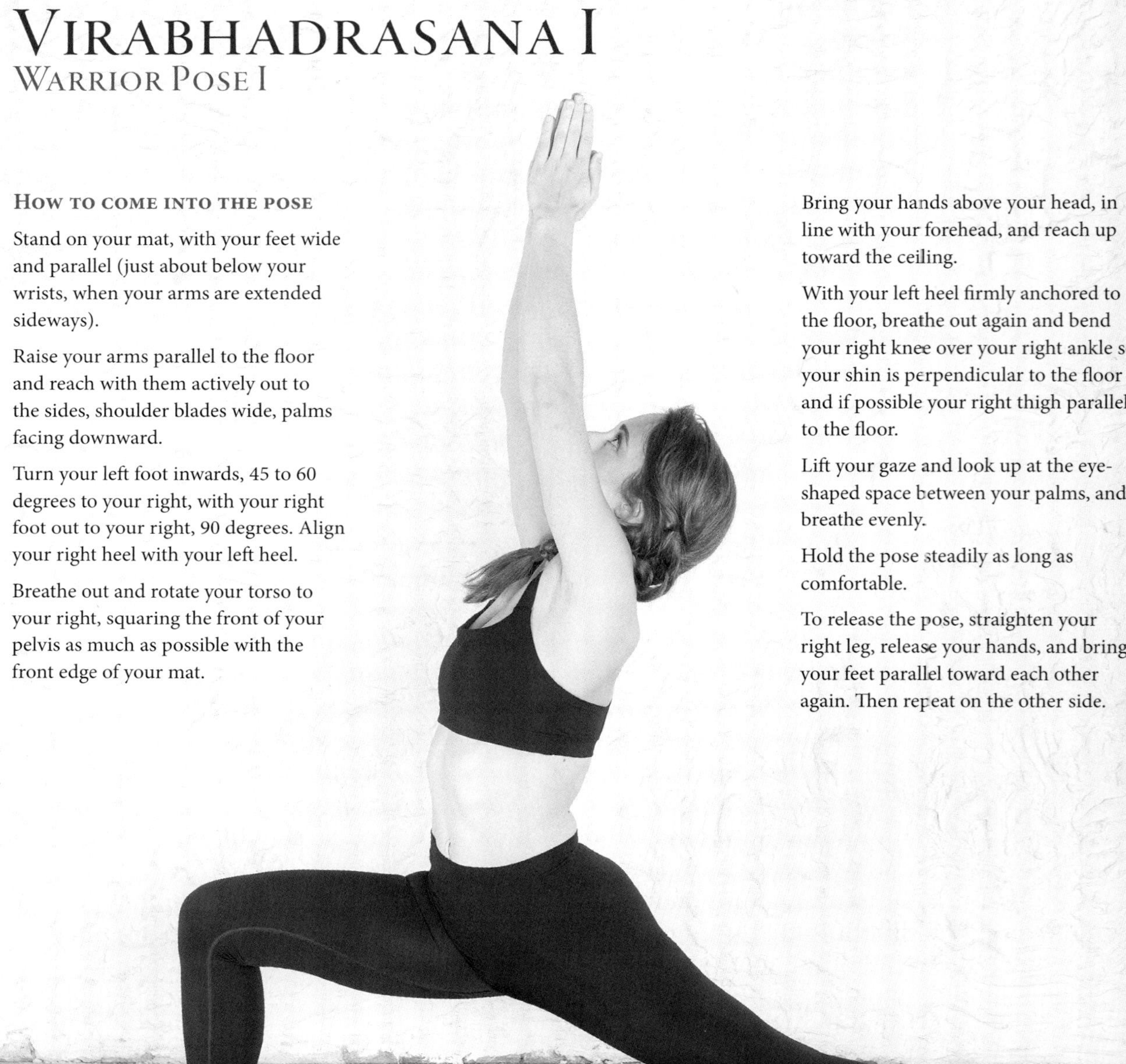

HOW TO COME INTO THE POSE

Stand on your mat, with your feet wide and parallel (just about below your wrists, when your arms are extended sideways).

Raise your arms parallel to the floor and reach with them actively out to the sides, shoulder blades wide, palms facing downward.

Turn your left foot inwards, 45 to 60 degrees to your right, with your right foot out to your right, 90 degrees. Align your right heel with your left heel.

Breathe out and rotate your torso to your right, squaring the front of your pelvis as much as possible with the front edge of your mat.

Bring your hands above your head, in line with your forehead, and reach up toward the ceiling.

With your left heel firmly anchored to the floor, breathe out again and bend your right knee over your right ankle so your shin is perpendicular to the floor and if possible your right thigh parallel to the floor.

Lift your gaze and look up at the eye-shaped space between your palms, and breathe evenly.

Hold the pose steadily as long as comfortable.

To release the pose, straighten your right leg, release your hands, and bring your feet parallel toward each other again. Then repeat on the other side.

Next pose

Continue with Mountain Pose or a variation thereof.

Alignment cues

The kneecap of the bent leg is slightly behind or right above the center of the ankle. Keep an angle of at least 90 degrees.

Aim to keep your hips as square as possible, while keeping your back heel firmly grounded into the floor.

Press down through the outer edge of your back foot, and keep your back leg straight.

Draw your shoulder blades downward toward your waist and keep the back of your neck elongated.

Contraindications & cautions

The same contraindications and cautions apply as in Tree Pose. Also be cautious in this pose if you have hamstring or groin issues.

Modifications & adjustments

If you feel unstable with a heel-to-heel alignment of your feet, you can go for a little gap between your heels.

If you have tightness or pain in your neck, look straight ahead.

If you have shoulder pain, you can keep your arms reaching sideways just below shoulder-blade level.

Variations

Baddha Virabhadrasana I

Humble-Warrior Pose

Come into Warrior I as described on the left. From there, interlock your hands behind your back and open your chest. Now bend forward and, hinging at your hips, reach with your nose toward the shin or ankle of your front (bent) leg.

Ashta Chandrasana

Eight-Point Crescent Moon Pose

Start in Downward-Facing Dog Pose. From here, step your right foot forward between your hands, making sure that your knee ends up over the heel. Keep your left leg straight, heel lifted off the floor and toes pushing firmly down into the floor. Raise your torso to upright. At the same time, sweep your arms wide to the sides and raise them overhead, palms together. Look straight ahead or up toward your hands, without dropping the head.

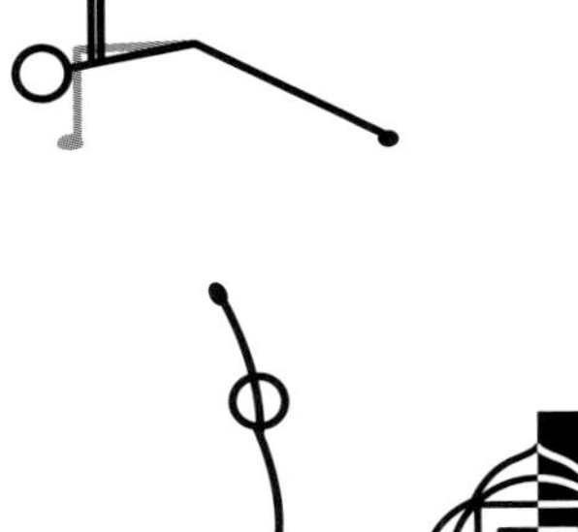

Virabhadrasana II
Warrior Pose II

How to come into the pose

Stand on your mat, with your feet wide and parallel (just about below your wrists, when your arms are extended sideways).

Raise your arms parallel to the floor and reach them actively out to the sides, shoulder blades wide, palms facing downward.

Keep the outer edge of your left foot parallel to the back of your mat and turn your right foot outward to your right, 90 degrees. Make sure to align your right heel with the arch of your left foot.

On an exhalation, bend your front knee. Align your knee directly over the ankle of your front foot.

Turn your head to gaze out across the tip of your right middle finger.

Look straight ahead and breathe evenly, and hold the pose steadily as long as comfortable.

To release the pose, straighten your right leg, release your hands, and bring your feet parallel to each other again. Then repeat on the other side.

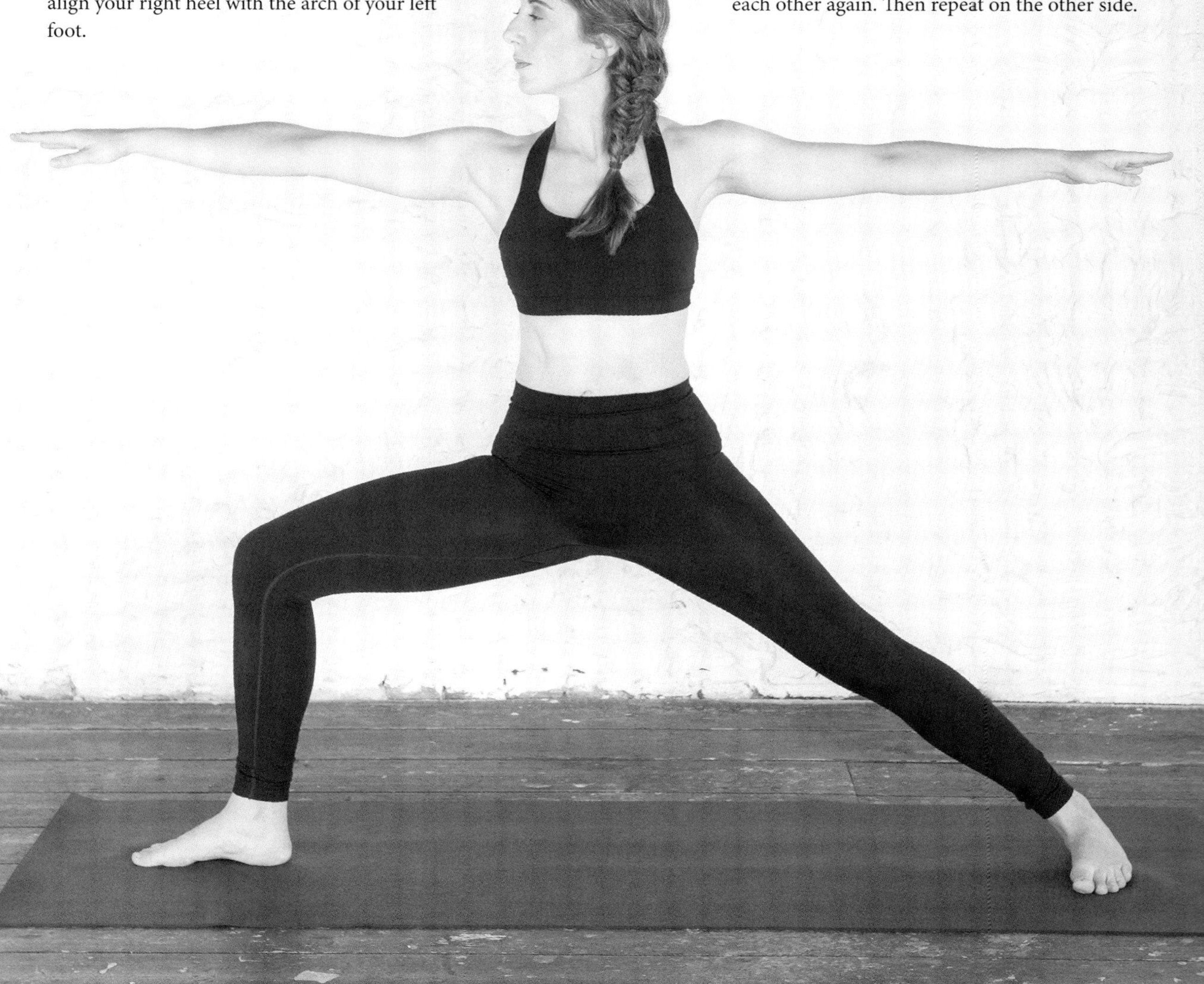

Next pose

Continue with Mountain Pose or a variation thereof.

Alignment cues

Keep your pelvis flat, with both hip joints facing toward the side of your mat (as far as possible without the front knee rolling in).

Your arms should be aligned directly over your legs. With your palms facing downward, reach actively from fingertip to fingertip.

Your front shin should be perpendicular to the floor. Sink your hips low, eventually bringing your front thigh parallel to the floor. Make sure your front shin stays vertical. Widen your stance as needed to make sure that your knee does not move forward past your ankle.

Press down through the outer edge of your back foot, while keeping your back leg straight.

Keep your torso perpendicular to the floor, with your head directly over your tailbone. Do not lean toward your front leg.

Broaden across your collarbones and lengthen the space between your shoulder blades

Contraindications & cautions

The same contraindications and cautions apply as in Tree Pose. Also be cautious in this pose if you have hamstring or groin issues.

Modifications & adjustments

If you feel unstable with a heel-to-arch alignment of your feet, you can go for a heel-to-heel alignment, or even allow a little gap between your heels.

Variations

Viparita Virabhadrasana II

Reverse Warrior Pose

Come into Warrior Pose II, as described on the left. On your next exhalation, drop your left hand to the back of your left thigh. On an inhalation, lift your right arm straight up, reaching your fingertips toward the ceiling. Your right biceps should be next to your right ear. Keep your front knee bent and your hips sinking low as you lengthen through the sides of your waist. Slide your back hand further down your leg and come into a slight backbend. Tilt your head slightly and bring your gaze to your right hand's fingertips. Keep your shoulders relaxed, chest lifting, and the sides of your waist elongated.

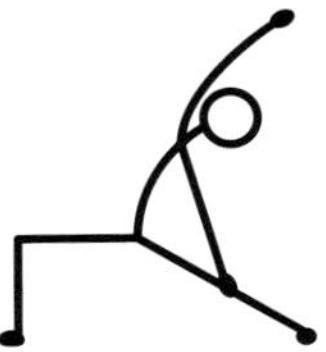

Baddha Virabhadrasana II

Bound Warrior Pose

Come into Warrior Pose II as described on the left. From there lower your right arm to rest your fingertips on the mat and place your right shoulder as low as you can against your right inner thigh. Reach your right arm back beneath your right hamstring. Now extend your left arm straight up toward the ceiling. Then, bend your elbow and bring your left arm behind you and clasp your hands behind your back. Do not allow your top shoulder to drop forward as you turn your head to look up at the ceiling.

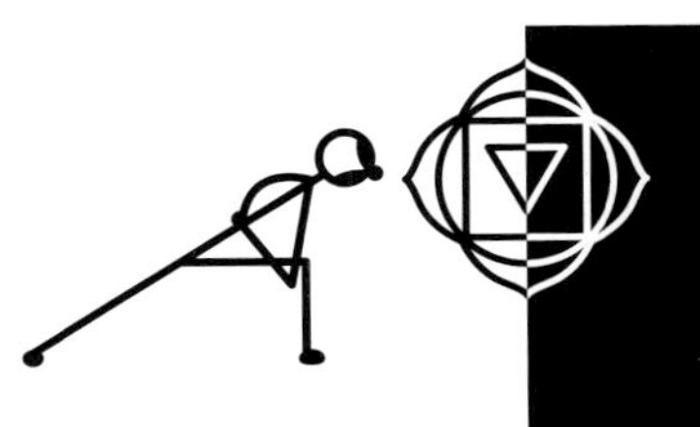

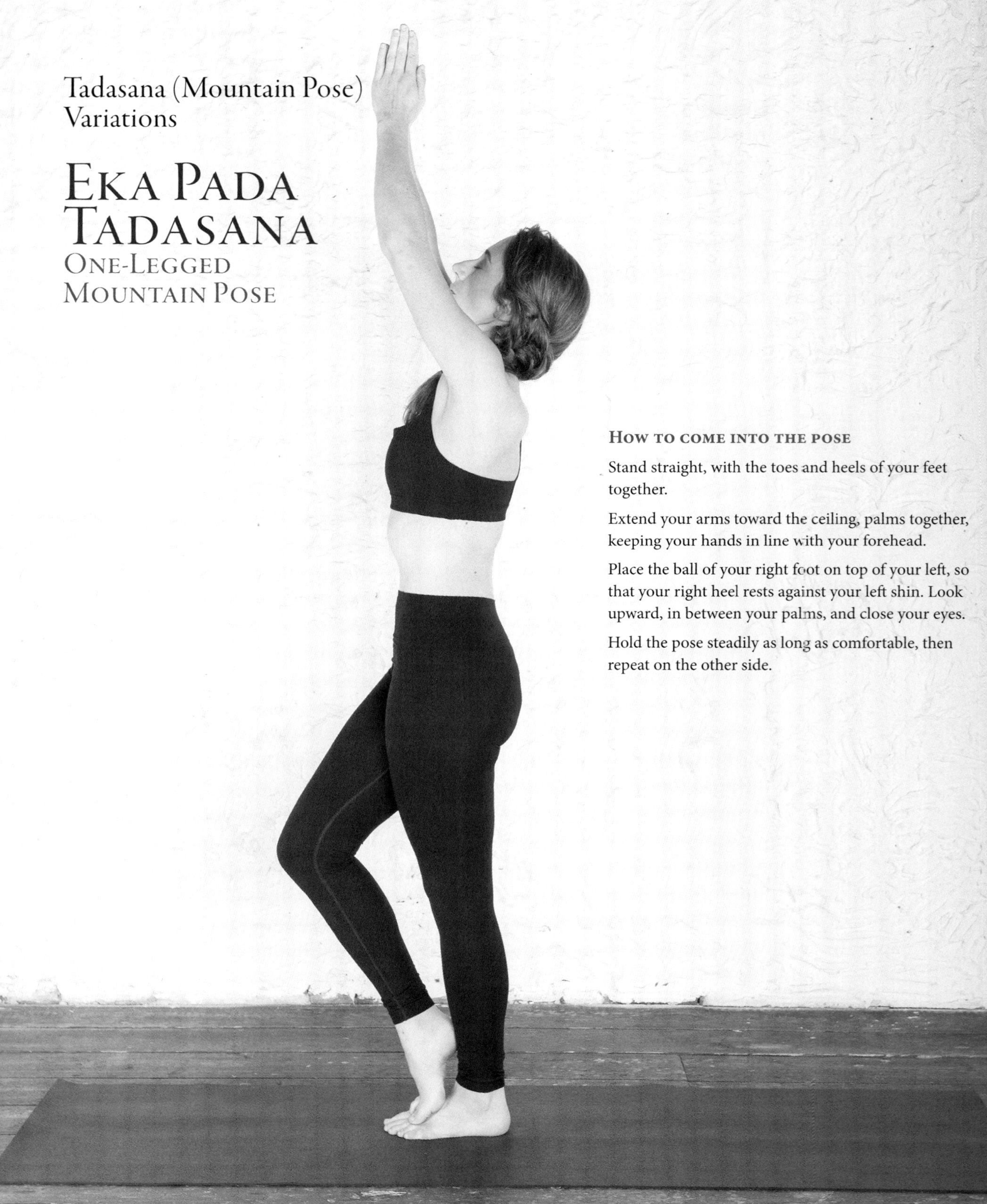

Tadasana (Mountain Pose) Variations

Eka Pada Tadasana

One-Legged Mountain Pose

How to come into the pose

Stand straight, with the toes and heels of your feet together.

Extend your arms toward the ceiling, palms together, keeping your hands in line with your forehead.

Place the ball of your right foot on top of your left, so that your right heel rests against your left shin. Look upward, in between your palms, and close your eyes.

Hold the pose steadily as long as comfortable, then repeat on the other side.

Next pose

Lie down in Corpse Pose for a final relaxation.

Alignment cues

Keep your inner thighs active.

Keep your core engaged and your spine in its natural curve. Avoid over-arching your lower back.

Your hands are in line with your forehead, and as you look upward keep your neck elongated.

Contraindications & cautions

There are no general contraindications for this pose. This pose, even though it appears to be simple, becomes difficult after 30 seconds. If you feel dizzy or start to sweat heavily, release the pose.

Modifications & adjustments

If balancing with eyes closed is too challenging, keep your eyes open and simply gaze at the eye-shaped space between your palms.

If the pose causes too much tension in your shoulders and neck, you can also keep your hands in Prayer position in front of your chest and look straight ahead.

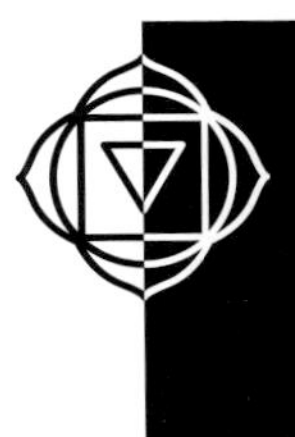

Utthita Tadasana

Five-Pointed Star Pose

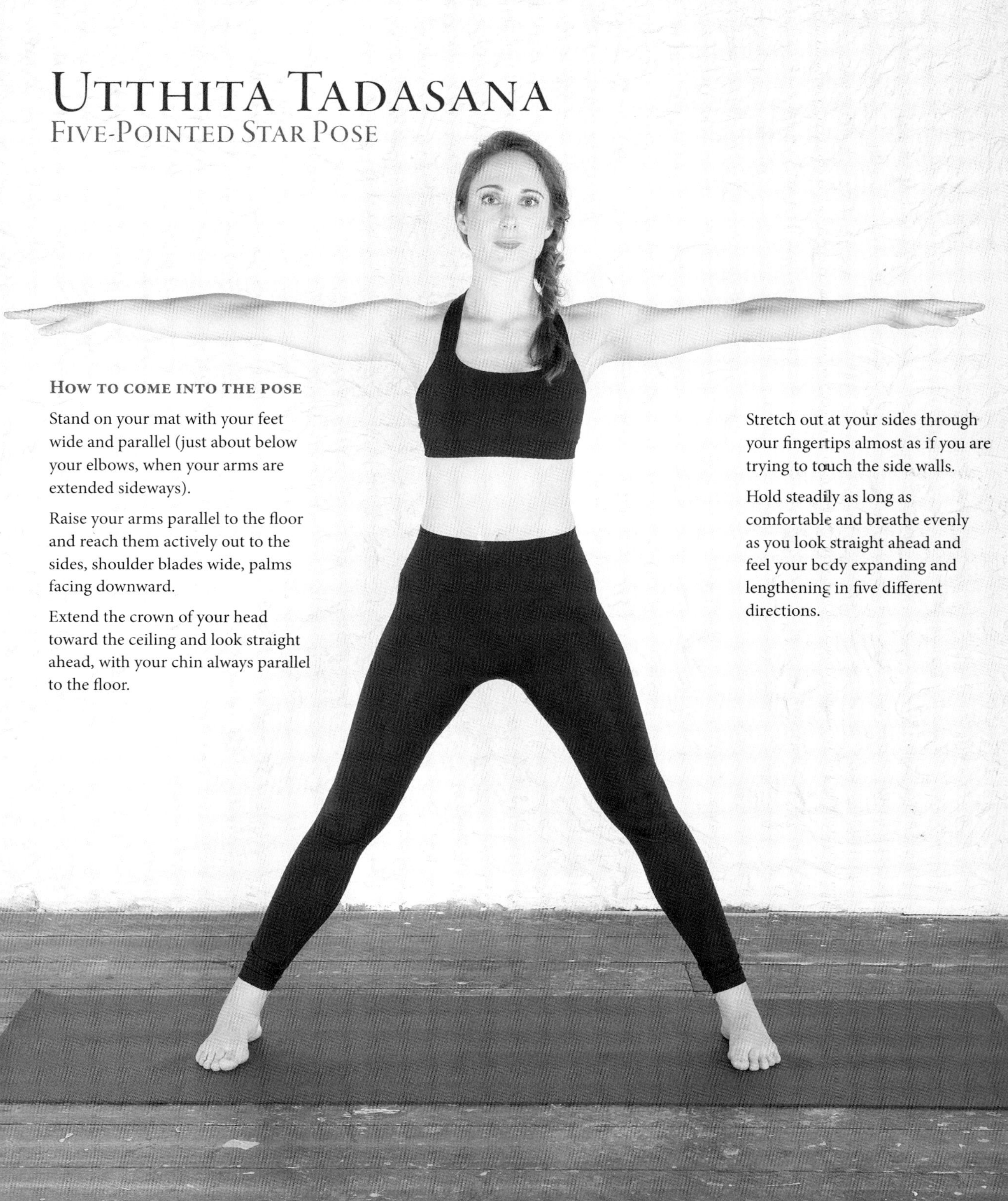

How to come into the pose

Stand on your mat with your feet wide and parallel (just about below your elbows, when your arms are extended sideways).

Raise your arms parallel to the floor and reach them actively out to the sides, shoulder blades wide, palms facing downward.

Extend the crown of your head toward the ceiling and look straight ahead, with your chin always parallel to the floor.

Stretch out at your sides through your fingertips almost as if you are trying to touch the side walls.

Hold steadily as long as comfortable and breathe evenly as you look straight ahead and feel your body expanding and lengthening in five different directions.

Next pose

Lie down in Corpse Pose for a final relaxation.

Alignment cues

Align your feet and heels parallel, then press your weight evenly across both feet.

Do not lock or hyperextend your knees; keep a micro-bend in them throughout the pose.

Keep your core engaged and your spine in its natural curve. Avoid over-arching your lower back.

Contraindications & cautions

There are no general contraindications for this pose. This pose, even though it looks simple, becomes difficult after 30 seconds. If you feel dizzy or start to sweat heavily, release the pose.

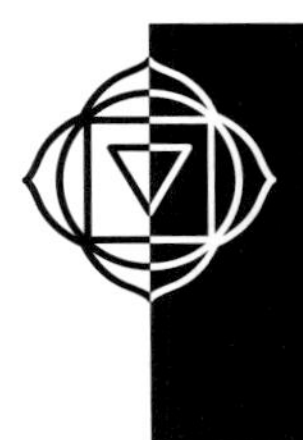

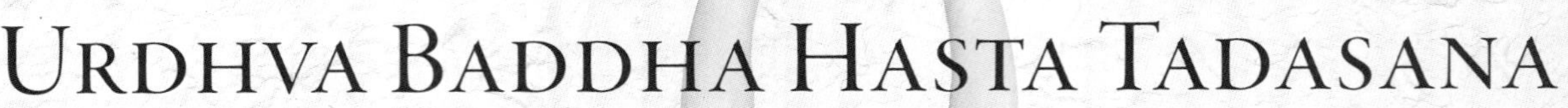

Urdhva Baddha Hasta Tadasana

Upward Bound-Hand Pose

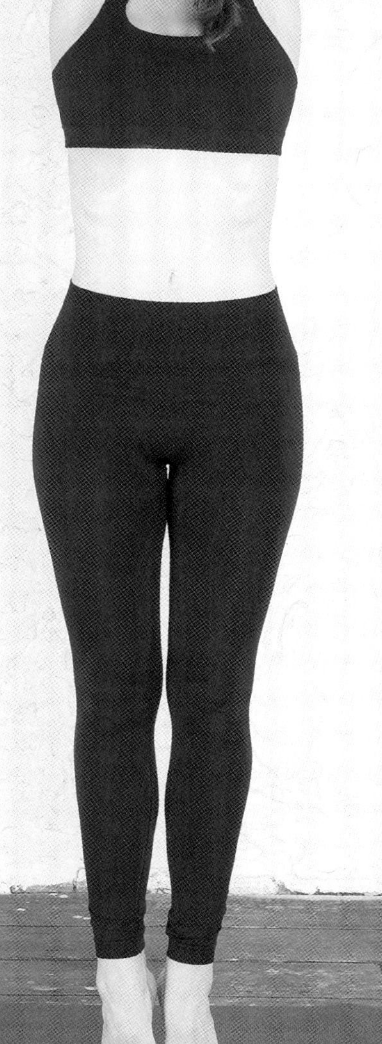

How to come into the pose

Stand on your mat, with your feet together.

Interlock your hands above your head, with palms facing upward.

Breathe in, stretch your hands as high up as you can, and allow your heels to lift off the floor.

Keep reaching up toward the ceiling and look diagonally up or straight ahead.

Hold steadily as long as comfortable and breathe evenly.

Next pose

Lie down in Corpse Pose for a final relaxation.

Alignment cues

Keep your heels pressed toward each other to stabilize your ankles.

Come up as high as you can on your toes.

In your effort to make yourself as tall as possible, your shoulders may lift up.

Keep your core engaged and your spine in its natural curve. Avoid over-arching your lower back.

Contraindications & cautions

There are no general contraindications for this pose. This pose, even though it looks simple, becomes heavy after 30 seconds. If you feel dizzy or start to sweat heavily, release the pose.

Modifications & adjustments

If balancing up on your toes is too challenging, keep your feet flat on the floor.

If the pose causes too much tension in your shoulders and neck, you can also keep your hands in Prayer position in front of your chest.

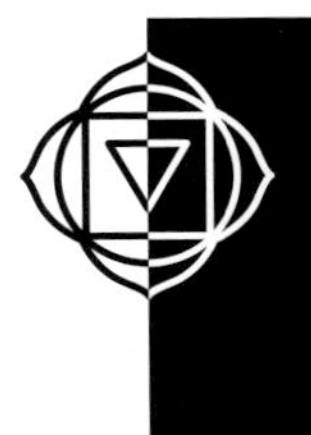

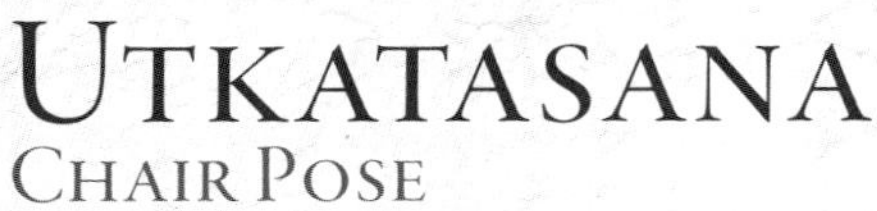

Utkatasana
Chair Pose

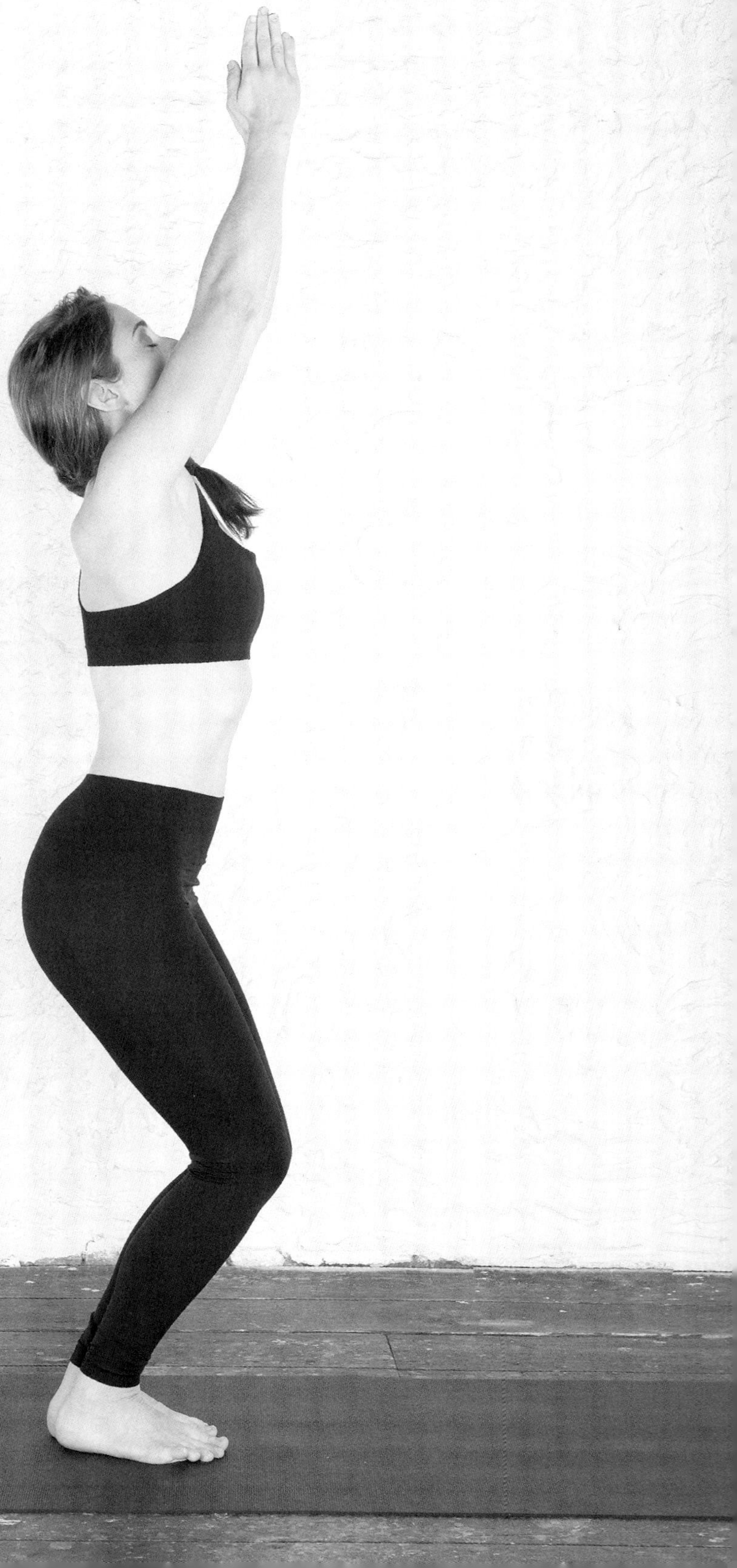

How to come into the pose

Come into a standing position with your feet together.

Breathe in and raise your hands up, palms together and in line with your forehead.

Breathe out and bend your knees as far as you can, while keeping your shoulders above your hips and your heels on the floor.

Tilt your head slightly and gaze at the eye-shaped space between your palms.

Keep creating the opposition between your hips reaching toward the floor and your fingertips reaching upward.

Hold steadily as long as comfortable and breathe evenly.

Next pose

Lie down in Corpse Pose for a final relaxation.

Alignment cues

Keep your shoulders above your pelvis and your pelvis above your heels. Avoid pushing your hips backward in your effort to go lower.

Draw your shoulder blades down toward your waist and your tailbone down to the floor, keeping your spine in its natural curve.

Look up in between your hands, but avoid dropping your head.

Contraindications & cautions

There are no general contraindications for this pose. This pose, even though it looks simple, becomes heavy after 30 seconds. If you feel dizzy or start to sweat heavily, release the pose.

Modifications & adjustments

To experience a little more mobility, you may keep your feet hip-width apart. In this case make sure to keep your knees parallel to each other.

If you have shoulder pain in this pose, bring your palms together in Prayer position, resting your thumbs at your sternum.

Variations

Parshva Utkatasana

Revolved Chair Pose

Come into Chair Pose, with your palms in front of your chest. Bend your knees further, allowing your pelvis to move behind your heels, and cross your right elbow over your left thigh. Twist your upper body so that your elbows are stacked above each other and look along your left elbow up toward the ceiling. Firmly press your palms against each other and broaden your shoulders and collarbones.

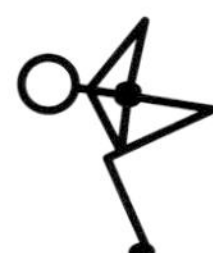

Utkata Konasana

Goddess Squat

Stand on your mat, with your feet just below your wrists when your arms are extended sideways. Turn your toes outwards and your heels, inwards, so that your feet land at a 45-degree angle. On an exhalation, bend your knees directly over your toes and lower your hips into a squat. Work toward bringing your thighs parallel to the floor, but do not force yourself into the squat. Bring your palms together in front of your chest in Prayer position and look straight ahead.

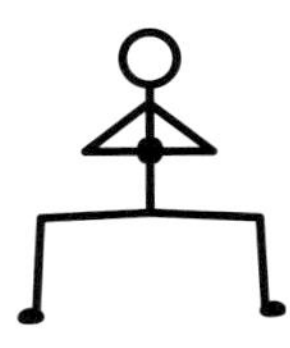

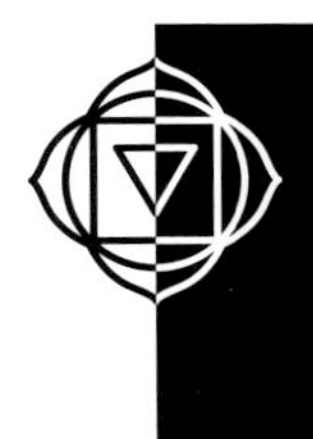

Classical Seated Postures

Vajrasana
Diamond Pose (aka Thunderbolt Pose)

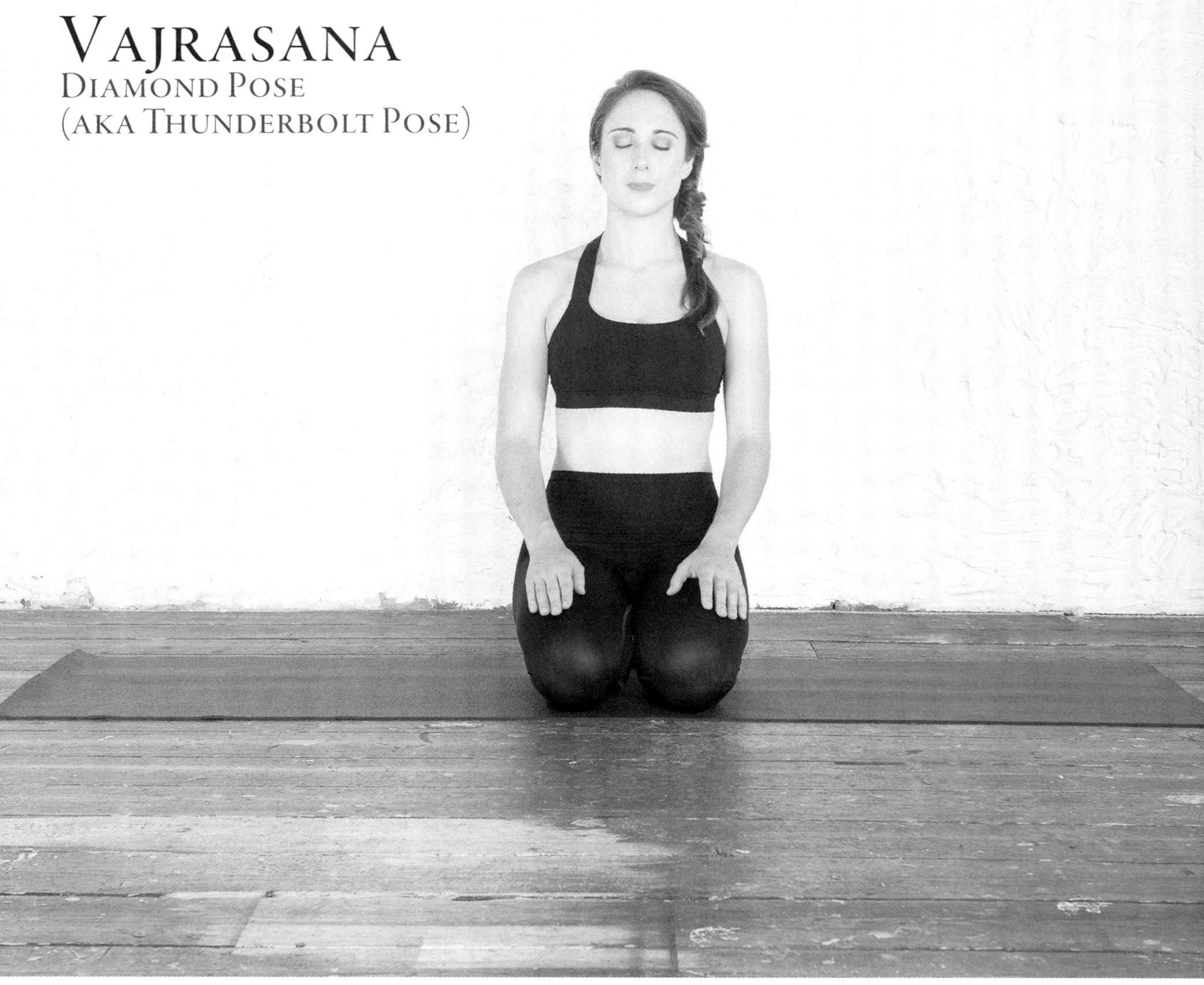

How to come into the pose

Start in a kneeling position, with your buttocks lifted off your legs.

Point your toes and press the tops of your toes firmly on the floor.

Come into a sitting position with your hips resting on your heels as you breathe out.

Let your hands rest on your thighs, palms facing downward. Relax your arms and close your eyes gently.

Alignment cues

Keep your spine, neck, and head in line, ears in line with your shoulders, hips, and heels.

Your weight is equally balanced between both sitting bones.

Keeping your thighs and heels together, avoid letting the heels drop outwards.

Your back is straight, chest open, shoulders relaxed.

Contraindications & cautions

- Knee issues
- Ankle issues

Modifications & adjustments

You can place a cushion or a folded blanket in between your buttocks and heels if you have difficulties sitting on your heels.

If you feel tension in your ankles, you can place a rolled blanket under your ankles before coming into the pose.

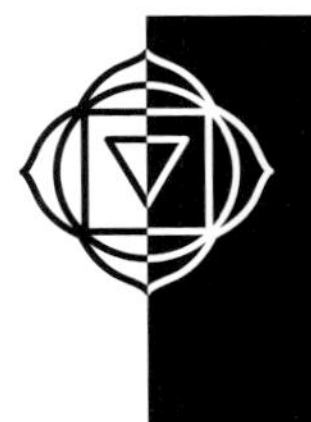

Sukhasana
Easy Sitting Pose

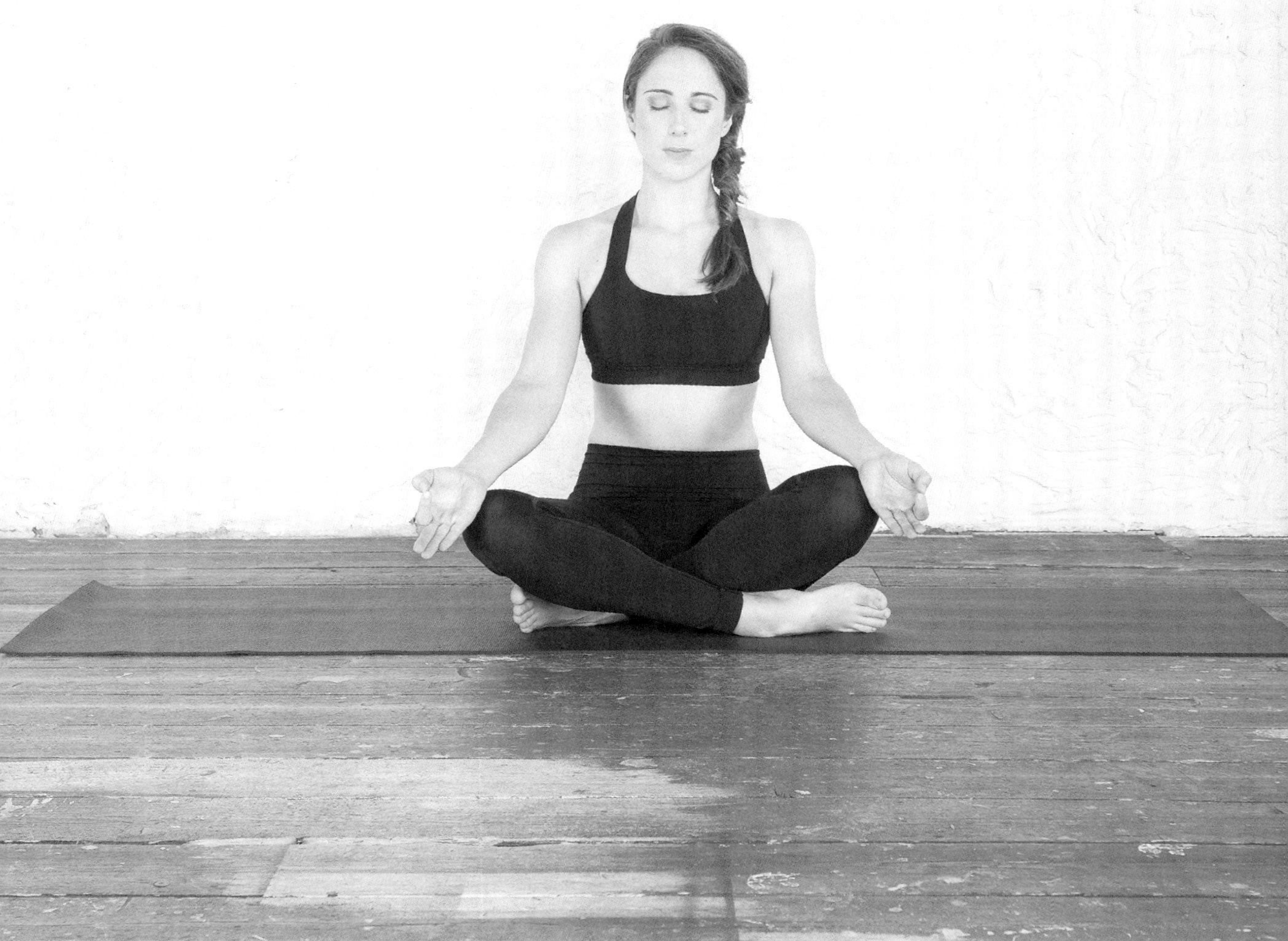

How to come into the pose

Start in a seated position, with your legs extended in front of you.

Cross your legs at the shins, and, keeping your knees wide, place each foot under the opposite knee.

Let your hands rest on your knees.

Keep your spine straight and look straight ahead with your eyes gently closed.

Alignment cues

Keep a constant opposition between your hips pushing into the ground and the crown of your head reaching upward.

Keep the spine in the back of the neck elongated.

Keep your weight equally divided between both sitting bones.

Cross your legs naturally—however feels most comfortable.

Contraindications & cautions

- Tight hips
- Knee issues
- Lower-back and spinal issues

Modifications & adjustments

If your pelvis is tilting and you are sitting on your tailbone instead of your sitting bones, you can sit on the edge of a cushion or blanket.

If your knees are far off the floor, support them as well with a folded blanket.

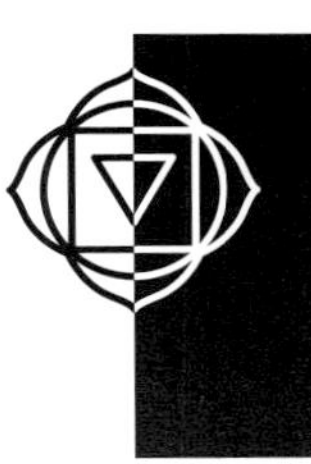

Ardha Padmasana
Half Lotus Pose

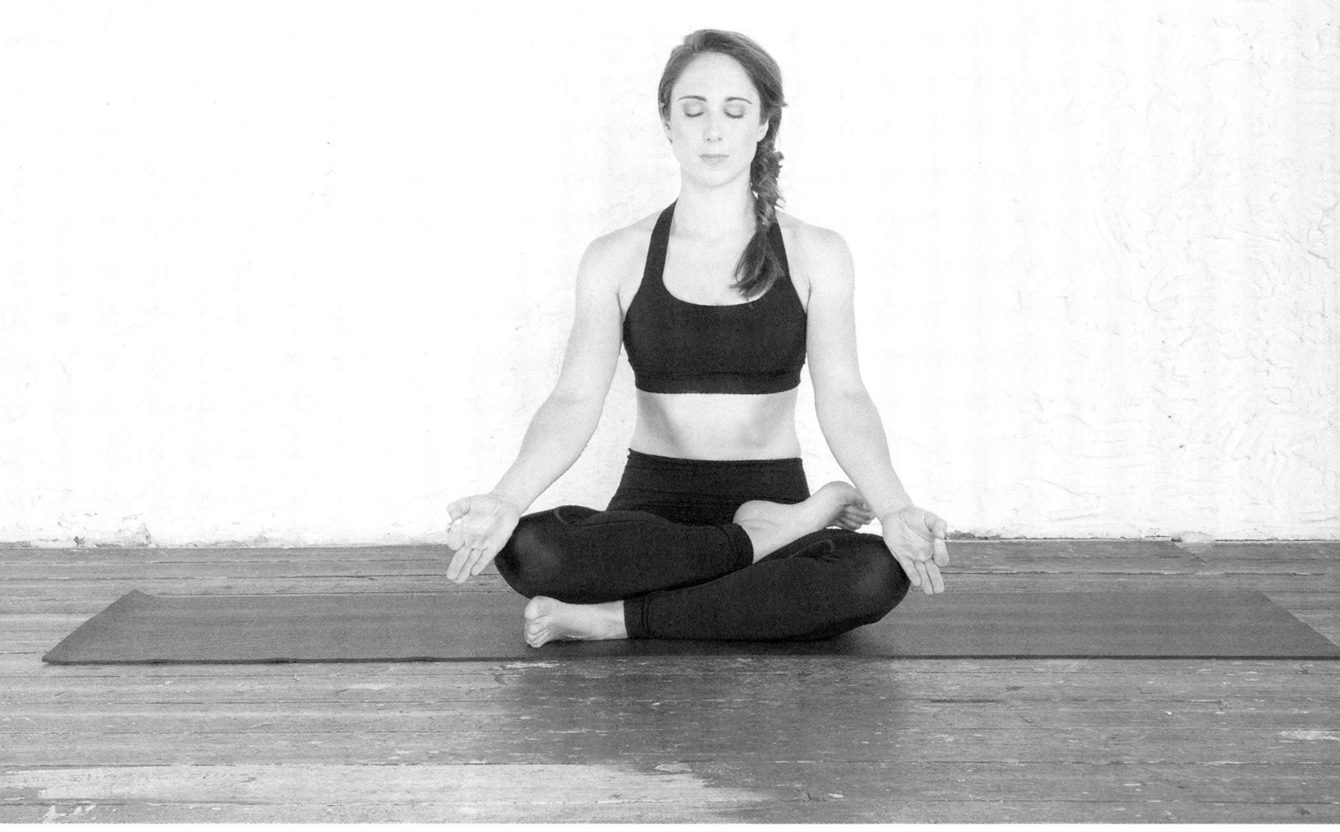

How to come into the pose

Start in a seated position on your mat, with your legs extended in front of you.

Bend your right leg and bring your right ankle to the crease of your left hip. Make sure that the top of your right foot is resting in the crease of your left hip and the sole of your foot is facing upward.

Bend your left leg and place your left ankle under your right knee.

Let your hands rest on your thighs, palms facing upward.

Keep your spine straight and close your eyes gently.

Alignment cues

Do not attempt this pose if you have to force your leg to cross over. Make sure to generate the rotation at your hip joint as you fold your leg into Half Lotus Pose, and avoid straining your knee!

Make sure you practice this pose on both sides.

Aim your heel to the crease of your opposite hip. Keep the upper foot active. You should not feel any pull or strain in your outer ankle.

Never push your upper knee down toward the floor, because that can injure your knee. Simply focus on releasing your leg at the groin.

Contraindications & cautions

- Ankle issues
- Tight hips
- Knee issues

Modifications & adjustments

If your pelvis is tilting and you are sitting on your tailbone instead of your sitting bones, you can sit on the edge of a cushion or blanket.

If your upper knee is not resting comfortably on your lower foot, use a folded blanket or a block to support your knee.

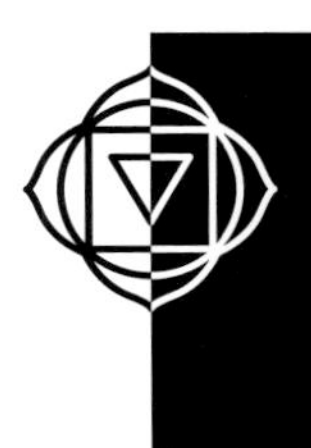

Padmasana
Lotus Pose

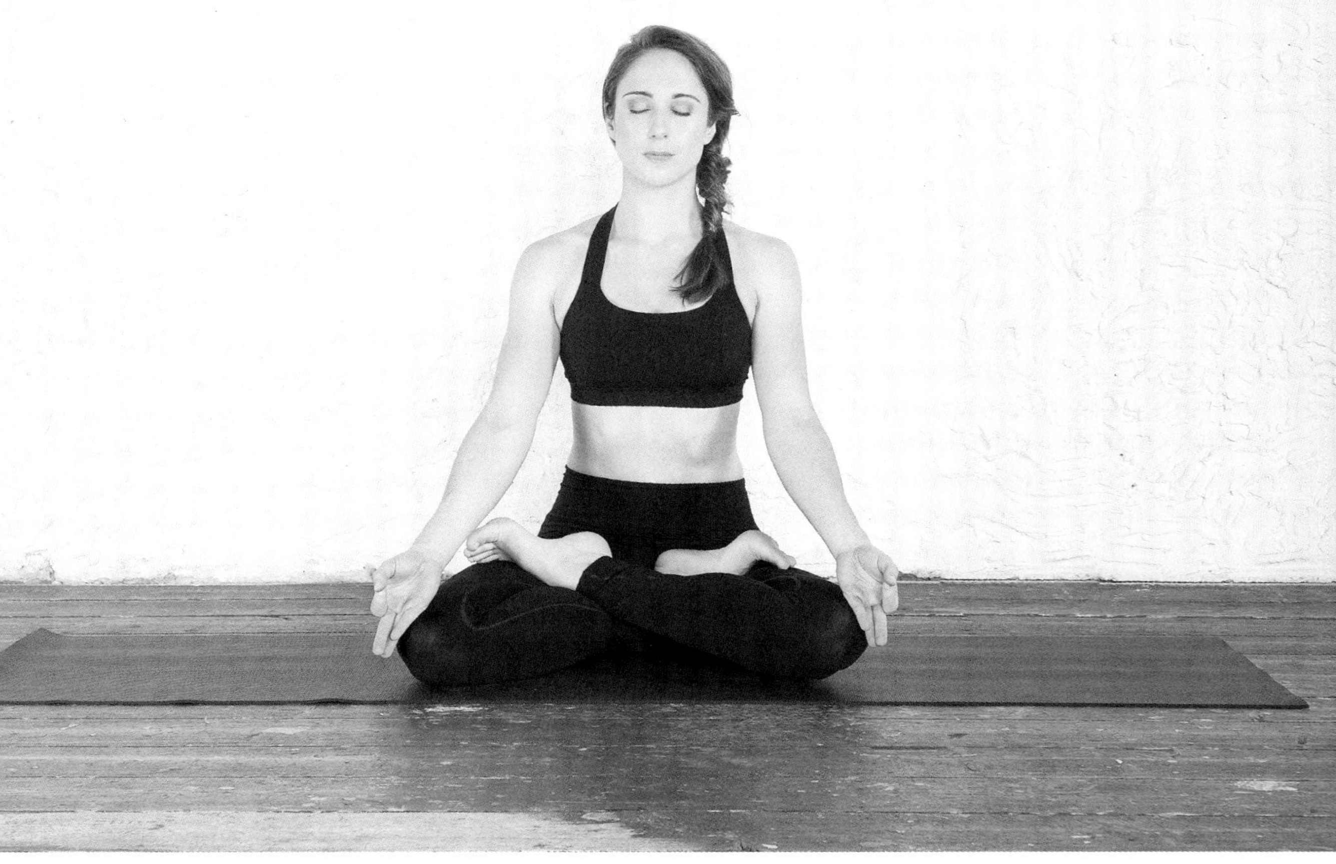

How to come into the pose

Start in a seated position on your mat, with your legs extended in front of you.

Bend your right leg and bring your right ankle to the crease of your left hip. Make sure that the top of your right foot is resting in the crease of your left hip and the sole of your foot is facing upward.

Bend your left leg, gently cross your left ankle over your right shin, and bring your left ankle to the crease of your right hip.

The top of your left foot is resting in the crease of your right hip, and the sole of your foot is facing upward.

Gently push your knees as close together as you can, pressing your sitting bones down on the floor and keeping your spine straight.

Close your eyes and breathe evenly, with your hands resting on your knees.

Then release the pose and repeat the same on the other side.

Alignment cues

Do not attempt this pose if you have to force your leg to cross over. Make sure to generate the rotation at your hip joints as you fold your legs into Lotus Pose, and avoid straining your knees.

Aim your heel to the crease of your opposite hip. You should not feel any pull or strain in your outer ankle.

Never push your upper knee down toward the floor, because that can injure your knee. Simply focus on releasing your leg at the groin.

Make sure you practice this pose on both sides.

Contraindications & cautions

- Ankle issues
- Tight hips
- Knee issues

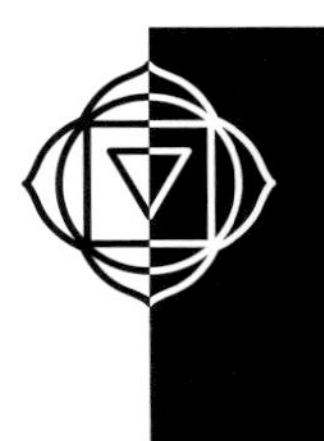

Swastikasana
Auspicious Pose

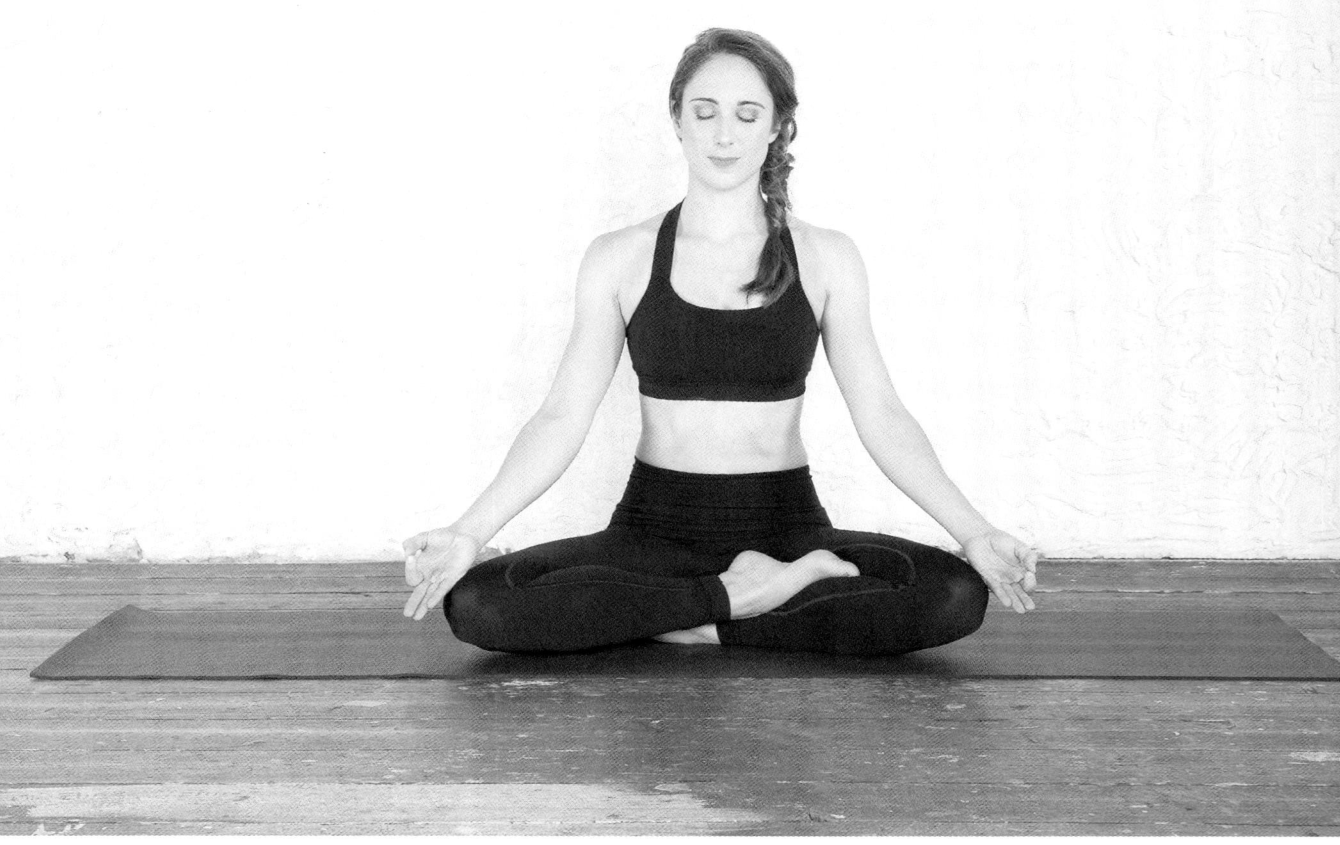

How to come into the pose

Start in a sitting position, with your legs extended in front of you.

Bend your right leg and place your right sole against the inside of your left thigh, placing your toes against the crease of your left knee.

Bend your left leg, cross your left ankle under your right leg, and place the sole of your left foot against your right inner thigh.

Hold the toes of your left foot, and gently pull them up so your toes are in the crease of your right knee.

Hold your knees on the floor and keep your spine straight, eyes gently closed.

Let your hands rest on your knees, palms facing upward, and breathe evenly.

Release the pose and repeat the same on the other side.

Alignment cues

Make sure to generate the rotation at your hip joint as you fold your legs into the pose. Do not torque your knee!

Avoid touching your heels to your perineum, but keep your toes tucked firmly in the crease of your knees.

Contraindications & cautions

- Ankle issues
- Tight hips
- Knee issues

Modifications & adjustments

If your knees are not resting comfortably on the floor, sitting on a folded blanket can make it easier.

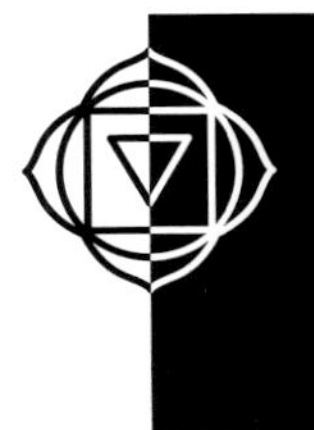

Siddhasana
Accomplished Pose

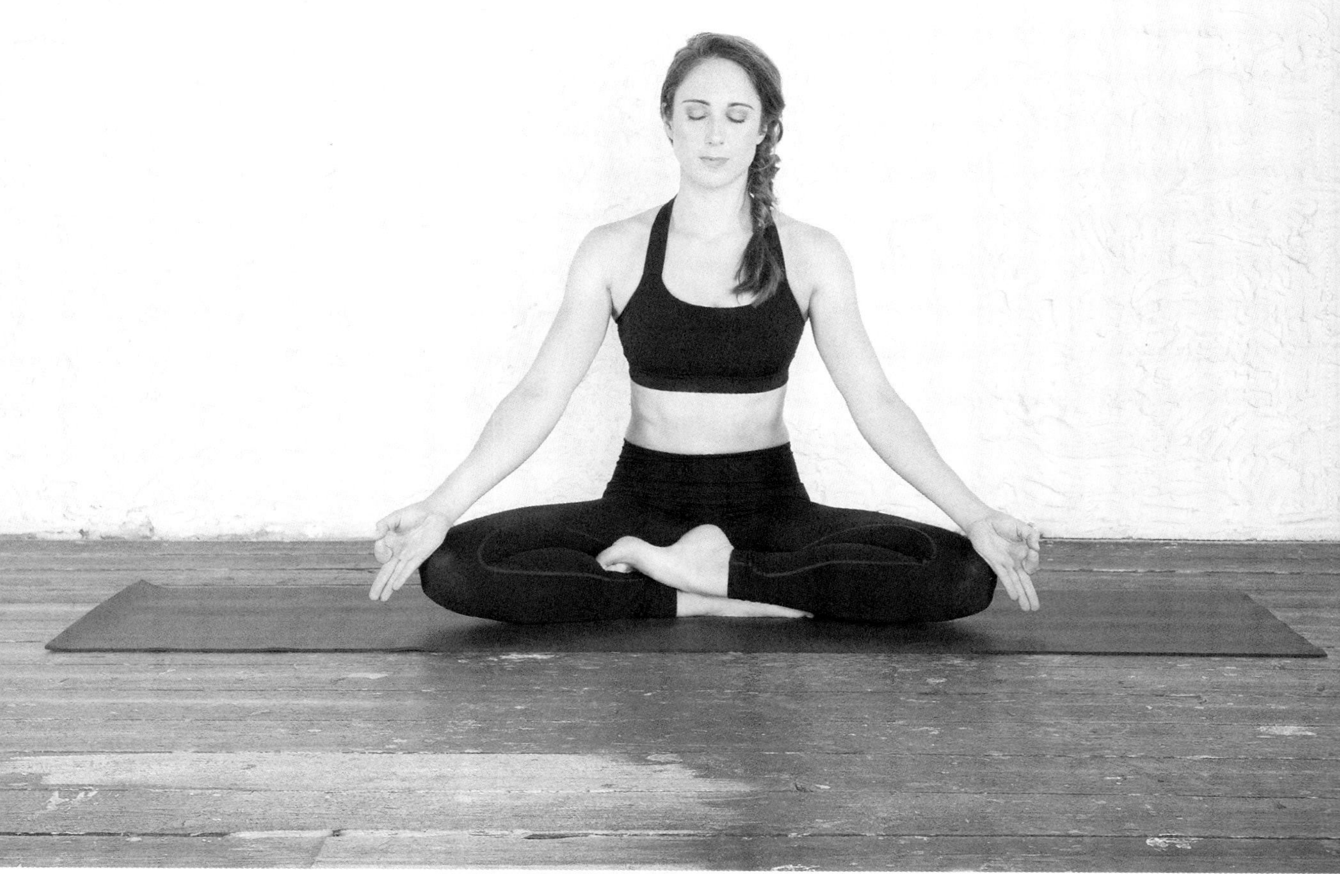

How to come into the pose

Start in a sitting position, with your legs extended in front of you.

Bend your right leg and place your right heel against your perineum.

Bend your left leg and place the outside of your left ankle over the inside of your right ankle.

Your left heel is touching the top of your pubic bone, and your knees are resting on the floor.

Let your hands rest on your thighs, and breathe evenly.

Keep your spine straight and gently close your eyes. Then release the pose and repeat the same on the other side.

Alignment cues

Make sure to generate the rotation at your hip joint as you fold your legs into the pose. Do not torque your knee!

Your ankles are resting on top of each other, and your heels are pressing against the perineum and the top of the pubic bone.

Contraindications & cautions

- Ankle issues
- Tight hips
- Knee issues

Modifications & adjustments

If your knees are not resting comfortably on the floor, sitting on a folded blanket can make it easier.

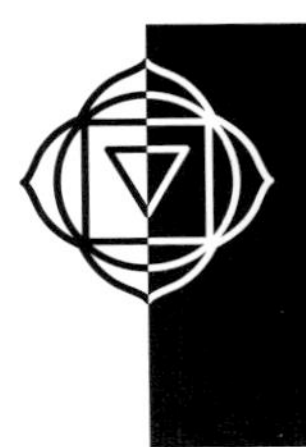

CHAPTER 18

SAMPLE SEQUENCES

Hip Opening (90 minutes)		
1	Initial Relaxation	5 min.
2	(Chanting Om)	
3	Kapalbhati	3 rounds (5 min.)
4	Anulom Vilom	5 min.
5	Shavasana	30–45 sec.
6	Surya Namaskara	6–8 rounds (10 min.)
7	Shavasana	1 min.
8	Yogic Bicycle	6–10 rep.
9	Shashankasana	30–45 sec.
10	Yoga Push-Ups	5 rep.
11	Shashankasana	30–45 sec.
12	Shirshasana	1 min.
13	Shashankasana	30–45 sec.
14	Vistrit Pada Sarvangasana (Legs in Butterfly)	1 min.
15	Halasana	30 sec.
16	Ardha Setu Bandhasana	30 sec.
17	Garbhasana	1 min. each side
18	Supta Padangusthasana I & II	1 min. each side
19	Supta Baddha Konasana	45 sec.
20	Ushtrasana	30–60 sec.
21	Adho Mukha Gomukhasana	1 min. each side
22	Ardha Baddha Padma Paschimottanasana	1 min.
23	Supta Virasana	1 min.
24	Makarasana	30–45 sec.
25	Bhujangasana	30–60 sec.
26	Makarasana	30–45 sec.
27	Vistrit Bhujangasana	30–45 sec.
28	Makarasana	30–45 sec.
29	Supta Eka Pada Kapotasana	90 sec. each side
30	Shashankasana	30–45 sec.
31	Malasana	1 min.
32	Prapadasana	15 sec. each side
33	Utthita Trikonasana	30 sec. each side
34	Utthita Hasta Padangusthasana I & II	20 sec. each side
35	Ardha Padma Vrkshasana	1 min. each side
36	Final Relaxation	15 min.
37	(Chanting Om Shanti)	

Chest and Heart Opening (90 minutes)

1	Initial Relaxation	5 min.
2	(Chanting Om)	
3	Kapalbhati	3 rounds (5 min.)
4	Anulom Vilom	5 min.
5	Shavasana	30–45 sec.
6	Surya Namaskara	6–8 rounds (10 min.)
7	Shavasana	1 min.
8	Paripurna Navasana	2 × 20 sec.
9	Shashankasana	30–45 sec.
10	Dolphin	5–10 rep.
11	Shashankasana	30–45 sec.
12	Vistrit Pada Shirshasana (Feet Toward Head)	1 min.
13	Shashankasana	30–45 sec.
14	Ushtrasana	30 sec.
15	Sukha Viparita Karani Mudra	30–60 sec.
16	Karnapidasana	45 sec.
17	Chakrasana	10–15 sec.
18	Pawanmuktasana	1 min.
19	Matsyasana	45 sec.
20	Shavasana	30–45 sec.
21	Pashchima Namaskarasana	1 min.
22	Marjaryasana I & II	1 min.
23	Adho Mukha Shvanasana	1 min.
24	Urdhva Mukha Shvanasana	30–45 sec.
25	Sashtang Pranam Asana	30–45 sec.
26	Salamba Ardha Shalabhasana	1 min. each side
27	Sashtang Pranam Asana	30–45 sec.
28	Dhanurasana	30–45 sec.
29	Shashankasana	30–45 sec.
30	Marichyasana A	30 sec. each side
31	Sukha Kakasana	30 sec.
32	Uttanasana	1 min.
33	Virabhadrasana I	30 sec. each side
34	Ashta Chandrasana	30 sec. each side
35	Tadasana	1 min.
36	Final Relaxation	15 min.
37	(Chanting Om Shanti)	

Intermediary – Working Toward a Peak Pose (90 minutes)

1	Initial Relaxation	5 min.
2	(Chanting Om)	
3	Kapalbhati	3 rounds (5 min.)
4	Anulom Vilom	5 min.

5	Shavasana	30–45 sec.
6	Surya Namaskara	6–8 rounds (10 min.)
7	Shavasana	1 min.
8	Pilates Splits	10–20 rep.
9	Happy Baby	1 min.
10	Spiderman Push-Ups	5–10 rep.
11	Shashankasana	30–45 sec.
12	Shirshasana	4 min.
13	Shashankasana	30–45 sec.
14	Ushtrasana	1 min.
15	Niralamba Sarvangasana	2 min.
16	Supta Konasana	1 min.
17	Eka Pada Chakrasana	10–15 sec. each side
18	Pawanmuktasana	1 min.
19	Uttanpadasana	30 sec.
20	Shavasana	30–45 sec.
21	Janu Shirshasana	1 min. each side
22	Paschimottanasana A	1 min.
23	Bhujangasana	1 min.
24	Makarasana	30–45 sec.
25	Shalabhasana	20 sec.
26	Makarasana	30–45 sec.
27	Sukha Hanumanasana	30–45 sec. each side
28	Shashankasana	30–45 sec.
29	Ardha Matsyendrasana	30 sec. each side
30	Chaturanga Dandasana	10–15 sec.
31	Eka Pada Koundinyasana (Peak I)	20 sec. each side
32	Padahastasana	1 min.
33	Svarga Dvijasana (Peak II)	20 sec. each side
34	Vrkshasana	2 min. each side
35	Final Relaxation	15 min.
36	(Chanting Om Shanti)	

Basic Sequence (75 minutes)		
1	Initial Relaxation	5 min.
2	(Chanting Om)	
3	Kapalbhati	3 rounds (5 min.)
4	Anulom Vilom	5 min.
5	Shavasana	30–45 sec.
6	Surya Namaskara	4–6 rounds (7 min.)
7	Shavasana	30–45 sec.
8	Double Leg Raises	6 rep.
9	Shavasana	30–45 sec.
10	Dolphin	10 rep.

11	Shashankasana	30–45 sec.
12	Shirshasana	1 min.
13	Shashankasana	30–45 sec.
14	Sarvangasana	1 min.
15	Halasana	30 sec.
16	Ardha Setu Bandhasana	30 sec.
17	Pawanmuktasana	30–45 sec.
18	Matsyasana	30 sec.
19	Shavasana	30–45 sec.
20	Paschimottanasana	1 min.
21	Purvottanasana	10 sec.
22	Makarasana	30–45 sec.
23	Bhujangasana	30–60 sec.
24	Makarasana	30–45 sec.
25	Dhanurasana	10–20 sec.
26	Shashankasana	30–45 sec.
27	Ardha Matsyendrasana	30 sec. each side
28	Sukha Kakasana	30 sec.
29	Trikonasana	30 sec. each side
30	Vrkshasana	1 min. each side
31	Final Relaxation	10 min.
32	(Chanting Om Shanti)	

Basic Sequence (60 minutes)		
1	Initial Relaxation	5 min.
2	(Chanting Om)	
3	Kapalbhati	2 rounds (3 min.)
4	Anulom Vilom	3 min.
5	Shavasana	30–45 sec.
6	Surya Namaskara	4–6 rounds (7 min.)
7	Shavasana	1 min.
8	Shashankasana	30–45 sec.
9	Shirshasana	1 min.
10	Shashankasana	30–45 sec.
11	Sarvangasana	1 min.
12	Halasana	30 sec.
13	Ardha Setu Bandhasana	30 sec.
14	Pawanmuktasana	30–45 sec.
15	Matsyasana	30 sec.
16	Shavasana	30–45 sec.
17	Paschimottanasana	1 min.
18	Purvottanasana	10 sec.
19	Makarasana	30–45 sec.
20	Bhujangasana	30–60 sec.
21	Makarasana	30–45 sec.

22	Dhanurasana	10–20 sec.
23	Shashankasana	30–45 sec.
24	Sukha Kakasana	30 sec.
25	Trikonasana	30 sec. each side
26	Vrkshasana	1 min. each side
27	Final Relaxation	10 min.
28	(Chanting Om Shanti)	

Basic Short Sequence (30 minutes)		
1	Initial Relaxation	2 min.
2	(Chanting Om)	
3	Anulom Vilom	10 rounds
4	Shavasana	30–45 sec.
5	Surya Namaskara	4 rounds (5 min.)
6	Shavasana	1 min.
7	Shashankasana	30–45 sec.
8	Shirshasana	1 min.
9	Shashankasana	30–45 sec.
10	Sarvangasana	1 min.
11	Ardha Setu Bandhasana	30 sec.
12	Pawanmuktasana	30–45 sec.
13	Sukha Gomukhasana	30 sec. each side
14	Paschimottanasana	1 min.
15	Bhujangasana	30 sec.
16	Dhanurasana	15 sec.
17	Sukha Kakasana	10 sec.
18	Trikonasana	20 sec. each side
19	Tadasana	1 min.
20	Final Relaxation	5 min.
21	(Chanting Om Shanti)	

"*If you want to learn something, read about it.*
If you want to understand something, write about it.
If you want to master something, teach it."

Yogi Bhajan

Asana Index

Sanskrit

English

Notes

1. As explained by James Mallinson in "A Response to Mark Singleton's Yoga Body" (Dec. 2011).

2. The Sanskrit texts mentioning mudras and bandhas are the *Amrtasiddhi*, the *Dattatreyayogasastra*, the *Vivekamartananda*, and the *Goraksha Shataka*.

3. For example the *Sarnghadarapaddhati*, 1363 AD.

4. Two other texts considered fundamental are the *Gheranda Samhita* and the *Shiva Samhita*. Another important text on Hatha Yoga, written at a later date by Srinivasabhatta Mahayogaindra, is the *Hatharatnavali*.

5. Mallinson, James. "Hatha Yoga." *Brill Encyclopedia of Hinduism* Volume 3, 2011.

6. C.C. Streeter, P.L. Gerbarg, R.B. Saper, D.A. Ciraulo, R.P. Brown. "Effects of yoga on the autonomic nervous system, gamma-aminobutyric-acid, and allostasis in epilepsy, depression, and post-traumatic stress disorder." *Medical Hypotheses* Volume 78, Issue 5 (May 2012): 571–579.

7. Robin, Mel. *A Physiological Handbook for Teachers of Yogasana*. Tucson, Arizona: Fenestra Books, 2002. Page 152.

8. Martin, Robert. *The Gravity Guiding System: Turning the Aging Process Upside Down*. Gravity Guidance Inc., 1982.

9. Peter Russell M.A., D.C.S. *The Brain Book*. Plume, 1984.

10. Luciano Bernardi, Alessandra Gabutti, Cesare Porta, Lucia Spicuzza. "Slow breathing reduces chemoreflex response to hypoxia and hypercapnia, and increases baroreflex sensitivity." *Jounal of Hypertension* (Dec. 2001).

11. Luciano Bernardi, Claudio Passino, Giammario Spadacini, Maurizio Bon, Luca Arcaini, Luca Malcovati, Gabriele Bandinelli, Annette Schneider, Cornelius Keyl, Paul Feil, Richard E. Greene, Carlo Bernasconi. "Reduced hypoxic ventilatory response with preserved blood oxygenation in yoga trainees and Himalayan Buddhist monks at altitude: Evidence of a different adaptive strategy?" *European Journal of Applied Psychology* Volume 99, Issue 5 (March 2007): 511–518.

12. Harish Johari. *Breath, Mind, and Consciousness*. Destiny Books, 1989. Page 7.

13. M.S. Chaya, A.V. Kurpad, H.R. Nagendra, R. Nagarathna. "The effect of long-term combined yoga practice on the basal metabolic rate of healthy adults." *BMC Complementary and Alternative Medicine* (2006).

14. Fontana, L., Klein, S., Hollozyy, J.O., Premachandra, B.N. "Effect of long-term calorie restriction with adequate protein and micronutrients on thyroid hormones." *The Journal of Clinical Endocrinology and Metabolism* Volume 91, Issue 8 (August 2006): 3232–3235.

15. Michael Ristow, Sebastian Schmeisser. "Extending life span by increasing oxidative stress." *Free Radical Biology and Medicine* Volume 51, Issue 2 (2011): 327–336.

16. Chin-Ming Jeng, Tzu-Chieh Cheng, Ching-Huei Kung, Hue-Chen Hsu. "Yoga and disc degenerative disease in cervical and lumbar spine: An MR imaging-based case control study." *European Spine Journal* Volume 20, Issue 3 (March 2011): 408–413.

17. Nisha Shantakumari, Shiefa Sequeira, Rasha El deeb. "Effects of a yoga intervention on lipid profiles of diabetes patients with dyslipidemia." *Indian Heart Journal* (March 2013): 127–131.

18. Francisca M. Vera, Juan M. Manzaneque, Enrique F. Maldonado, Gabriel A. Carranque, Francisco M. Rodriguez, Maria J. Blanca, Miguel Morell. "Subjective Sleep Quality and hormonal modulation in long-term yoga practitioners." *Biological Psychology* Volume 81 (2009): 164–168.

Resources

Avison, Joanna Sarah.
Yoga: Fascia, Anatomy and Movement. UK: Handspring Publishing, 2015.

Broad, William J.
The Science of Yoga: The Risks and Rewards. New York: Simon & Schuster, 2012.

Bangali Baba (translated by).
Yogasutra Patanjali: With the Commentary of Vyasa. Delhi: Motilal Banarsidass Publishers Private Limited, 2010.

Buhnemann, Gudrun.
Eighty-Four Asanas in Yoga: A Survey of Traditions. New Delhi: D.K. Printworld (P) Ltd., 2007.

Coulter, David H.
Anatomy of Hatha Yoga: A Manual for Students, Teachers, and Practitioners. Delhi: Motilal Banarsidass Publishers Private Limited, 2004.

Easwaran, Eknath (translated by).
The Upanishads, Second Edition. Berkeley, CA: Nilgiri Press, 2007.

Harvey, Alison.
A Pathway to Health: How Visceral Manipulation Can Help You. Berkeley, CA: North Atlantic Books, 2010.

Keil, David.
Functional Anatomy of Yoga: A Guide for Practitioners and Teachers. Chichester, UK: Lotus Publishing, 2014.

McCall, Timothy.
Yoga as Medicine: The Yogic Prescription for Health and Healing. New York: Bantam Dell, 2007.

Rai Bahadur Srisa Chandra Vasu (translated by).
The Gheranda Samhita. New Delhi: Munshiram Manoharlal Publishers Pvt. Ltd., 2007.

Rai Bahadur Srisa Chandra Vasu (translated by).
The Siva Samhita. New Delhi: Munshiram Manoharlal Publishers Pvt. Ltd., 2008.

Robin, Mel.
A 21st-Century Yogasanalia: Celebrating the Integration of Yoga, Science, and Medicine. Wheatmark Inc., 2017.

Satyananda Saraswati.
Asana Pranayama Mudra Bandha. Munger, India: Bihar School of Yoga, 2008.

Swami Vishnu-devananda.
The Complete Illustrated Book of Yoga. New York: Three Rivers Press, 1988.

Sinh, Panham (translated by).
The Hatha Yoga Pradipika. New Delhi: Munshiram Manoharlal Publishers Pvt. Ltd., 2007.

About the Authors

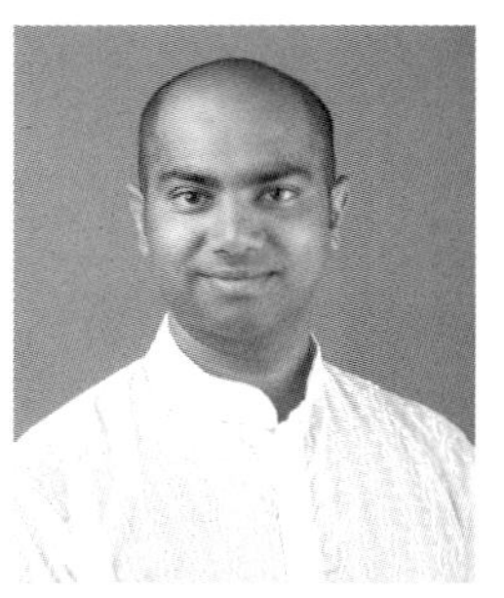

Ram Jain

Ram is founding director of the Arhanta Yoga Ashrams (India and the Netherlands). Since 2009, the Arhanta Yoga Ashrams have become renowned internationally for their professional yoga teacher training courses, and have trained thousands of yoga teachers from all over the world.

Born in New Delhi, India, in a traditional and spiritual family, his yoga and Vedic philosophy education started at the age of eight years as a part of his primary school education. He has in-depth knowledge of classical Hatha Yoga and is also well versed in ancient Indian scriptures. Since the start of his teaching career in 1998, he has worked with many different anatomy and physiology experts and has developed unique teaching, adjustment, and modification techniques.

Presently, he is the lead teacher for various teacher training programs, ranging from Hatha Yoga, Yin Yoga, and Vinyasa Yoga to meditation and Yoga Nidra. He teaches for several months a year in India and the rest of the year in the Netherlands.

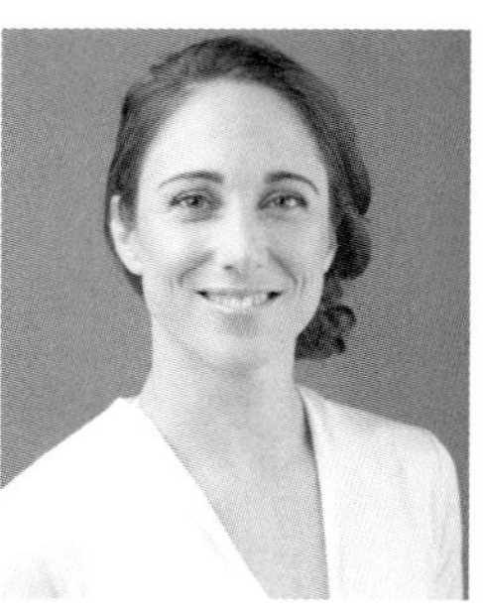

Michèle Hauswirth

Michèle was born and raised in Switzerland. Since early adolescence she has been fascinated by art, bodywork, the body-mind connection, and alternative therapies. Following her strong inclination for art and physical expression, she emigrated to the Netherlands at the age of 19 to study modern dance. Soon after, she was exposed to the teachings and practice of yoga and was immediately mesmerized. Hauswirth has been teaching yoga since 2007 and training yoga teachers since 2011 at the Arhanta Yoga Ashrams in India and the Netherlands.

Starting off with physical challenges, she transformed her body, mastering many advanced asanas with her regular practice and discipline. By following a diligent self-practice, working with many different teachers, styles, and techniques, she gained a profound understanding of physiology and movement techniques. This, in combination with her extensive teaching experience, gave her an understanding of the importance of structure and sequencing for a holistic yoga asana practice.

“

Hatha Yoga: A Comprehensive Guide *is a great tool to get a deeper insight on the essence of yoga. The very down-to-earth approach and professional expertise of the authors make it very approachable and easy to apply."*

Alexandre Beauchard, yoga teacher and owner of *Buddha Balance*

“

It was a pleasure to read this book, as it creates a bridge between the traditional Indian understanding of what yoga is and how this old wisdom can be of great use in our modern lives. Hatha Yoga: A Comprehensive Guide *is built up with great clarity and structure, and each asana is described in detail, including its benefits as well as contraindications. I am convinced that this book will open many minds to the value that a traditional yoga practice can bring to our lives."*

Dagmar Schöndorf, M.D., yoga teacher, acupuncturist and medical psychotherapist

“

As a yoga teacher and dedicated yoga practitioner, I find this by far the best and most complete book on Hatha Yoga that I have ever read. Hatha Yoga: A Comprehensive Guide *is an extremely comprehensive tool for sequencing yoga practices. The book guides you to understand the deeper layers of yoga in such a clear and comprehensive way that it is a pleasure to read. It is a guide and a tool that will serve self-practitioners and yoga teachers alike on their personal and professional yoga path."*

Suzanne Janssens-Kievit, founder and owner of *The Yoga Villa*

“

This is the best book about yoga that I have ever read; it's practical and to the point. It provides sound knowledge on the physiological effects of practicing yoga, helping the western mind to understand why yoga works. I enjoyed the simplicity and clarity of the writing, making it very easy to read and understand. It also provides a step-by-step guide on asanas and how to create asana sequences that work. The perfect guide to have at hand for teachers as well as self-practitioners."

Maria Aguirregomozcorta, M.D. Neurology, yoga teacher

"

Easy to understand but far more illuminative than other books on yoga, Hatha Yoga: A Comprehensive Guide *is a must-read for yoga teachers of all styles. It's scientific while still honoring the spirituality of yoga, and offers little-known wisdom that you can only learn in the best yoga teacher training program. When it comes to learning how to actually teach Hatha Yoga, no other book compares."*

Julie Bernier, yoga teacher and registered ayurvedic practitioner,
author of *Yoga for Health and Happiness*

"

A very important book. This approach will give the teacher or ardent practitioner a well-grounded way to format their practice. Chakra-based sequencing provides a yogic understanding of asana that moves beyond the gross, dense or superficial. I highly recommend it!"

Nathan Anderson, lead yoga teacher trainer at *Yoga NOHO, Los Angeles*

"

Hatha Yoga: A Comprehensive Guide *is a comprehensive tool for students as well as teachers. I like to think of it as an encyclopedia to the Hatha Yoga practice."*

Helena Schouenborg, yoga teacher, addiction & health counselor